Cannabis sativa Cultivation, Production, and Applications in Pharmaceuticals and Cosmetics

Rafiq Lone
Central University of Kashmir, India

Aabid Hussain Mir
University of Kashmir, India

Javid Manzoor
Jiwaji University, India

IGI Global
PUBLISHER of TIMELY KNOWLEDGE

A volume in the Advances in Medical Diagnosis, Treatment, and Care (AMDTC) Book Series

Published in the United States of America by
IGI Global
Engineering Science Reference (an imprint of IGI Global)
701 E. Chocolate Avenue
Hershey PA, USA 17033
Tel: 717-533-8845
Fax: 717-533-8661
E-mail: cust@igi-global.com
Web site: http://www.igi-global.com

Library of Congress Cataloging-in-Publication Data

Names: Lone, Rafiq, 1982- editor. | Mir, A. H. (Aabid Hussain), editor. | Manzoor, Javid, 1987- editor.
Title: Cannabis sativa cultivation, production, and applications in pharmaceuticals and cosmetics / edited by Rafiq Lone, Aabid Mir, Javid Manzoor.
Description: Hershey, PA : Medical Information Science Reference, [2022] | Includes bibliographical references and index. | Summary: "Cannabis sativa has a long history but has not been exploited for beneficial uses. This plant can solve many problems in the present most importantly in pharmaceutical and cosmetic industry. Biosprorospecting of this very important plant can generate economic upliftment of weaker sections of the society and states if properly used under rule and regulations. This book will discusses in detail the current research conducted in the field of Cannabis Sativus so that to make it more useful and sustainable for the future. It will focuses on the exploration of Cannabis Sativus phytoconstituents in various fields especially in pharmaceutical and cosmetic industry. This book will cover topics such as commercial products and their use in pharmaceutical industry"-- Provided by publisher.
Identifiers: LCCN 2022042967 (print) | LCCN 2022042968 (ebook) | ISBN 9781668457184 (hardcover) | ISBN 9781668457191 (ebook)
Subjects: MESH: Cannabis | Cannabinoids--therapeutic use | Phytotherapy
Classification: LCC RM666.C266 (print) | LCC RM666.C266 (ebook) | NLM QV 766.5.C2 | DDC 615.7/827--dc23/eng/20221026
LC record available at https://lccn.loc.gov/2022042967
LC ebook record available at https://lccn.loc.gov/2022042968

This book is published in the IGI Global book series Advances in Medical Diagnosis, Treatment, and Care (AMDTC) (ISSN: 2475-6628; eISSN: 2475-6636)

British Cataloguing in Publication Data
A Cataloguing in Publication record for this book is available from the British Library.

For electronic access to this publication, please contact: eresources@igi-global.com.

Advances in Medical Diagnosis, Treatment, and Care (AMDTC) Book Series

ISSN:2475-6628
EISSN:2475-6636

Mission

Advancements in medicine have prolonged the life expectancy of individuals all over the world. Once life-threatening conditions have become significantly easier to treat and even cure in many cases. Continued research in the medical field will further improve the quality of life, longevity, and wellbeing of individuals.

The **Advances in Medical Diagnosis, Treatment, and Care (AMDTC)** book series seeks to highlight publications on innovative treatment methodologies, diagnosis tools and techniques, and best practices for patient care. Comprised of comprehensive resources aimed to assist professionals in the medical field apply the latest innovations in the identification and management of medical conditions as well as patient care and interaction, the books within the AMDTC series are relevant to the research and practical needs of medical practitioners, researchers, students, and hospital administrators.

Coverage

- Experimental Medicine
- Medical Procedures
- Critical Care
- Patient-Centered Care
- Disease Management
- Patient Interaction
- Emergency Medicine
- Chronic Conditions
- Medical Testing
- Internal Medicine

IGI Global is currently accepting manuscripts for publication within this series. To submit a proposal for a volume in this series, please contact our Acquisition Editors at Acquisitions@igi-global.com or visit: http://www.igi-global.com/publish/.

The Advances in Medical Diagnosis, Treatment, and Care (AMDTC) Book Series (ISSN 2475-6628) is published by IGI Global, 701 E. Chocolate Avenue, Hershey, PA 17033-1240, USA, www.igi-global.com. This series is composed of titles available for purchase individually; each title is edited to be contextually exclusive from any other title within the series. For pricing and ordering information please visit http://www.igi-global.com/book-series/advances-medical-diagnosis-treatment-care/129618. Postmaster: Send all address changes to above address.

Titles in this Series

For a list of additional titles in this series, please visit: www.igi-global.com/book-series/advances-medical-diagnosis-treatment-care/129618

Medical Cannabis and the Effects of Cannabinoids on Fighting Cancer, Multiple Sclerosis, Epilepsy, Parkinson's, and Other Neurodegenerative Diseases
Rana R. Zeine (Kean University, USA) and Brian W. Teasdale (Kean University, USA)
Medical Information Science Reference • © 2023 • 406pp • H/C (ISBN: 9781668456521) • US $345.00

Perspectives on Coping Strategies for Menstrual and Premenstrual Distress
B.S. Parimal (The Maharaja Sayajirao University of Baroda, India) and Kavita Gupta (The Maharaja Sayajirao University of Baroda, India)
Medical Information Science Reference • © 2023 • 344pp • H/C (ISBN: 9781668450888) • US $325.00

Pharmacological Benefits of Natural Agents
Narayanaswamy Radhakrishnan (St. Peter's Institute of Higher Education and Research (SPIHER), India) Srinivasan Vasantha (St. Peter's Institute of Higher Education and Research (SPIHER), India) and Ashok Kumar Pandurangan (B.S. Abdur Rahman Crescent Institute of Science and Technology, India)
Medical Information Science Reference • © 2023 • 335pp • H/C (ISBN: 9781668467374) • US $325.00

Cases on Multimorbidity and Its Impact on Elderly Patients
Adil Hamad Alharthi (King Fahad Armed Forces Hospital, Saudi Arabia)
Medical Information Science Reference • © 2023 • 300pp • H/C (ISBN: 9781668423547) • US $325.00

Handbook of Research on Advanced Phytochemicals and Plant-Based Drug Discovery
Ajeet Singh (ICAR-Indian Institute of Wheat and Barley Research, India)
Medical Information Science Reference • © 2022 • 722pp • H/C (ISBN: 9781668451298) • US $545.00

AI Applications for Disease Diagnosis and Treatment
Rajae El Ouazzani (Moulay Ismail University of Meknes, Morocco) Mohammed Fattah (Moulay Ismail University of Meknes, Morocco) and Nabil Benamar (Moulay Ismail University of Meknes, Morocco)
Medical Information Science Reference • © 2022 • 332pp • H/C (ISBN: 9781668423042) • US $435.00

Historical and Epidemiological Analyses on the Impact of Infectious Disease on Society
Edward Greenberg (Cigna, USA)
Medical Information Science Reference • © 2022 • 261pp • H/C (ISBN: 9781799886891) • US $325.00

IGI Global
PUBLISHER of TIMELY KNOWLEDGE

701 East Chocolate Avenue, Hershey, PA 17033, USA
Tel: 717-533-8845 x100 • Fax: 717-533-8661
E-Mail: cust@igi-global.com • www.igi-global.com

Table of Contents

Foreword xii

Preface xiii

Chapter 1
Cannabis sativa: History, Cultivation, and Medicine 1
Anuradha Sharma, Government Degree College, Bhaderwah, India
Malti Rajput, PSPS Government PG College for Women, India
Javid Manzoor, Shri JJT University, India

Chapter 2
Historical Evolution of *Cannabis sativa* Transmogrifying Utilizations 29
Irfan Bashir, University of Kashmir, Srinagar, India
Sameena Bashir, University of Kashmir, Srinagar, India

Chapter 3
Cultivation of Cannabis: Medicinal, Social, and Legal Aspects 43
Khursheed Ahmad Wani, Government Degree College Thindim Kreeri, Baramulla, India
Syed Javid Andrabi, SP College, Srinagar, India
Javid Manzoor, Government Degree PG College, Bhaderwah, India
Heena Qadir, Government Degree College, Awantipora, India
Kounsar Jan, Government Degree College Thindim Kreeri, Baramulla, India

Chapter 4
Medicinal Uses of *Cannabis sativa* and Its Derivatives 52
Zahid Nabi, Central University of Jammu, India
Javaid Manzoor Lone, JJT University, Jhunjhunu, India
Anuradha Sharma, Government Degree College, Bhaderwah, India

Chapter 5
Cannabis sativa: A Versatile Herb – An Overview on Pharmaceutical and Cosmetic Applications 63
Priyanka Joshi Jain, Principal K.M. Kundnani College of Pharmacy, University of Mumbai, India
Nikhil Prem Rajnani, Principal K.M. Kundnani College of Pharmacy, University of Mumbai, India
Nalini Satish Kurup, Principal K.M. Kundnani College of Pharmacy, University of Mumbai, India

Chapter 6
Role of *Cannabis sativa L.* in the Cosmetic Industry: Opportunities and Challenges.......................... 81
Anup Kumar Sarkar, Dukhulal Nibaran Chandra College, India
Sanjoy Sadhukhan, Raiganj University, India

Chapter 7
Bioactive Properties and Food Applications of *Cannabis sativa* and Applications of Its Molecular Modeling.. 101
Sefa Celik, Istanbul University, Turkey
Elif Cakir, Istanbul Aydin University, Turkey
Alev Er, Istanbul University, Turkey

Chapter 8
Cannabis sativa: A Miracle Plant for Remediation of Soil Pollutants 115
Khursheed Ahmad Wani, Government Degree College Thindim Kreeri, Baramulla, India
Shivom Singh, ITM University, India
Siraj Yousuf, Government Degree College, Bijbehara, India

Chapter 9
Heavy Metals and Pesticides on Contaminants of Concern in Cannabis 129
Asma Zafar, University of Kashmir, India
Sheema Zaffar, University of Kashmir, India
Ab Qayoom Mir, Government Degree College, Hajin, India
Irfan Jamila, Government Degree College for Women, Srinagar, India
Waseem Yaseen, Government Degree College, Kangan, India

Chapter 10
Cannabis sativa and Its Ability to Combat Climate Change: Unravelling Sustainable Benefits of Cannabis and Its Derivatives.. 143
Zahid Nabi, Central University of Jammu, India
Shivali Kundan, Central University of Jammu, India
Neha Verma, Central University of Jammu, India
Dinesh Kumar, Central University of Jammu, India

Chapter 11
Marijuana, i.e., *Cannabis sativa*: The Quandary of Being an Amalgamate of a Useful and Abusive Medicinal Herb 153
Javid Manzoor, Shri JJT University, India
Sajood Ahmad Bhat, Government Degree College, Bhaderwah, India
Anuradha Sharma, Government Degree College, Bhaderwah, India

Compilation of References 172

About the Contributors 223

Index... 226

Detailed Table of Contents

Foreword xii

Preface xiii

Chapter 1
Cannabis sativa: History, Cultivation, and Medicine 1
Anuradha Sharma, Government Degree College, Bhaderwah, India
Malti Rajput, PSPS Government PG College for Women, India
Javid Manzoor, Shri JJT University, India

Cannabis sativa is a widely dispersed plant that may be found in a broad range of habitats, elevations, and climatic conditions all over the globe. It is a member of the Cannabis genus. Historically, it has been used by humans for more than 5000 years, making it one of the oldest plant sources of food and textile fibres. Originating in Western Asia and Egypt, the cultivation of Cannabis sativa for textile fibre later spread to Europe, and in 1606, the cultivation of hemp was brought to North America, where it has remained since. For the majority of the 18th and 19th centuries, hemp had an important economic role in Europe, primarily in the manufacturing of ropes and textiles. Cannabis sativa L. (marijuana; Cannabaceae) is a popular plant with extensive distribution that produces fibre and food, as well as a psychoactive drug. Hemp seed has traditionally been harvested for the oil that can be derived from it and used in a variety of applications, including culinary and the production of soaps, paints, lubricants, and cosmetics. Furthermore, hemp has long been used as a medical plant.

Chapter 2
Historical Evolution of *Cannabis sativa* Transmogrifying Utilizations 29
Irfan Bashir, University of Kashmir, Srinagar, India
Sameena Bashir, University of Kashmir, Srinagar, India

Cannabis sativa is known in India as hemp, ganja, and bhang. Its domestication date is unclear. According to archaeological evidence, hemp was known in the past, with the earliest mentions coming from China and India. Excellent hemp study could help us objectively examine humans' particular interaction with the plant. Different civilizations use the plant in a number of ways. In ancient India, the plant was largely used to make textiles and other therapeutic remedies. Company officials were concerned that its use would lead to insanity during colonial times. According to the 1893-1894 hemp drug committee report, the East India Company officials' perspectives had evolved. They passed a slew of hemp-related legislation and imposed new taxes. According to the commission's findings, Bhang has no biological or societal implications. How did colonial rulers who were against consuming it yet saw it as a good source of fibre change their minds? It is hoped to better understand how perceptions, misperceptions, politics, and rules shape attitudes toward drug use.

Chapter 3
Cultivation of Cannabis: Medicinal, Social, and Legal Aspects.. 43
Khursheed Ahmad Wani, Government Degree College Thindim Kreeri, Baramulla, India
Syed Javid Andrabi, SP College, Srinagar, India
Javid Manzoor, Government Degree PG College, Bhaderwah, India
Heena Qadir, Government Degree College, Awantipora, India
Kounsar Jan, Government Degree College Thindim Kreeri, Baramulla, India

Interest in growing cannabis for medical and recreational purposes is increasing worldwide. This study reviews the cultivation of cannabis, its medicinal significance, and its social impacts. It is believed that cannabis has many medicinal properties that could prove very useful for the managing different disease, and at the same time it has many harmful effects that expose it to many legal and social aspects. Cannabis contains a psychoactive compound called tetrahydrocannabinols (THC) that creates a psychogenic effect. It can be consumed through the respiratory tract and digestive tract through smoking and oral ingesting, respectively. In contrast, cannabidiol (CBD), another component derived from cannabis, is a non-psychoactive cannabinoid that has gained popularity for its medicinal values and as a supplement.

Chapter 4
Medicinal Uses of *Cannabis sativa* and Its Derivatives 52
Zahid Nabi, Central University of Jammu, India
Javaid Manzoor Lone, JJT University, Jhunjhunu, India
Anuradha Sharma, Government Degree College, Bhaderwah, India

Cannabis Sativas has found applications in medical industry since time immemorial. With the evolution of time marijuana plant Cannabis sativa, its derivatives, cannabinoids, have grown increasingly popular as a potential treatment for various diseases which include ailments of heart, skin, and other vital organs. Products extracted from Cannabis have found their usage in various stages of medical treatment. Various ailments can be cured by the giving the patient required dose of cannabis or hemp oil. Moreover, Cannabis reduces chronic pain, increases lung capacity, helps lose weight and regulates diabetes.

Chapter 5
Cannabis sativa: A Versatile Herb – An Overview on Pharmaceutical and Cosmetic Applications... 63
Priyanka Joshi Jain, Principal K.M. Kundnani College of Pharmacy, University of Mumbai, India
Nikhil Prem Rajnani, Principal K.M. Kundnani College of Pharmacy, University of Mumbai, India
Nalini Satish Kurup, Principal K.M. Kundnani College of Pharmacy, University of Mumbai, India

Cannabis sativa (Hemp) is an herbaceous species used in foods and beverages, cosmetics, pharmaceuticals, nutraceuticals, etc. It has two active constituents: Tetrahydrocannabinol and Cannabidiol. Cannabinoids suppress uncontrolled growth of cancerous cells, provide pain relief to HIV patients, and help with neurogenic symptoms. Cannabis extracts have exhibited more effectiveness against various bacteria and yeast. Improvement in skin hydration and skin elasticity was observed. Excessive sebum production and proliferation of sebocytes is normalized. Hemp extracts arrest the anagen phase of the hair cycle to cause reversal of the temporal and vertex thinning in Androgenetic alopecia. It has antioxidant potential as well as an anti-ageing effect. Owing to the variability in legislation in different countries, Cannabis sativa poses challenges in research. This chapter discusses the diverse applications of this double-edged herb.

Chapter 6
Role of *Cannabis sativa L.* in the Cosmetic Industry: Opportunities and Challenges.......................... 81
Anup Kumar Sarkar, Dukhulal Nibaran Chandra College, India
Sanjoy Sadhukhan, Raiganj University, India

Cannabis sativa L. is a flowering plant in the family Cannabaceae, and has been cultivated since ancient times for its fibres, oils, resins, dried inflorescences, and leaves. It can be used for a variety of industrial purposes. Over the years, the therapeutic and pharmacological efficacy of its phytoconstituents is shown in a variety of human diseases and health. The use and exploitation of the plant have sparked controversy; however, there are recent legalizations of its use for medical and other purposes in many countries within the corresponding legislative framework. In addition to this legalization, C. sativa is encouraging the very rapid growth of the cannabis oriented pharmaceutical industry. This chapter summarized recent developments in the science of C. sativa and its products about their industrial application, while also addressing gaps in the existing knowledge and future research directions for this high-value multi-use, and potential industrial plant with universal benefits.

Chapter 7
Bioactive Properties and Food Applications of *Cannabis sativa* and Applications of Its Molecular Modeling.. 101
Sefa Celik, Istanbul University, Turkey
Elif Cakir, Istanbul Aydin University, Turkey
Alev Er, Istanbul University, Turkey

In addition to being the oldest cultivated plant from past to present as a raw material source, Cannabis sativa L. is a strategically characteristic plant used for food, medicine, cosmetics, and pharmacological purposes. Molecular modeling is an important means for elucidating molecular structures and plays an important role in the design and development of new pharmaceuticals. This chapter includes the beneficial properties of the primary and secondary metabolites contained in cannabis such as foaming, emulsifying, gelling, film formation; antioxidant, antimicrobial activities and bakery products by means of their superior nutritional values, snack products, dairy products, processed meat products, in beverages such as coffees, teas, soda and functional food ingredients in many other areas of the food industry, nutritional supplements, usability in the development of new food formulations on hemp and molecular modeling studies on constituents of cannabis sativa.

Chapter 8
Cannabis sativa: A Miracle Plant for Remediation of Soil Pollutants 115
Khursheed Ahmad Wani, Government Degree College Thindim Kreeri, Baramulla, India
Shivom Singh, ITM University, India
Siraj Yousuf, Government Degree College, Bijbehara, India

Phytoremediation is a plant-based technology that is both cost-effective and environmentally beneficial, and it is classified as an in-situ modification method. Using phytoremediation, on the other hand, results in the restoration of the preservation site's biological activity, physical structure, and chemical properties. Heavy metals can be found in a variety of places in the environment. Because most of these compounds are water soluble, they circulate quickly across the environment. Heavy metals and other pollutants in high concentrations can impair the body's physiology and biochemistry, resulting in health problems. This chapter will review the literature available in different data bases on Cannabis sativa for possible remediation of pollutants from different ecosystems.

Chapter 9
Heavy Metals and Pesticides on Contaminants of Concern in Cannabis 129
Asma Zafar, University of Kashmir, India
Sheema Zaffar, University of Kashmir, India
Ab Qayoom Mir, Government Degree College, Hajin, India
Irfan Jamila, Government Degree College for Women, Srinagar, India
Waseem Yaseen, Government Degree College, Kangan, India

Cannabis is cultivated in different parts of the world for different purposes. Potential dangers from microbiological contamination exist for cannabis users. Opportunistic infections in immunocompromised patients can be brought on by bacteria and fungi. Allergies and asthma can be brought on by even dead germs. Shigla toxin and aflatoxins are two examples of microbial overload-related toxins that might be problematic, though it's unlikely. There is currently work being done to identify the diverse microbiome that the cannabis plant supports. Because of how readily heavy metals bioaccumulate in the tissues of cannabis, hemp crops have been employed in bioremediation. Because heavy metals are linked to a wide range of human ailments, it is important to keep them to a minimum in crops grown for human consumption. The chapter discusses interlinkage of heavy metals and pesticides associated with cannabis.

Chapter 10
Cannabis sativa and Its Ability to Combat Climate Change: Unravelling Sustainable Benefits of Cannabis and Its Derivatives.. 143
Zahid Nabi, Central University of Jammu, India
Shivali Kundan, Central University of Jammu, India
Neha Verma, Central University of Jammu, India
Dinesh Kumar, Central University of Jammu, India

Cannabis sativa plant is a multifunctional crop having multiple uses, including for food, fibre, fuel, and construction materials. This makes it a valuable resource for farmers, as it provides multiple income streams and reduces the need for mono-cropping. In addition, hemp has the potential to play a significant role in promoting carbon sequestration and sustainable land use practices. By using hemp for carbon sequestration, for harvesting bioenergy and making of bioplastics, we can help to mitigate the effects of climate change, improve soil health, and promote sustainable agriculture practices. With continued research and investment, this chapter assess different possibilities that could be explored to harvest environmental benefits of Cannabis sativa.

Chapter 11
Marijuana, i.e., *Cannabis sativa*: The Quandary of Being an Amalgamate of a Useful and Abusive Medicinal Herb 153
Javid Manzoor, Shri JJT University, India
Sajood Ahmad Bhat, Government Degree College, Bhaderwah, India
Anuradha Sharma, Government Degree College, Bhaderwah, India

Cannabis sativa, popularly known as "marijuana," poses a problem since it may have both beneficial and harmful effects. Cannabis has long been used for medicinal and recreational purposes, which demonstrates its value as a plant. Instead of this, enough evidence suggests that abusing this wonder herb can have negative effects on a number of organs and organ systems, such as the pulmonary system, the body's defense system, the cardiovascular system, etc. Additionally, it may affect both male and female potency and may also have clastogenic effects. Yet, it cannot be ruled out that there are some benefits to using marijuana responsibly, since it has been shown to be a miraculous treatment for atrophy, acute pain, a loss of muscular tone, motion sickness, and insomnia. This chapter will attempt to provide a thorough understanding of the various health effects of the herb and its extracted active bioactive ingredients.

Compilation of References 172

About the Contributors 223

Index 226

Foreword

Cannabis sativa although maligned in terms of its use as an addictive agent, recently secured the attention of pharmaceutical properties. Needless to mention, this miraculous herb has now turned out to be the cynosure of researchers across globe and in fact governments at local level are trying to formulate policies for controlled cultivation of the erstwhile maligned plant.

Despite the fact that some states have already legalised cannabis, many others are in the midst of the process and are grappling with a tangled web of questions, such as how to ensure the safe production of cannabis while protecting employees, how to ensure equitable marketing, and how to regulate growers, processors, and retailers.

To address these critical issues and lay the groundwork for the safe regulation of cannabis, present work titled *Cannabis* sativa *Cultivation, Production, and Applications in Pharmaceuticals and Cosmetics* will be quite useful to formulate policies in this regard.

Given the voluminous chapters contributed by scholars all across the world, it is felt that this book would comprehensively provide pathway and regulation mechanisms for the policy makers.

I hope this book would come handy to everyone in terms of contents and wealth of information

S. M. Zuber
Department of Zoology, Government Degree College, Bijbehara, India

Preface

Cannabis sativa has been widely cultivated as a source of bast fibres and/or seeds. The plant is native to India and Persia, but over the last 6000 years, it has been cultivated in nearly all temperate and tropical countries of the world and is likely to be one of the oldest non-food crops known. Historically, hemp fibres were used for the production of rope, cordage, fabrics and paper. During the 18th and 19th centuries hemp had a significant commercial role in europe for the production of ropes and textiles. Hemp seed has historically been harvested for the oil that can be crushed from it for use in culinaries and manufactures such as soaps, paints, lubricants and cosmetics. In addition, hemp has been grown as a medicinal plant and investigations into the uses of hemp as a therapeutic and medicinal plant continue.

This book discusses these consequences in further detail and presents the research conducted to make this Cannabis sativus useful and sustainable for the future. It focuses on the exploration of Cannabis sativus phytoconstituents in various fields especially in pharmaceutical and cosmetic industry. This book covers topics such as commercial productsand use in medicinal field.

Cannabis sativa has a history but has not been exploited for beneficial uses fully. This plant can solve many problems in the nowadays, most importantly in pharmaceutical and cosmetic industry. Bioprospecting of this very important plant can generate economic upliftment of weaker sections of the society and states if properly used under rules and regulations.

The book will be an excellent reference for PG students of Plant sciences, Biotechnology, Agricultural Sciences, food scientists, technologists, chemists, new product developers, researchers, academics, professionals working in the food industry, and pharmacologists, pharmacists and clinicians interested in nutrition and metabolism.

The book has received 11 chapters from scholars across the globe.

Chapter 1 deals with the history of the palnt. *Cannabis sativa* is a widely dispersed plant that may be found in a broad range of habitats, elevations, and climatic conditions all over the globe. It is a member of the Cannabis genus. Historically, it has been used by humans for more than 5000 years, making it one of the oldest plant sources of food and textile fibres.

Chapter 2 details the evolutionary history of the palnt. *Cannabis sativa* is known in India as hemp, ganja, and bhang. Its domestication date is unclear. According to archaeological evidence, hemp was known in the past, with the earliest mentions coming from China and India.

Chapter 3 reviews the cultivation of cannabis, its medicinal significance and social impacts. of cannabis cultivation. It is believed that cannabis has many medicinal properties that could prove very useful for the managing different disease and at the same time it has many harmful effects that expose it to many legal and social aspects.

Chapter 4 argued that Cannabis Sativas has found applications in medical industry since time immemorial. With the evolution of time marijuana plant *Cannabis sativa* and its derivatives, cannabinoids, have grown increasingly popular as a potential treatment for various diseases which include ailments of heart, skin, and other vital organs.

Chapter 5 advocated that *Cannabis sativa* (Hemp) is an herbaceous species used in foods and beverages, cosmetics, pharmaceuticals, nutraceuticals etc. It has two active constituents Tetrahydrocannabinol and Cannabidiol. Cannabinoids suppress uncontrolled growth of cancerous cells, provide pain relief to HIV patients and help with neurogenic symptoms Cannabis extracts have exhibited more effectiveness against various bacteria and yeast. Improvement in skin hydration and skin elasticity was observed. Excessive sebum production and proliferation of sebocytes is normalized.

Chapter 6 summarized recent developments in the science of C. sativa and its products about their industrial application, while also addressing gaps in our existing knowledge and future research directions for this high-value multi-use and potential industrial plant with universal benefits.

Chapter 7 includes besides the beneficial properties of the primary and secondary metabolites contained in cannabis such as foaming, emulsifying, gelling, film formation; antioxidant, antimicrobial activities and bakery products by means of their superior nutritional values, snack products, dairy products, processed meat products, in beverages such as coffees, teas, soda and functional food ingredients in many other areas of the food industry, nutritional supplements, usability in the development of new food formulations on hemp and molecular modeling studies on constituents of Cannab*is sativa*.

Chapter 8 reviewed the literature available in different data bases on *Cannabis sativa* for possible remediation of pollutants from different ecosystems. Heavy metals and other pollutants in high concentrations can impair the body's physiology and biochemistry, resulting in health problems. This chapter will review the literature available in different data bases on *Cannabis sativa* for possible remediation of pollutants from different ecosystems.

Chapter 9 discusses interlinkage of heavy metals and pesticides associated with cannabis. Cannabis is cultivated in different parts of the world for different purposes. Potential dangers from microbiological contamination exist for cannabis users. Opportunistic infections in immunocompromised patients can be brought on by bacteria and fungi. Allergies and asthma can be brought on by even dead germs. Shigla toxin and aflatoxins are two examples of microbial overload-related toxins that might be problematic, though it's unlikely.

Chapter 10 is a multifunctional crop having multiple uses, including for food, fibre, fuel, and construction materials. This makes it a valuable resource for farmers, as it provides multiple income streams and reduces the need for mono-cropping. In addition, hemp has the potential to play a significant role in promoting carbon sequestration and sustainable land use practices. By using hemp for carbon sequestration, for harvesting bioenergy and making of bioplastics we can help to mitigate the effects of climate change, improve soil health, and promote sustainable agriculture practices. With continued research and investment.

Chapter 11 attempts to provide a thorough understanding of the various health effects of the herb and its extracted active bioactive ingredients. Yet, it cannot be ruled out that there are some benefits to using marijuana responsibly, since it has been shown to be a miraculous treatment for atrophy, acute pain, a loss of muscular tone, motion sickness, and insomnia. I hope this book would be quite useful for academicians, researchers, and industrialists.

Rafiq Lone
Central University of Kashmir, India

Aabid Hussain Mir
University of Kashmir, India

Javid Manzoor
Jiwaji University, India

Chapter 1
Cannabis sativa: History, Cultivation, and Medicine

Anuradha Sharma
Government Degree College, Bhaderwah, India

Malti Rajput
PSPS Government PG College for Women, India

Javid Manzoor
https://orcid.org/0000-0002-2821-206X
Shri JJT University, India

ABSTRACT

Cannabis sativa is a widely dispersed plant that may be found in a broad range of habitats, elevations, and climatic conditions all over the globe. It is a member of the Cannabis genus. Historically, it has been used by humans for more than 5000 years, making it one of the oldest plant sources of food and textile fibres. Originating in Western Asia and Egypt, the cultivation of Cannabis sativa for textile fibre later spread to Europe, and in 1606, the cultivation of hemp was brought to North America, where it has remained since. For the majority of the 18th and 19th centuries, hemp had an important economic role in Europe, primarily in the manufacturing of ropes and textiles. Cannabis sativa L. (marijuana; Cannabaceae) is a popular plant with extensive distribution that produces fibre and food, as well as a psychoactive drug. Hemp seed has traditionally been harvested for the oil that can be derived from it and used in a variety of applications, including culinary and the production of soaps, paints, lubricants, and cosmetics. Furthermore, hemp has long been used as a medical plant.

INTRODUCTION

Cannabis sativa L. (C. sativa), popularly known as Indian hemp, is a herbaceous annual plant that has been grown since ancient times in Central Asia (India and China) (Russo et al., 2008). Cannabis sativa is perhaps the most well-known plant ever found by mankind, and it has a long history of complicated

DOI: 10.4018/978-1-6684-5718-4.ch001

metabolic biology and interesting physiology (Zwenger, 2014). Cannabis sativa (often known as "Cannabis") is an angiosperm in the Cannabaceae family. Cannabis sativa has been farmed for more than 5000 years for fibres and seed oil (Lash, 2010, Leizer et al., 2000), as well as medical (Clarke and Merlin, 2013; Zuardi, 2006) and recreational usage (Small, 2017). (Burstein, 1997 and Cota et. al., 2003). Cannabis fibres are one of its most commonly used products; in fact, for thousands of years, the plant was valued more for its fibre production than for any other application (Small, 2017). Cannabis fibres are extracted from the plant's stem and used to make fabrics, ropes, canvas, home furnishings, and industrial items (Montonya, 2016). Cannabis seeds are eaten, fed to animals, and used to make seed oil for food and cosmetics. Cannabis seeds have a high concentration of two essential fatty acids (EFAs), linolenic acid (omega-3) and linoleic acid (omega-6) (Callaway, 2004). Cannabis seeds are also high in all (important) amino acids, fibre, vitamins A, D, E, and C, thiamine, and riboflavin, as well as minerals including phosphorus, iron, potassium, and calcium (Leyva, 2011). Cannabis seeds and oil have remained popular in the food and cosmetics sectors of Asia, Europe, and America because to its high nutritional content (Lawrence, 2019).

Cannabis sativa extract has been used in Arabic-Islamic medicine for its numerous curative properties such as diuretic, anti-emetic, anti-epileptic, anti-inflammatory, anti-parasitic, antipyretic, anti-bacteria, anti-tumor, vernucide and vermifuge, dermatic, carminative, and painkilling properties; the most commonly used part was seeds; and the common methods of preparation were seeds' oil and juice from the leaves (Lozano, 2001). Regardless, Cannabis leaves alone have the potential to cure over 25 different kinds of ailments (Kala et al., 2004), and other plant components including as seeds, flowers, and roots are also being employed.

Cannabis sativa is a wonder plant having about 500 chemical entities (Radwan et al., 2009), including over 100 phytocannabinoids and 120 terpenes (Calvi et al., 2018), of which fewer than 30 biosynthetic pathways have been identified (Booth and Bohlmann 2019). Small and Cronquist (Small and Cronquist, 1976) classified the hemp varieties wherein a concentration of 0.3% (dry weight) of Δ9-tetrahydrocannabinol (THC) is proposed to be a chemical demarcation between marijuana and hemp. Plants with THC concentration of $<$0.3% are considered as hemp (ðber-type) while those containing THC of ^{3}0.3% are considered as marijuana (drugtype) (Small and Cronquist, 1976; Cascini et. al., 2019)

Cannabis is well recognised for its narcotic and medicinal properties. However, it has a wide range of additional uses. It is employed in a variety of sectors such as food, cosmetics, energy, and textiles (Schultes et. al., 2001; Lawrence, 2019; Chaffey, 2001; Callaway, 2004). Cannabis has also been studied for its possible application in bioremediation of polluted soils. Cannabis demonstrated high tolerance to heavy metals such as cadmium (Shi and Cai, 2009; Ahmad et al., 2015; Husain et al., 2019), copper, and nickel (Ahmad et al., 2015; Husain et al., 2019), as well as effective atrazine absorption from soil (Wang, 2021), making the plant an effective bioremediation agent for heavy metals. Hemp is also more environmentally friendly and generates higher quality paper than forest sources (Kamat et. al., 2002). Cannabis is also an excellent source of biofuels (Finnan et. al., 2013; Das et. al., 2017). As a result, hemp has been determined to be a superior alternative for fossil fuels than biodiesel and bioethanol derived from OSR and sugar beet, respectively (Finnan et. al., 2013).

Aside from uses in the building and automotive sectors, hemp fibres are appealing due to their inherent antibacterial properties. Hemp bast fibres have been characterised as antibacterial (Hao et al., 2014; Khan et al., 2015), and they have been used to make an antibacterial finishing agent (Bao et al., 2014), surgical devices (Gu, 2006), and functionalized textiles (Cassano et al., 2013). This feature is related to the chemical makeup of hemp bast fibres: both free and esterified sterols and triterpenes, including

-sitosterol and -amyrin, have been identified (Gutierrez and delRio, 2005). These chemicals are known to have antibacterial effects (Kiprono et al., 2000; Ibrahim, 2012).

Although cannabis is proven to be medical, it is also regarded an illegal narcotic because to the strong psychoactivity of its phytocannabinoid, THC. THC has been shown in studies to negatively impact brain development in young people (Arseneault et. al., 2002). THC has also been linked to the later development of mental illnesses such as schizophrenia (Andreasson et. al., 1987; Barkus et. al., 2010; Trezza et. al., 2008; Gleason et. al., 2012; Renard et. al., 2018; Lubman et. al., 2015). As a narcotic, hemp is eaten either alone or in the form of a beverage. It is most often used for smoking, although excessive smoking is dangerous and may lead to insanity. In different countries, Indian hemp is known as Bang (Egypt), Bhang, Charas, Ganja (India), Bhango, Gaanjaa (Nepal), Canamo indico, Hachis, Marihuana (Spain), Canapa indica, Marihuana (Italy), Marihuana, Marihuana (France), Da ma cao, Da ma ren, Huo ma, Xian ma (United Kingdom)

Cannabis is a contentious plant. The plant's narcotic element necessitates its continued illegality, but its beneficial qualities are difficult to overlook. Cannabis prohibition started in the early decades of the twentieth century (Figure5).

Figure 1. Major events in the legal history of Cannabis

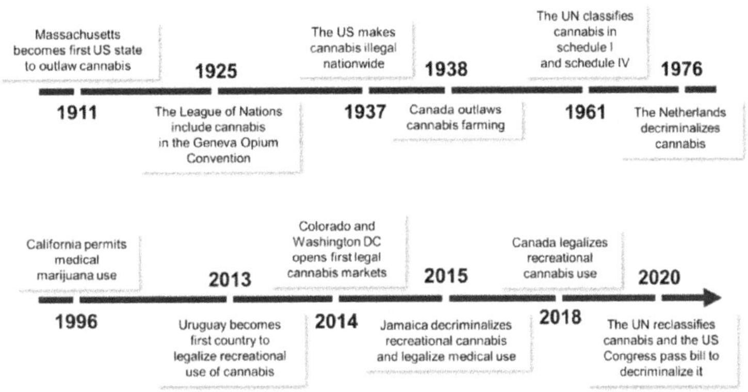

Cannabis is said to be the most widely used illegal substance in the world (UNODC, 2019). The continual changes in Cannabis's legal status, as well as the increasing global population, make it unlikely that non-medical cannabis usage will decline. Countries started reconsidering their regulatory legislation as they gained a better grasp of the nature of Cannabis phytochemistry (Figure 1). Uruguay was the first nation to legalise cannabis for medicinal and recreational use in 2013. (Seddon and Floodgate, 2020). However, only Canada, Uruguay, Malta, and the Netherlands have allowed recreational cannabis usage, while a few other nations have just decriminalised it. Despite its illegality, various breeding and pharmaceutical initiatives are now underway across the globe to cultivate medical Cannabis for pharmaceutical preparation with high standardised quality (de Meijer et al., 2003; Vanhove et al., 2011). However, this chapter will concentrate on the historical viewpoint of Cannabis, including its genesis and dissemination, various cultivation and breeding forms, and medical usage.

HISTORY

Historically, Central Asia and South-East Asia have been postulated as plausible areas for C. sativa's natural origin and/or primary domestication, and are likely to have played an important part in its development (Stevens et al., 2016; Jiang et al., 2006). Archaeologists excavating the Yanghai Tombs in northwest China in the early 2000s discovered the burial of a shaman buried 2,700 years ago, which is the earliest tangible proof of pharmacologically active cannabis. There discovered a stockpile of well-preserved C. sativa in the tomb. The presence of the psychoactive tetrahydrocannabinol (THC) was later verified by investigation of the plant remnants (Russo et. al., 2008).

The earliest evidence of cannabis usage in medicine was discovered in a fourth-century grave in a cave in Beit Shemesh, 30 kilometres west of Jerusalem. In 1989, archaeologists digging the cave discovered the remains of a 14-year-old girl who died during delivery. There were charred plant residues on her belly, which chemical investigation revealed contained THC. The archaeologists found that cannabis had been burned in a vessel and that the girl had breathed cannabis smoke during her labour (Pain, 2015)

Furthermore, multiple Neolithic pieces of evidence discovered in Taiwan imply that C. sativa was employed for a variety of uses 12,000 years ago (Li, 1974) and played an important part in early cordage and textile making. In fact, it has been described as the oldest known farmed fibre plant (Cherney and Small, 2016), and it is still used as a component of fishing nets today (Savo et. al., 2013). Clarke and Merlin contended that the finding of C. sativa psychoactivity was an inadvertent occurrence (Merlin, 2003; Clarke and Merlin, 2013).

According to the western-centric perspective of the American researchers, the unintentional burning of C. sativa plants caused by natural phenomena may have exposed its psychoactive properties. Indeed, by viewing prehistoric human communities, we might speculate on how they interacted with their surroundings. Luna L. E. stated in the 1980s that a group of Peruvian shamans from Iquitos considered medicinal herbs (Luna, 1984). During shamanic ceremonies, they utilised ayahuasca, a psychedelic-producing drink based on Banisteriopsis caapi and Psychotria viridis. These plants were regarded "teachers" because shamans could utilise them to treat their village's diseases while fasting and singing certain tunes. This "plant-teacher" approach has been discussed by numerous scholars throughout the globe (VanPool, 2009; Mafimisebi and Oguntade, 2010; Jauregui et al., 2011; Gagliano, 2013; Armijos et al., 2014) and might explain the employment of C. sativa in early human religious rites.

Since then, numerous types of C. sativa have been developed, with some plants selected as cultivars, mostly used to create textile fibres, and others, particularly as medications for religious rites. Several faiths have acknowledged C. sativa as a holy plant throughout the millennia (Touwn, 1981). Indeed, it is mentioned in the holy books of Asian nations as a plant with mystical properties and is used in religious rites. Hinduism and tantric Buddhism lineages in India and Tibet employed C. sativa flowers and resins to aid meditation and contact with spirits (Schultes et. al., 1992). According to Buddhist mythology, Siddhartha Gautama's primary source of food during his six years of austerity was Bhang, a specific C. sativa concoction (Touwn, 1981).

According to some writers, the term Cannabis appeared in Semitic languages such as Hebrew and occurs multiple times in the Old Testament. In fact, the usage of C. sativa as incense and holy oil is mentioned in Exodus, Isaiah, Jeremiah, and Ezekiel (Bennett, 2011; Abel, 1980).

C. sativa was first used medicinally some 5000 years ago, when Emperor Chen Nung, known as the "Father of Chinese Agriculture," compiled the first Chinese pharmacopoeia (Abel, 1980). C. sativa was given for tiredness, rheumatism, and malaria in this ancient literature (Abel, 1980). Furthermore, Chinese doctors mostly employed C. sativa seeds for their vegetal oils and proteins. C. sativa seeds are high in -linoleic acid (Anwara et al., 2006), which doctors prescribe for eczema and psoriasis, as well as oral usage for inflammatory illnesses (Jeong et. al., 2014). Furthermore, the use of C. sativa as a medicine is widely documented on Assyrian claytablets (Anderson and Scurlock, 2005) and the Egyptian Ebers Papyrus, both of which date from about 3000 years ago (Epstein, 2010). The Greeks and Romans were likewise familiar with C. sativa (Mercuri et. al., 2002).

Herodotus (about 400 B.C.) recorded its usage among Indians, while Diodorus Siculus (around 60 B.C.) said that ancient Egyptian ladies took C. sativa to relieve pain and enhance their mood (Carod-Artal, 2013). Furthermore, the Roman writer Pliny the Elder described the use of C. sativa roots for pain relief (Ryz et. al., 2017). Pedacius Dioscorides, a Greek physician, classified several plants, including C. sativa, and detailed their medicinal properties about the same time (Riddle, 2011). Galen, a Roman physician who was immensely influential in the Ancient and Middle Ages, also published some observations regarding C. sativa. He recounted a tradition among Roman elites, in particular, of concluding their meal with a cannabis-based dessert (Butrica, 2002).

Cannabis usage was connected with impoverished socioeconomic situations in mediaeval Arabic society. A tale of "Old Man of the Mountains" and Hasan's followers, the "ashishin," as described in Marco Polo's chronicles is an example (Fleischhauer, 1956). C. sativa in its different varieties was known in mediaeval Europe. Italians, in particular, pioneered large-scale cultivation and marketing of the plant in the Mediterranean region. C. sativa, on the other hand, was unknown in the Americas until the arrival and settlement of the first European immigrants. During this time, C. sativa was largely employed for the strength and resilience of its fibres. Indeed, the botanical types appropriate for textile manufacture were mostly introduced by the Spanish and English colonies in the Americas. Furthermore, although considerable amounts of C. sativa were sold in Europe during the Modern Age, they were solely meant for industrial trade.

Nonetheless, C. sativa has some inebriating properties in magic and traditional medicine (Benet, 1975). In 1484, Pope Innocent VIII issued a papal bull banning witchcraft and the use of Cannabis sativa (Kors and Peters, 2000). Furthermore, several herbalist treatises of the time debated the medicinal usefulness of C. sativa seeds and flowers. Travelogues written by explorers, sea captains, affluent travellers, priests, and merchants heading to Africa and the East Indies in the following centuries taught Europeans a variety of applications for C. sativa (Abel, 1980). With the invasion of India, the sensuous applications of C. sativa were more well recognised throughout the European continent. Two Portuguese physicians, Garcia da Orta and CristobalAcosta, reported on the effects of C. sativa, which included euphoria, sedation, hunger stimulation, hallucinations, and aphrodisiac effects (Lee, 2013).

Furthermore, under the East India Company's British colonisation, C. sativa was sold throughout Asia in a number of formulations such as Bhang, Ganja, or Charas. Ganja and Charas are flower and resin preparations with high psychedelic content (O'Shaughnessy, 1843). Bhang, on the other hand, has a modest psychotropic effect equivalent to that of several Western alcoholic beverages. Also, around the middle of the eighteenth century, the Swedish scientist Carl Linnaeus worked on authoring the Species Plantarum, coining the term Cannabis sativa for the first time. Other botanists started to argue the presence of various varieties of Cannabis based on size, form, and resin content as a result of the diaries of Indies travellers. Jean Lamarck, in instance, reserved the appellation Cannabis sativa for the European plant and Cannabis indica for the cultivars of Indian provenance (Small and Cronquist, 1976). The mystique of the Orient that dominated the nineteenth century also gave rise to private hashish user groups. Many Romantic artists and authors, including Théophile Gautier, Charles Baudelaire, Honoré de Balzac, Alexandre Dumas, and Gustave Flaubert, visited these societies (Levinthal, 2012). Jacques Joseph Moreau, a French physician, investigated the effects of C. sativa on mental disease in 1830. (Moreau, 1973). He believed that the voluptuous use of C. sativa may produce experiences similar to hallucinations and delusions in insane patients (Moreau, 1973).

Furthermore, in nineteenth-century English medicine, C. sativa was introduced as an analgesic, anti-inflammatory, anti-emetic, and anti-convulsant (Aldrich, 1997). Despite the benefits described above, it was strongly prohibited in the twentieth century due to its remarkable psychoactive effects, and it was removed from the British Pharmacopoeia in 1932 and included as a prohibited substance for therapeutic use in the Misuse of Drugs Regulation Act of the United Kingdom in 1971. (Hall, 2008).

Due to federal statute "The Marijuana Tax Act," production, possession, or transfer of Cannabis sativa was prohibited in the United States in 1937. (Bonnie and Whitebread, 1974). Despite these prohibitions, shamans and healers continued to utilise C. sativa as a local and traditional medicine, there was considerable pharmacological study on its chemical components, and there were various socio-cultural discussions over it. Many indigenous groups throughout the globe now employ C. sativa derivatives to treat a variety of ailments. C. sativa leaves are used for wound healing in the Miandam district of Swat, North Pakistan; powdered leaves are used as an anodyne, sedative, tonic, and narcotic (Akhtar et. al., 2013). C. sativa is used by small ethnic groups in remote regions in Nepal, Arunachal Pradesh, and Haryana to treat gastrointestinal illnesses, pain, and snake bites in humans and cattle (Panghal et. al., 2010; Kunwar et. al., 2010; Namsa et. al., 2011; Abbasi et. al., 2013). Furthermore, C. sativa is used as an ethno veterinary treatment by certain cattle producers in Uganda and Kenya (Gakuubi and Wanzala, 2012; Nabukenya et. al., 2014). Finally, even among certain isolated Caucasian ethnic groups, the historic usage of cannabis as a traditional treatment is still practised (Bussmann et. al., 2016).

In terms of pharmacology, Gaoni and Mechoulam paved the ground for cannabinoid research in 1964 by isolating and synthesising the major phytocannabinoid, D9-THC (Mechoulam and Gaoni, 1965). Pfizer focused on the creation of synthetic cannabinoid receptor ligands in the 1980s (Pertwee, 2006). Following that, the cannabinoid type-1 (CB1) receptor was found in 1990, followed by the cannabinoid type-2 (CB2) receptor in 1993. (Pertwee, 2006). Furthermore, two endogenous CB receptor ligands, arachidonoyl ethanolamine and 2-arachidonylglycerol, were identified in the 1990s (Pertwee, 2006). Finally, Di Marzo and colleagues created the phrase "endocannabinoid system" about the same time, which includes endogenous ligands, receptors, and production and degradation enzymes (Di Marzo et. al., 1994). All of these findings and studies on Cannabis sativa have led to the discovery of novel synthetic compounds capable of modulating the endocannabinoid system in inflammation, pain, and metabolic functions (Lazzari et. al., 2011, 2012, 2017; Mastinu et. al., 2012, 2013, 2018; Manca et. al., 2013; Tambaro et. al., 2014; Bonini et. al., 2016).

Even now, many western nations are divided about the legal position of C. sativa (Mc Ginty et. al., 2017). Many individuals see the ability to use C. sativa for medicinal or recreational purposes as a victory for civil rights, while others see it as a serious social issue. Those who have used C. sativa claim that it has: heightened the senses; increased acoustic perception; calmed emotions; facilitated communication; fostered creative ideas by allowing "thinking outside the box" and hence boosted inventiveness (Kowal et. al., 2015).

Terrance McKenna, an American ethnobotanist, proposed that the usage of C.sativa by humans may have accelerated the creation of language and communication, hence favouring the transition to civilization (McKenna, 1992). Furthermore, certain schools of thought suggested that ingesting psychedelic chemicals in a properly regulated setting might result in a medically safe experience that causes deep, long-lasting psychological and behavioural changes (Nichols, 2016). Indeed, psychedelic-assisted psychotherapy provides a solution to the issue of innovative psychiatric medicine development (PAP). To present, there are promising clinical studies using PAP in combination with LSD, MDMA, ketamine, psilocybin, and ibogaine as a therapy for alcoholism, nicotine addiction, terminal disease anxiety, and persistent post-traumatic stress disorder (Schenberg, 2018).

Several research on C. sativa have shown that it helps remove dreams of stressful situations and enhance sleep (Pedersen and Sandberg, 2013; Babson et. al., 2017). War veterans, in particular, characterised C. sativa usage as more effective and less complicated by adverse effects when compared to alcohol or other psycho drugs (Betthauser et. al., 2015). C. sativa, in fact, may be used as part of a psychotherapy approach to help introspection and direct confrontation of the roots of psychological trauma. These encouraging findings in the pharmacological and psychological effects of cannabis may be used by legislators to weigh the legalisation of C. sativa. Still, production and sale of C. sativa are banned in many countries, which encourages smuggling and makes finding standardised extracts difficult (Dragone et. al., 2018). As a result, a medically supervised and chemically standardised usage of C. sativa may be the legal solution today.

A League of Nations-mediated international convention to restrict the opium trade was expanded at the last minute to include cannabis. Signatories agreed to govern the cannabis trade and prohibit trafficking. The 1961 United Nations Single Convention on Narcotic Drugs tightened even further, and a decade later, the UN Convention on Psychotropic Substances rendered cannabis study all but impossible; only approved persons in supervised facilities could operate with it. Sativex (nabiximols), the first cannabis-based medicine approved in Canada, is a mouth spray of whole-cannabis extract having equal levels of THC and cannabidiol. The spray was created by GW Pharmaceuticals, which was founded by Geoffrey Guy and Brian Whittle in response to the UK report. Today, nabiximols is licenced in 27 countries to treat spasticity in MS patients (Russo et. al., 2008)

CULTIVATION

Methods of Cannabis Propagation

Domestication of cannabis started more than 12,000 years ago in East Asia (Ren et. al., 2021). Cannabis was first utilised as a versatile plant until about 4000 years ago, when selection for either medicine or fibre production started (Ren et. al., 2021). Cannabis is being grown in both outdoor and indoor agricultural methods. The cultivation location is heavily influenced by the intended final result. Less valued items, such as fibres and seed oils, are often grown on open fields (Monthony et. al., 2021). Outdoor farming for high-value Cannabis products, such as those used for medical or recreational reasons, is also possible. However, greenhouses or indoor production facilities are often employed to optimise the quality and quantity of the plant's final output (Monthony et. al., 2021). Cannabis may be grown utilising seeds, clonal propagation, or tissue culture techniques in open or closed agricultural settings (Figure 3). Clonal propagation is the primary technique of propagation in indoor controlled farming systems, and it is often accomplished by stem cuttings (Adhikary et. al., 2021; Monthony et. al., 2021). Desired traits are preserved for future generations by propagating the successful mother plant (Chandra et. al., 2017). However, there have been multiple reports of clonal propagation limits. These include the necessity for a big area to keep the ideal mother plants, the high chance of diseases and pests, and the difficulty in keeping auto-flowering kinds in a vegetative condition (Monthony et. al., 2021).

Tissue culture techniques are employed instead of clonal propagation to reduce the constraints of clonal propagation. Several research have been undertaken throughout the years to establish the best conditions for Cannabis tissue culture growth (Adams et. al., 2021 and Hesami et. al., 2021). The majority of in vitro investigations utilising diverse combinations of cytokinins and auxins resulted in effective callus production (Figure 3E) of various Cannabis explants (Adhikary et. al., 2021; Monthony et. al., 2021). Recently, (Galan-vila et al., 2021) demonstrated in vitro direct regeneration from hypocotyls, cotyledons, and leaves of 7-day-old Cannabis seedlings. According to the research, hypocotyls were the best responding explant, with a greater percentage of regeneration (53.3%). However, research on indirect Cannabis regeneration through callus tissues is contradictory. Some investigations have shown that callus tissues can regenerate (Zhang et. al., 2021; Slusarkiewicz-Jarzina et. al., 2005; Wielgus et. al., 2008; Lata et. al., 2010; Hussain, 2014; Movahedi et. al., 2014; Hesami et. al., 2021). However, several results imply a lack of consistent and rigorous techniques for cannabis indirect regeneration (Adhikary et. al., 2021; Monthony et. al., 2021; Smykalova et. al., 201). Nonetheless, a recent work (Zhang et al., 2021) revealed effective indirect regeneration from calli of various hemp explants, with the best shoot regeneration rate of 7.1% attained from calli produced from embryo hypocotyl of immature grains. Furthermore, overexpression of genes involved in shoot organogenesis boosted regeneration efficiency by 1.7 times (Zhang et. al., 2021). Despite these accomplishments, further research is needed to develop better indirect regeneration rates for hemp and marijuana. It is also critical to do research to determine the best conditions for in vitro cannabis development. Sucrose concentration, light intensity, and light spectrum have been discovered to influence several characteristics of Cannabis development, including shoot length, root length, shot number, node number, and canopy area (Pepe et. al., 2021).

Different Cultivation and Breeding Forms

Seed Selecting and Germination

High effectiveness to standardize hydroponic indoor growing, cannabis seeds are sown in tiny jiffy pots. Germination begins in 3-7 days. Well-developed seedlings were moved to a smaller container for optimal vegetative development. Plants were moved to a multi-flow hydroponics system fitted with a nutrient reservoir and an electronic timer to manage the flow of nutrients after sufficient root and biomass growth (Chandra et al., 2010). Cannabis females with the highest vitality to become mothers should be maintained under continual vegetative light, generally HID lights for 24 hours and hydroponic solution, to provide you with the necessary propagation stock.

Selecting and Cloning

Potter et al. (2004) reported using “clones” to keep the genotype genetically similar for each successive generation of plants as its mother plant. Clones are rooted cuttings that have been propagated asexually or vegetatively. These clones were put into seedling trays with tiny culture media and nutrients from a hydroponic solution. For the first month, all clones were subjected to consistent vegetative light, typically HID lamps, 95-100% relative humidity (RH), and temperatures of 27 C. Root creation began in two to three weeks, and after the roots reached a suitable size, they were transferred into a larger hydroponic system with new circumstances for faster growth (Cervantes, 2006; Chandra et. al., 2010).

Vegetative Period

During this stage, all clones were housed in a grow chamber under comparable environmental conditions (light, temperature, RH, and CO2 concentration) for indoor culture throughout the growth period. Full spectrum 1,000-watt HID bulbs installed above the plants supplied light for these plants. To reduce heating caused by HID lights, a hot air suction fan installed around 3-4 feet between plants and bulb was continually maintained. By adjusting the distance between plant and light source, photosynthetically active radiation (PAR) of about 700 $^{+}$-25μmol m^{-2} s^{-1} maintained at the pot level. Using an automatic electric timer photoperiod regulated to maintain vegetative (18 h/day) stage. Grow room temperature and humidity kept nearly constant at ~ 60 F and ~ 60% respectively throughout the growing period. Plants were fertilised with a vegetative fertiliser mix during their acclimation and vegetative development, and they developed a 50-centimeter-long, robust root system by the end of this period (Potter, 2004; Chandra et. al., 2010).

Flowering Period

Induced flowering after 12 hours of light exposure in an ideal nutritional environment. In 7-14 days, the plant will begin to produce flowers with female pistils, at which point the inflorescences will have grown larger and more cannabinoids will have been produced. The rate of cannabinoids production drops dramatically during week 8 of flowering, when the stigma and trichomes begin to senesce and become an organ/brown colour (Potter, 2004; Chandra et. al., 2010).

In Vitro Micropropagation

Direct organogenesis is considered the most dependable technique of clonal multiplication because it maintains genetic homogeneity across progenies (Chandra et al., 2010). Despite this, few publications have been published documenting the regeneration techniques created for various Cannabis genotypes and explant sources. Fisse and colleagues (1981) devised a technique for inducing from Cannabis calli. These cultures, however, were observed to be unresponsive to shoot development. Mandolino and Ranalli (1999) demonstrated shoot regeneration from calli, however Feeney and Punja (2003) failed to produce hemp plantlets, either directly or indirectly, from callus or suspension cultures. Lata et al. (2008; 2010a,b) created a high frequency plant regeneration system using callus and nodal segments produced from leaf tissue and kept in a brief immersion bioreactor for high yield shoot multiplication.

Synthetic Seed Technology

Some plants have been known to produce synthetic seeds and regenerate plantlets (Sicurani et. al., 2001; Brischia et. al., 2002; Hao and Deng, 2003). Some papers discuss the encapsulation of vegetative propagates such as axillary buds or shoot tips, which might be employed for bulk clonal propagation as well as long-term germplasm conservation (Mathur et. al., 1989; Pattnaik and Chand, 2000). Synthetic seed technology might be a helpful tool for cost-effective large-scale clonal replication and germplasm conservation of C. sativa's screened and chosen top germplasm (Chandra et al., 2010). C. sativa nodal segments comprising axillary buds were encapsulated in sodium alginate with calcium chloride dihydrate from several shoot cultures (CaCl2.2 H2O) Regrowth and conversion following encapsulation were studied in vitro and in vivo for various planting substrates (Lata et. al., 2008; 2009).

PHARMACOLOGICAL ASPECTS OF *CANNABIS SATIVA*

Cannabinoids in Animal kingdom

The primary endocannabinoids ligands found in the Animal kingdom are N-arachidonoylethanolamine (AEA) and 2-arachidonoyl glycerol (2AG) (McPartland, 2004). AEA and 2-AG are synthesised from arachidonate-containing cell membrane phospholipids and released promptly. Fatty acid amide hydrolase (FAAH) and monoacylglycerol lipase (MAGL) are AEA and 2-AG degradation enzymes that modulate cannabinoidergic tone through hydrolysis. Cannabinoid type-1 (CB1) receptor and cannabinoid type-2 (CB2) receptor are the two primary endocannabinoid receptors (Mechoulam et. al., 1998). The endocannabinoid system (ECS) is found in all animals with a nervous system, including Hydra, as well as mammals, birds, amphibians, fish, and numerous echinoderms and mussels (Salzet et. al., 2000). However, ECS has not been discovered in all terrestrial invertebrates. There have been few reports of cannabis receptors and/or enzymes in insects. They discovered that C. sativa may cause neurological and behavioural abnormalities in insects, thus agronomists have long used its extracts as insect repellents (McPartland et. al., 2001). The ECS has a significant neuromodulatory effect in mammals (Mechoulam et. al., 1998). Mice with CB1 receptor deletions had altered nociceptive responses, severe hypomobility, and significantly increased mortality (Zimmer et al., 1999). Cannabinoid receptors are around ten times more abundant in human brains than opioid receptors (Sim et. al., 1996). CB1 receptors, in particular, are widely expressed in the hippocampus, basal ganglia, amygdala, cortical areas, and cerebellum, all of which are involved in mood, cognitive functioning, and motor control (Tsou et. al., 1998). Lower levels have been discovered in other brain locations, such as the brainstem, which houses the regulatory centres for breathing and heart function (Akerman et. al., 2013). CB1 receptors have also been found in the colon, liver, adipose tissue, and immune cells (Jourdan et. al., 2010). CB2 receptor expression in the brain is substantially lower under normal conditions compared to CB1 receptors; nevertheless, during inflammation, CB2 receptor levels dramatically rise in microglia and other glial cells (Savonenko et. al., 2015). Given the expression of cannabinoid receptors in the neurological system and the interactions of cannabinoids with neurotransmitters such as dopamine, glutamate, serotonin, and gamma-aminobutyric acid, cannabis may have significant medicinal potential (Thompson et. al., 2003). A vast variety of cannabinoid compounds capable of modulating the CB1, CB2 receptors, and the metabolism of the endocannabinoids, AEA and2 AG, have been discovered and described in recent decades (Rampa et. al., 2012; Giacoppo et. al., 2014). These findings highlight the physiological significance of the endocannabinoid system.

Cannabinoids and Diseases

The usage of various C. sativa preparations (both natural and synthetic) is related with treatment techniques for a variety of disorders. Certainly, because of the ECS's widespread location in the brain and periphery, its activation or inhibition governs a variety of pathologic processes (Mastinu et. al., 2018).

The ECS has a role in a variety of illnesses, including metabolic and neuroinflammatory ailments. Cannabinoids, in particular, affect hunger/satiety and neuro inflammation in the brain, and in the periphery, they are implicated in the peripheral metabolic processes of the liver, fat, and muscles, as well as the anti-inflammatory response in blood cells (Mastinu et. al., 2018). Nonetheless, cannabinoids are linked with an increased risk of short-term side effects such as asthenia, balance issues, confusion, dizziness, disorientation, diarrhoea, euphoria, sleepiness, dry mouth, tiredness, hallucination, nausea, somnolence, vomiting, and anxiety (Lim et al., 2017).

Pain

The pharmacological potential of C. sativa was assessed in a meta-analysis conducted by Whiting and colleagues (Whiting et al., 2015), which found evidence in favour of the use of cannabinoids for the treatment of chronic neuropathic or cancer pain (smoked D9THC and nabiximols) (Solowij and Battisti, 2008). PrNMI, a synthetic peripherally limited cannabinoid molecule, was shown to be efficient in decreasing chemotherapy-induced peripheral neuropathy in a rat model of cisplatin-induced neuropathic pain, and this action was mediated through CB1 receptors activation (Mulpuri et. al., 2018). Mellar Davies recently published a review on the topic of cannabinoids and pain management, wherein he emphasises the analgesic potential with reduced cannabimimetic side effects and good therapeutic index of peripherally restricted cannabinoids, regionally administered cannabinoids, bifunctional cannabinoid ligands, cannabinoid enzyme inhibitors, endocannabinoids that do not interact with classic cannabinoid receptors, cannabinoid (Davis, 2014). Several methods exist for gaining the analgesic benefits of cannabinoids without experiencing the psychoactive effects, such as the use of peripherally restricted CB1 receptor agonists, selective CB2 receptor agonists, inhibitors of endocannabinoid catabolism or uptake, and the modulation of other non-CB1/CB2 receptor targets of cannabinoids, such as TRPV1, GPR55, and PPARs (Starowicz and Finn, 2017).

Colitis

C. sativa formulations have been used to treat gut disorders such as gastrointestinal discomfort, gastroenteritis, and diarrhoea (Couch et. al., 2018). Phytocannabinoids may reduce inflammation in the stomach by primarily activating the CB2 receptor and promote wound healing by activating the CB1 receptor. Several publications have observed that isolated C. sativa components such as CBC, CBD, and CBG have beneficial effects in animal models of inflammatory bowel disease following an inflammatory insult (Naftali et. al., 2014; Pagano et. al., 2016, Hasenoehrl et. al., 2017). Furthermore, Nallathambi and colleagues discovered that D9-THCA had anti-inflammatory action on colon epithelial cells (Nallathambi et. al., 2017).

Spasticity

More than 85% of persons with multiple sclerosis (MS) have spasticity. Baclofen, tizanidine, diazepam, and botulinum toxin are now utilised to treat MS-related spasticity (Flachenecker et. al., 2014). These drugs are not always totally effective, and their usage or dosage may be restricted due to negative effects (Soelberg Sorensen, 2017). As a result, the usage of C. sativa among MS patients is expanding over the globe. Indeed, multiple studies have shown that the pharmaceutical use of cannabis may help with MS-related spasticity (Koppel et. al., 2014; Nielsen et. al., 2018; Allan et. al., 2018). Nabiximols (Sativex oral spray, which has been approved by regulatory agencies in Canada, New Zealand, and several European countries), oral cannabis extract, and synthetic tetrahydrocannabinol were found to be effective in reducing patient-reported symptoms of spasticity and pain in MS patients who had not responded well to other drugs. Nabiximols, in particular, is typically well accepted by MS patients, with a minimal misuse potential, little risk of psychotropic effects, and no evidence of dosage tolerance (Keating, 2017). Furthermore, the improvements in spasticity, health-related quality of life, and daily living activities reported in MS patients were long-lasting (Keating, 2017). However, several writers have raised concerns about the use of C. sativa derivatives in MS patients (Pavisian et al., 2014; Rudroff and Honce, 2017; Rice and Cameron, 2018; Herzog et al., 2018). To begin, adverse effects such as an increased chance of developing psychosis, changes in working memory, executive function, and other cognitive processes have been identified. Second, because to differences in legal status between Europe and the United States, cannabis derivatives utilised in research do not necessarily belong to the same varieties/cultivars, raising the issue of which strain is the best. As a result, the use of C. sativa derivatives in MS-associated spasticity will need further large, multicenter, randomised, placebo-controlled trials.

Nausea and Vomiting

C. sativa has long been recognised for its ability to reduce or prevent nausea and vomiting caused by a range of factors. This has resulted in substantial research revealing a vital function for cannabis derivatives in nausea and vomiting treatments (Sharkey et. al., 2014). Several C. sativa compounds are available for the treatment of nausea and vomiting due to the dispersion of the endocannabinoid system in the gut. The FDA (Food and Drug Administration) authorised nabilone, a synthetic analogue of D9-THC, in 1985 for the treatment of chemotherapy-induced nausea and vomiting that had not responded to standard antiemetic medicines (dopamine receptor 2 (D2) antagonists) (Sharkey et al., 2014; Whiting et al., 2015). Indeed, nabilone medication reduces nausea and vomiting episodes in chemotherapy patients as compared to metoclopramide (D2 antagonist) (Sharkey et al., 2014, Badowsky, 2017). Furthermore, cancer patients treated with dronabinol, a synthetic analogue of D9-THC, had less acute nausea and a much shorter duration than those treated with prochlorperazine (D2 antagonist) (Badowski, 2017). However, certain adverse effects have been reported for these C. sativa compounds as well (Tafelski et. al., 2016, Schussel et. al., 2018). As a result, additional research is required to determine the safety of cannabis for nausea and vomiting therapy.

Anorexia

Cannabinoids influence total body weight by interfering with many central and peripheral regulatory circuits that regulate energy balance (Horn et. al., 2018; Mastinu et. al., 2018). Increased expression of the CB1 receptor has been discovered in the insular cortex, inferior temporal and frontal lobes of persons suffering from anorexia and bulimia nervosa, indicating an impairment in the processing of interceptive, gustatory, and reward-related behaviour (Gérard et al., 2011). Subchronic treatment with both the natural D9-THC and the synthetic CB1/CB2 receptor agonist CP-55,940 was able to significantly reduce body weight loss and running wheel activity in an activity-based anorexia rat model, while also increasing leptin signalling and decreasing corticosterone plasma levels (Scherma et. al., 2017). Several studies suggest the use of pharmacological CB1 signalling activation to help patients with mental disorders such as anorexia nervosa or bulimia, as well as patients with cancer anorexia-cachexia, regain body weight (Koch, 2017; Andries et. al., 2014). Some clinical studies have shown that dronabinol, a CB1/CB2 agonist, may help patients with anorexia nervosa and cancer anorexia-cachexia syndrome recover body weight (Andries et. al., 2014; Inui, 2002).

Sleep Disorders

Cannabis and cannabinoids have sparked medical attention in the past several decades due to its possible use in sleep problems. Indeed, certain cannabis components may improve sleep quality by affecting specific sleep modifications. CBD, in particular, may offer therapeutic promise for the treatment of REM sleep behaviour disorder insomnia and excessive daytime drowsiness. D9-THC may reduce sleep latency, however long-term use may worsen sleep quality (Chait, 1990; Barratt et. al., 1974; Freemon, 1982). Short-term nabilone and dronabinol treatment may be beneficial in obstructive sleep apnea by modulating serotonin tone (Ramar et al., 2018; Calik and Carley, 2017); nabilone may also be useful in reducing nightmares associated with post-traumatic stress disorder and improving sleep in patients with chronic pain (Babson et. al., 2017).

Tourette Syndrome

Cannabinoids may be useful in the treatment of Tourette's syndrome. Indeed, certain clinical investigations found that chronic cannabis or dronabinol therapy improved vocal blocking tics and concomitant Tourette syndrome linked diseases in individuals with treatment-resistant Tourette syndrome (Jakubovski and Müller-Vahl, 2017; Abi-Jaoude et al., 2017).

Anxiety

Cannabis has been shown in recent research to have both anxiogenic and anxiolytic effects. Because C. sativa includes both D9-THC and CBD, they have different psychoactive properties: low doses of D9-THC are anxiolytic, but large doses are anxiogenic, while CBD has anxiolytic effects in both animals and humans owing to its impact on limbic and paralimbic regions (Whiting et. al., 2015). This calming effect of CBD may explain why many individuals suffering from anxiety disorders utilise cannabis as "self-medication" to alleviate their symptoms (Lim et. al., 2017). These findings imply that CBD may be beneficial for anxiety disorders, but further research is needed to confirm these findings (Crippa et al., 2009).

CONCLUSION

Cannabis sativa spp. is a remarkable multi-component natural resource that is employed in a variety of applications, including nutritional supplements, textiles, construction materials, body care items, food, and medications, to mention a few. It has been grown for millennia to take use of the plant's arsenal of beneficial natural chemicals. This chapter investigates the chemical ingredients of the plant that are responsible for its medicinal qualities and investigates effective compounds as nutraceuticals. A qualitative and quantitative examination of these components reveals significant patterns for both fiber-type hemp and medicinal C. sativa. The history, cultivation, and medical applications of C. sativa are discussed in detail.

REFERENCES

Russo, E. B., Jiang, H. E., Li, X., Sutton, A., Carboni, A., del Bianco, F., Mandolino, G., Potter, D. J., Zhao, Y. X., Bera, S., Zhang, Y. B., Lü, E. G., Ferguson, D. K., Hueber, F., Zhao, L. C., Liu, C. J., Wang, Y. F., & Li, C. S. (2008). Phytochemical and genetic analyses of ancient cannabis from Central Asia. *Journal of Experimental Botany, 59*(15), 4171–4182. doi:10.1093/jxb/ern260 PMID:19036842

Zwenger, S.R. *(2014). The biotechnology of* Cannabis sativa. *2.* Extreme Publications Inc.

Lash, R. (2010). Industrial Hemp: The crop for the seventh generation. *Am Indian Law Rev., 27*(1), 313–356. doi:10.2307/20070692

Leizer, C., Ribnicky, D., Poulev, A., Dushenkov, S., & Raskin, I. (2000). The composition of hemp seed oil and its potential as an important source of nutrition. *J Nutraceuticals Funct Med Foods. 2*(4), 35–53. doi:10.1300/J133v02n04_04

Clarke, R. C., & Merlin, M. (2013). *Cannabis: evolution and ethnobotany*. University of California Press.

Zuardi, A. W. (2006). History of cannabis as a medicine: A review. *The British Journal of Psychiatry, 28*(2), 153–157. doi:10.1590/S1516-44462006000200015 PMID:16810401

Small, E. (2017). Classification of Cannabis sativa L. in Relation to agricultural, biotechnological, medical, and recreational utilization. In S. Chandra, H. Lata, & M. ElSohly (Eds.), *Cannabis sativa L. - Botany and Biotechnology*. Springer. doi:10.1007/978-3-319-54564-6_1

Burstein, S. (1997). Marijuana as a medicine. *Nature, 386*(6623), 320. doi:10.1038/386320d0 PMID:9121543

Cota, D., Marsicano, G., Luts, B., Vicennati, V., Stalla, G. K., Pasquali, R., & Pagotto, U. (2003). Endogenous cannabinoid system as a modulator of food intake. *International Journal of Obesity and Related Metabolic Disorders, 27*(3), 289–301. doi:10.1038j.ijo.0802250 PMID:12629555

Small, E. (2017). Classiðcation of Cannabissativa L. in relation to Agricultural, Biotechnology and Recreational Utilization. In S. Chandra, H. Lata, & M. ElSohly (Eds.), *Cannabis sativa L. Botany and Biotechnology*. Springer. doi:10.1007/978-3-319-54564-6_1

Montonya, D. (2016). *Hemp as Fibre and Food? Regulatory Developments and Current Issues; Breaðng Paper*. Parliamentary Research Service.

Leyva, D. R., McCullough, R. S., & Pierce, G. N. (2011). Medicinal Use of Hempseeds (Cannabis sativa L.): Effects on Platelet Aggregation. In V. R. Preedy, R. R. Watson, & V. B. Patel (Eds.), *Nuts and Seeds in Health and Diseases Prevention*. Elsevier. doi:10.1016/B978-0-12-375688-6.10074-X

Callaway, J. C. (2004). Hempseed as a nutritional resource: An overview. *Euphytica, 140*(1-2), 65–72. doi:10.100710681-004-4811-6

Lawrence, R. G. (2019). *Pot in Pans: A History of Eating Cannabis*. The Rowman & Littleðeld Publishing Group.

Lozano, I. (2001, January). (201). The therapeutic use of Cannabis sativa (L.) in Arabic medicine. *Journal of Cannabis Therapeutics*, *1*(1), 63–70. doi:10.1300/J175v01n01_05

Kala CP, Farooquee NA, Dhar U. (2004). Prioritization of medicinal plants on the basis of available knowledge, existing practices and use value status in Uttaranchal. *India Biodiv Conser. 13*(2), 453–469. doi:: BIOC.0000006511.67354.7f. doi:10.1023/B

Radwan, M. M., Elsohly, M. A., Slade, D., Ahmed, S. A., Khan, I. A., & Ross, S. A. (2009). Biologically active cannabinoids from high-potency Cannabis sativa. *Journal of Natural Products*, *72*(5), 906–911. doi:10.1021/np900067k PMID:19344127

Calvi, L., Pavlović, R., Panseri, S., Giupponi, L., Leoni, V., & Giorgi, A. (2018). Quality traits of medical Cannabis sativa L. inflorescences and derived products based on comprehensive mass-spectrometry analytical investigation. Recent Advances in Cannabinoid Research. IntechOpen.

Booth, J. K., & Bohlmann, J. (2019). Terpenes in Cannabis sativa - from plant genome to humans. *Plant Science*, *284*, 67–72. doi:10.1016/j.plantsci.2019.03.022 PMID:31084880

Small, E., & Cronquist, A. (1976). A Practical and Natural Taxonomy for Cannabis. *Taxon*, *25*(4), 405–435. doi:10.2307/1220524

Cascini, F., Farcomeni, A., Migliorini, D., Baldassarri, L., Boschi, I., Martello, S., Amaducci, S., Lucini, L., & Bernardi, J. (2019). Highly Predictive Genetic Markers Distinguish Drug-Type from Fiber-Type Cannabis sativa L. *Plants*, *8*(11), 496. doi:10.3390/plants8110496 PMID:31718081

Chaffey, N. (2001). Hemp on the move. *Trends in Plant Science*, *6*, 505.

Shi, G., & Cai, Q. (2009). Cadmium tolerance and accumulation in eight potential energy crops. *Biotechnology Advances*, *27*(5), 555–561. doi:10.1016/j.biotechadv.2009.04.006 PMID:19393309

Ahmad, R., Tehsin, Z., Malik, S. T., Asad, S. A., Shahzad, M., Bilal, M., Shah, M. M., & Khan, S. A. (2015). S.A. Phytoremediation Potential of Hemp (Cannabis sativa L.): Identiðcation and Characterization of Heavy Metals Responsive Genes. *Clean-Soil Air Water*, *44*(2), 195–201. doi:10.1002/clen.201500117

Husain, R., Weeden, H., Bogush, D., Deguchi, M., Soliman, M., Potlakayala, S., Katam, R., Goldman, S., & Rudrabhatla, S. (2019). Enhanced tolerance of industrial hemp (Cannabis sativa L.) plants on abandoned mine land soil leads to overexpression of cannabinoids. *PLoS One*, *14*(8), e0221570. doi:10.1371/journal.pone.0221570 PMID:31465423

Wang, X., Li, Q. X., Heidel, M., Wu, Z., Yoshimoto, A., Leong, G., Pan, D., & Ako, H. (2021). Comparative evaluation of industrial hemp varieties: Field experiments and phytoremediation in Hawaii. *Industrial Crops and Products*, *170*, 113683. doi:10.1016/j.indcrop.2021.113683

Finnan, J., & Styles, D. (2013). Hemp: A more sustainable annual energy crop for climate and energy policy. *Energy Policy*, *58*, 152–162. doi:10.1016/j.enpol.2013.02.046

Das, L., Liu, E., Saeed, A., Williams, D. W., Hu, H., Li, C., Ray, A. E., & Shi, J. (2017). Industrial hemp as a potential bioenergy crop in comparison with kenaf, switchgrass and biomass sorghum. *Bioresource Technology*, *244*, 641–649. doi:10.1016/j.biortech.2017.08.008 PMID:28810219

Arseneault, L., Cannon, M., Poulton, R., Murray, R., Caspi, A., & Mofðtt, T. E. (2002). Cannabis use in adolescence and risk for adult psychosis: Longitudinal prospective study. *BMJ (Clinical Research Ed.)*, *325*(7374), 1212–1213. doi:10.1136/bmj.325.7374.1212 PMID:12446537

Andreasson, S., Allebeck, P., Engström, A., & Rydberg, U. (1987). Cannabis and schizophrenia. A longitudinal study of Swedish conscripts. *Lancet*, *330*(8574), 1483–1486. doi:10.1016/S0140-6736(87)92620-1 PMID:2892048

Barkus, E., & Murray, R. M. (2010). Substance use in adolescence and psychosis: Clarifying the relationship. *Annual Review of Clinical Psychology*, *6*(1), 365–389. doi:10.1146/annurev.clinpsy.121208.131220 PMID:20192802

Trezza, V., Cuomo, V., & Vanderschuren, L. J. (2008). Cannabis and the developing brain: Insights from behavior. *European Journal of Pharmacology*, *585*(2-3), 441–452. doi:10.1016/j.ejphar.2008.01.058 PMID:18413273

Gleason, K. A., Birnbaum, S. G., Shukla, A., & Ghose, S. (2012). Susceptibility of the adolescent brain to cannabinoids: Long-term hippocampal effects and relevance to schizophrenia. *Translational Psychiatry*, *2*(11), e199. doi:10.1038/tp.2012.122 PMID:23188199

Renard, J., Rushlow, W. J., & LaViolette, S. R. (2018). Effects of Adolescent THC Exposure on the Prefrontal GABAergic System: Implications for Schizophrenia-Related Psychopathology. *Frontiers in Psychiatry*, *9*, 281. doi:10.3389/fpsyt.2018.00281 PMID:30013490

Lubman, D. I., Cheetham, A., & Yücel, M. (2015). Cannabis and adolescent brain development. *Pharmacology & Therapeutics*, *148*, 1–16. doi:10.1016/j.pharmthera.2014.11.009 PMID:25460036

Hao X. M., Yang Y., An L. X., Wang J. M., Han L. (2014). Study on antibacterial mechanism of hemp fiber. *Adv. Mat. Res.* doi:10.4028/www.scientific.net/AMR.887-888.610

Khan, B. A., Wang, J., Warner, P., & Wang, H. (2015). Antibacterial properties of hemp hurd powder against *E. coli*. *Journal of Applied Polymer Science*, *132*(10), 41588. doi:10.1002/app.41588

Bao, Q., Liu, H., Fu, K., Zhang, C., Wang, C., & Feng, Y. (2014). *Hemp Bast Fiber Extract with Antibacterial Activity, Preparation Method, and Application of Hemp Bast Fiber Extract.* Patent publication number CN104018343A. Washington, DC: U.S. Patent and Trademark Office.

Gu, L. F. (2006). *Surgical Sewing Free Zipper Made of Antibiotic Material Hemp Fiber.* Patent publication number CN 2829641 Y. Washington, DC: U.S. Patent and Trademark Office.

Cassano, R., Trombino, S., Ferrarelli, T., Nicoletta, F. P., Mauro, M. V., Giraldi, C., & Picci, N. (2013). Hemp fiber (*Cannabis sativa* L.) derivatives with antibacterial and chelating properties. *Cellulose (London, England)*, *20*(1), 547–557. doi:10.100710570-012-9804-3

Gutiérrez, A., & del Río, J. C. (2005). Chemical characterization of pitch deposits produced in the manufacturing of high-quality paper pulps from hemp fibers. *Bioresource Technology*, *96*(13), 1445–1450. doi:10.1016/j.biortech.2004.12.008 PMID:15939271

Kiprono, P. C., Kaberia, F., Keriko, J. M., & Karanja, J. N. (2000). The in vitro anti-fungal and anti-bacterial activities of beta-sitosterol from *Senecio lyratus* (Asteraceae). *Z. Naturforsch. C*, *55*(5-6), 485–488. doi:10.1515/znc-2000-5-629 PMID:10928565

Ibrahim, T. A. (2012). Chemical composition and biological activity of extracts from Salvia bicolor Desf. growing in Egypt. *Molecules (Basel, Switzerland)*, *17*(10), 11315–11334. doi:10.3390/molecules171011315 PMID:23011275

UNODC. (2019). *World Drug Report. Cannabis and Hallucinogens*. UNODC.

de Meijer, E. P., Bagatta, M., Carboni, A., Crucitti, P., Moliterni, V. M., Ranalli, P., & Mandolino, G. (2003). The inheritance of chemical phenotype in Cannabis sativa L. *Genetics*, *163*(1), 335–346. doi:10.1093/genetics/163.1.335 PMID:12586720

Vanhove, W., Van Damme, P., & Meert, N. (2011). Factors determining yield and quality of illicit indoor cannabis (Cannabis spp.) production. *Forensic Science International*, *212*(1–3), 158–163. doi:10.1016/j.forsciint.2011.06.006 PMID:21737218

Seddon, T., & Floodgate, W. (2020). *Regulating Cannabis: A Global Review and Future Directions*. Palgrave Macmillan. doi:10.1007/978-3-030-52927-7

Stevens, C. J., Murphy, C., Roberts, R., Lucas, L., Silva, F., & Fuller, D. Q. (2016). Between China and South Asia: A middle Asian corridor of crop dispersal and agricultural innovation in the bronze age. *The Holocene*, *26*(10), 1541–1555. doi:10.1177/0959683616650268 PMID:27942165

Jiang, H. E., Li, X., Zhao, Y. X., Ferguson, D. K., Hueber, F., Bera, S., Wang, Y. F., Zhao, L. C., Liu, C. J., & Li, C. S. (2006). A new insight into Cannabis sativa (Cannabaceae) utilization from 2500-year-old Yanghai Tombs, Xinjiang, China. *Journal of Ethnopharmacology*, *108*(3), 414–422. doi:10.1016/j.jep.2006.05.034 PMID:16879937

Russo, E. B., Jiang, H. E., Li, X., Sutton, A., Carboni, A., Del Bianco, F., Mandolino, G., Potter, D. J., Zhao, Y.-X., Bera, S., Zhang, Y.-B., Lü, E.-G., Ferguson, D. K., Hueber, F., Zhao, L.-C., Liu, C.-J., Wang, Y.-F., & Li, C.-S. (2008). Phytochemical and genetic analyses of ancient cannabis from Central Asia. *Journal of Experimental Botany*, *59*(15), 4171–4182. doi:10.1093/jxb/ern260 PMID:19036842

Pain, S. (2015). A potted history. *Nature*, *525*(7570), S10–S11. doi:10.1038/525S10a PMID:26398731

Li, H. (1974). Anarchaeological and historical account of Cannabis in China. *Economic Botany*, *28*(4), 437–448. doi:10.1007/BF02862859

Cherney, J. H., & Small, E. (2016). Industrial hemp in North America:production,politicsand potential. *Agronomy (Basel)*, *6*(4), 58. doi:10.3390/agronomy6040058

Savo, V., La Rocca, A., Caneva, G., Rapallo, F., & Cornara, L. (2013). Plants used in artisanal ðsheries on the Western Mediterranean coasts of Italy. *Journal of Ethnobiology and Ethnomedicine*, *9*(1), 9. doi:10.1186/1746-4269-9-9 PMID:23356937

Merlin, M.D., (2003). Archaeological evidence for the tradition of psychoactive plant use in the old world. *Econ. Bot. 57*, 295–323. doi: 057[0295:AEFTTO]2.0.CO;2. doi:10.1663/0013-0001(2003)

Clarke, R. C., & Merlin, M. D. (2013). *Cannabis, Evolution and Ethnobotany*. University of California press.

Luna, L. E. (1984). The concept of plants as teachers among four mestizo shamans of Iquitos, northeastern Peru. *Journal of Ethnopharmacology, 11*(2), 135–156. doi:10.1016/0378-8741(84)90036-9 PMID:6492831

VanPool, C.S., (2009). The signs of the sacred: identifying shamans using archaeological evidence. *J. Anthropol. Archaeol.* 28, 177–190. doi:. 02.003. doi:10.1016/j.jaa.2009

Maðmisebi, T. E., & Oguntade, A. E. (2010). Preparation and use of plant medicines for farmers' health in Southwest Nigeria: Socio-cultural, magico-religious and economic aspects. *Journal of Ethnobiology and Ethnomedicine*, *6*(1), 1. doi:10.1186/1746-4269-6-1 PMID:20089149

Jauregui, X., Clavo, Z. M., Jovel, E. M., & Pardo-de-Santayana, M. (2011). "Plantas con madre": plants that teach and guide in the shamanic initiation process in the EastCentral Peruvian Amazon. *J. Ethnopharmacol. 134*, 739–752. doi:1016/j.jep.2011.01.042.

Gagliano, M. (2013). Persons as plants: ecopsychology and the return to the dream of nature. Landsc.: *J. Int. Cent. Landsc. Lang. 5*(2). áhttp://ro.ecu.edu.au/landscapes/ vol5/iss2/14ñ.

Armijos, C., Cota, I., & González, S. (2014). Traditional medicine applied by the Saraguro yachakkuna: A preliminary approach to the use of sacred and psychoactive plant species in the southern region of Ecuador. *Journal of Ethnobiology and Ethnomedicine*, *10*(1), 26. doi:10.1186/1746-4269-10-26 PMID:24565054

Touwn, M. (1981). The religious and medicinal uses of Cannabis in China, India and Tibet. *Journal of Psychoactive Drugs*, *13*(1), 23–34. doi:10.1080/02791072.1981.10471447 PMID:7024492

Schultes, R. E., Hoffman, A., & Ratsch, C. (1992). *Plants of the Gods – Their Sacred, Healing and Hallucinogenic Powers*. Healing Arts Press.

Bennett, C. (2011). Early/Ancient History. In J. Holland (Ed.), *The Pot Book: A Complete Guide to Cannabis* (pp. 17–26). Its Role in Medicine, Politics, Science, and Culture.

Abel, E. L. (1980). *Marijuana: The First Twelve Thousand Years*. Springer. doi:10.1007/978-1-4899-2189-5

Epstein, H. A. (2010). A natural approach to soothing atopic skin. *Skinmed*, *8*, 95–97. PMID:20527141

Anderson, B. R., & Scurlock, J. (2005). *Diagnoses in Assyrian and Babylonian Medicine*. University of Illinois Press.

Mercuri, A., Accorsi, C., & Bandini Mazzanti, M. (2002). The long history of Cannabis and its cultivation by theRomans in central Italy,shown by pollen recordsfromLago Albano and Lago di Nemi. *Vegetation History and Archaeobotany*, *11*(4), 263–276. doi:10.1007003340200039

Anwara, F., Latifa, S., Ashrafb, M., (2006). Analytical Characterization of Hemp (Cannabis sativa) *Seed Oil from Different Agro-Ecological Zones of Pakistan, 83*, 323–329. áhttps://doi:. doi:10.1007/s11746-006-1207-xñ

Jeong, M., Cho, J., Shin, J. I., Jeon, Y. J., Kim, J. H., Lee, S. J., Kim, E. S., & Lee, K. (2014). Hempseed oil induces reactive oxygen species- and C/EBP homologous proteinmediated apoptosis in MH7A human rheumatoid arthritis ðbroblast-like synovial cells. *Journal of Ethnopharmacology*, *154*(3), 745–752. doi:10.1016/j.jep.2014.04.052 PMID:24814038

Pepe, M., Hesami, M., Small, F., & Jones, A. M. P. (2021). A.M.P. Comparative Analysis of Machine Learning and Evolutionary Optimization Algorithms for Precision Micropropagation of Cannabis sativa: Prediction and Validation of in vitro Shoot Growth and Development Based on the Optimization of Light and Carbohydrate Sources. *Front. Plant Sci.*, *12*, 757869. doi:10.3389/fpls.2021.757869 PMID:34745189

Zhang, X., Xu, G., Cheng, C., Lei, L., Sun, J., Xu, Y., Deng, C., Dai, Z., Yang, Z., Chen, X., Liu, C., Tang, Q., & Su, J. (2021). Establishment of an Agrobacterium –mediated genetic transformation and CRISPR/Cas9-mediatedtargetedmutagenesisinHemp (CannabissativaL.). *Plant Biotechnology Journal*, *19*(10), 1979–1987. doi:10.1111/pbi.13611 PMID:33960612

Slusarkiewicz-Jarzina, A., Ponitka, A., & Kaczmarek, Z. (2005). Inñuence of cultivar, explant source and plant growth regulator on callus induction and plant regeneration of Cannabis sativa L. *Acta Biologica Cracoviensia. Series; Botanica*, *47*, 145–151.

Wielgus, K., Luwanska, A., Lassocinski, W., & Kaczmarek, Z. (2008). Estimation of Cannabissativa L. Tissue Culture Conditions Essential for Callus Induction and Plant Regeneration. *Journal of Natural Fibers*, *5*(3), 199–207. doi:10.1080/15440470801976045

Lata, H., Chandra, S., Khan, I. A., & ElSohly, M. (2010). ElSohly, M.A. High Frequency Plant Regeneration from Leaf Derived Callus of HighΔ9Tetrahydrocannabinol Yielding Cannabis sativa L. *Planta Medica*, *76*(14), 1629–1633. doi:10.1055-0030-1249773 PMID:20354950

Hussain, S. H. F. (2014). *Cannabinoids production in Cannabis sativa L. An In Vitro Approach.* [Ph.D. Thesis, Technischen Universitat Dortmund, Dortmund, Germany].

Movahedi, M., Ghasemi-Omran, V., & Torabi, S. (2014). The effect of different concentrations of TDZ and BA on in vitro regeneration of Iranian cannabis (Cannabis sativa) using cotyledon and epicotyl explants. *J. Plant Mol. Breed.*, *3*, 20–27.

Hesami, M., & Jones, A. M. P. (2021). Modeling and optimizing callus growth and development in Cannabis sativa using random forest and support vector machine in combination with a genetic algorithm. *Applied Microbiology and Biotechnology*, *105*(12), 5201–5212. doi:10.100700253-021-11375-y PMID:34086118

Smýkalová, I., Vrbová, M., Cvečková, M., Plačková, L., Žukauskaitė, A., Zatloukal, M., Hrdlička, J., Plíhalová, L., Doležal, K., & Griga, M. (2019). Cvecˇková, M.; Placˇková, L.; Žukauskait˙e, A.; Zatloukal, M.; Hrdlicˇka, J.; Plíhalová, L.; Doležal, K.; Griga, M. The effects of novel synthetic cytokinin derivatives and endogenous cytokinins on the in vitro growth responses of hemp (Cannabis sativa L.) explants. *Plant Cell, Tissue and Organ Culture*, *139*(2), 381–394. doi:10.100711240-019-01693-5

Fisse, J., Braut, F., Cosson, L., & Paris, M. (1981). E ´tude in vitro des capacite ´s organoge ´ne ´tiques de tissus de Cannabis sativa L.; Effet de diffe ´rentes substances de croissance [In vitro study of the organoge netic capacities of Cannabis sativa L. tissues; Effect of different growth substances]. *Plantes Me ´dicinales et Phytotherapie*, *15*, 217–223.

Mandolino, G., & Ranalli, P. (1999). Advances in biotechnological approaches for hemp breeding and industry. In P. Ranalli (Ed.), *Advances in hemp research* (pp. 185–212). The Haworth Press.

Feeney, M., & Punja, Z. K. (2003). Tissue culture and Agrobacterium-mediated transformation of hemp (Cannabis sativa L.). *In Vitro Cellular & Developmental Biology. Plant*, *39*(6), 578–585. doi:10.1079/IVP2003454

Lata, H., Chandra, S., Khan, I. A., & ElSohly, M. A. (2008). Propagation of Cannabis sativa L. using synthetic seed technology. *Planta Medica*, *74*(3), 328–328. doi:10.1055-2008-1075214

Lata, H., Chandra, S., Khan, I., & ElSohly, M. (2010a). Cannabis sativa L. Micropropagation in temporary immersion bioreactor system. *Planta Medica*, *76*(05, P9). doi:10.1055-0030-1251771

Lata, H., Chandra, S., Khan, I. A., & ElSohly, M. A. (2010b). High frequency plant regeneration from leaf derived callus of high delta (9)-tetrahydrocannabinol yielding Cannabis sativa L. *Planta Medica*, *76*(14), 1629–1633. doi:10.1055-0030-1249773 PMID:20354950

Sicurani, M., Piccioni, E., & Standardi, A. (2001). Micropropagation and preparation of synthetic seed in M.26 apple rootstock I: Attempts towards saving labor in the production of adventitious shoot tips suitable for encapsulation. *Plant Cell Tiss Org*, *66*(3), 207–216. doi:10.1023/A:1010627720368

Brischia, R., Piccioni, E., & Standardi, A. (2002). Micropropagation and synthetic seed in M.26 apple rootstock (II): A new protocol for production of encapsulated differentiating propagules. *Plant Cell Tiss Org*, *68*(2), 137–141. doi:10.1023/A:1013802723018

Hao, Y. J., & Deng, X. X. (2003). Genetically stable regeneration of apple plants from slow growth. *Plant Cell Tiss Org*, *72*(3), 253–260. doi:10.1023/A:1022388728497

Mathur, J., Ahuja, P. S., Lal, N., & Mathur, A. K. (1989). Propagation of Valeriana-Wallichii Dc using encapsulated apical and axial shoot buds. *Plant Science*, *60*(1), 111–116. doi:10.1016/0168-9452(89)90050-2

Pattnaik, S., & Chand, P. K. (2000). Morphogenic response of the alginate encapsulated axillary buds from in vitro shoot cultures of six mulberries. *Plant Cell Tiss Org*, *60*(3), 177–185. doi:10.1023/A:1006424626433

Lata, H., Chandra, S., Khan, I. A., & ElSohly, M. A. (2009). Propagation through alginate encapsulation of axillary buds of Cannabis sativa L. an important medicinal plant. *Physiology and Molecular Biology of Plants*, *15*(1), 79–86. doi:10.100712298-009-0008-8 PMID:23572915

Ren, G.; Zhang, X.; Li, Y.; Ridout, K.; Serrano-Serrano, M.L.; Yang, Y.; Liu, A.; Ravikanth, G.; Nawaz, M.A.; Mumtaz, A.S.; et al. (2021). Large-scale whole-genome resequencing unravels the domestication history of Cannabis sativa. *Sci. Adv.*,7, eabg 2286.

Monthony, A. S., Page, S. R., Hesami, M., & Jones, A. M. P. (2021). A.M.P. The Past, Present and Future of Cannabis sativa Tissue Culture. *Plants*, *10*(1), 185. doi:10.3390/plants10010185 PMID:33478171

Adhikary, D., Kulkarni, M., El Mezawy, A., Mobini, S., Elhiti, M., Gjuric, R., Ray, A., Polowick, P., Slaski, J. J., Jones, M. P., & Bhowmik, P. (2021). Medical Cannabis and Industrial Hemp Tissue Culture: Present Status and Future Potential. *Front. PlantSci., 12*, 627240. doi:10.3389/fpls.2021.627240 PMID:33747008

Chandra, S., Lata, H., ElSohly, M. A., Walker, L. A., & Potter, D. (2017). Cannabis cultivation: Methodological issues for obtaining medicalgrade product. *Epilepsy & Behavior, 70*, 302–312. doi:10.1016/j.yebeh.2016.11.029 PMID:28202406

Adams, T. K., & Masondo, N. A. (2021). Malatsi, P.; Makunga, N.P.Cannabissativa: FromTherapeutic Uses to Micropropagation and Beyond. *Plants, 10*, 2078. doi:10.3390/plants10102078 PMID:34685890

Hesami, M., Baiton, A., Alizadeh, M., Pepe, M., Torkamaneh, D., & Jones, A. M. P. (2021). Advances and Perspectives in Tissue Culture and Genetic Engineering of Cannabis. *International Journal of Molecular Sciences, 22*(11), 5671. doi:10.3390/ijms22115671 PMID:34073522

Galán-Ávila, A., Gramazio, P., Ron, M., Prohens, J., & Herraiz, F. J. (2021). A novel and rapid method for Agrobacterium-mediated production of stably transformed Cannabis sativa L. plants. *Industrial Crops and Products, 170*, 113691. doi:10.1016/j.indcrop.2021.113691

Chandra, S. H., Lata, I., Khan, A., & ElSohly, M. A. (2010). Propagation of elite Cannabis sativa for the production of Δ9-Tetrahydrocannabinol (THC) using biotechnological tools. In A. Rajesh (Ed.), *Medicinal plant biotechnology* (pp. 98–114). CABI. doi:10.1079/9781845936785.0098

Potter, D. J. (2004). Growth and morphology of medicinal Cannabis. In G. W. Guy, B. A. Whittle, & P. J. Robson (Eds.), *The medicinal uses of Cannabis and Cannabinoids* (pp. 17–54). Pharmaceutical Press.

Cervantes, J. (2006). *Marijuana horticulture: The indoor/outdoor medical grower's bible.* Van Patten.

Abbasi, A. M., Khan, S. M., Ahmad, M., Khan, M. A., Quave, C. L., & Pieroni, A. (2013). Botanical ethnoveterinary therapies in three districts of the Lesser Himalayas of Pakistan. *Journal of Ethnobiology and Ethnomedicine, 9*(1), 84. doi:10.1186/1746-4269-9-84 PMID:24359615

Abel, E. L. (1980). *Marijuana: The First Twelve Thousand Years.* Springer., doi:10.1007/978-1-4899-2189-5

Abi-Jaoude, E., Chen, L., Cheung, P., Bhikram, T., Sandor, P. (2017). Preliminary evidence on cannabis effectiveness and tolerability for adults with tourette syndrome. *J. Neuropsychiatry Clin. Neurosci.* 29, 391–400. doi:. neuropsych.16110310. doi:10.1176/appi

Akerman, S., Holland, P. R., Lasalandra, M. P., & Goadsby, P. J. (2013). Endocannabinoids in the brainstem modulate dural trigeminovascular nociceptive traffic via CB1 and "triptan" receptors: Implications in migraine. *The Journal of Neuroscience: The Official Journal of the Society for Neuroscience, 33*(37), 14869–14877. doi:10.1523/JNEUROSCI.0943-13.2013 PMID:24027286

Akhtar, N., Rashid, A., Murad, W., & Bergmeier, E. (2013). Diversity and use of ethnomedicinalplantsint heregionofSwat,NorthPakistan. *Journal of Ethnobiology and Ethnomedicine, 9*(1), 25. doi:10.1186/1746-4269-9-25 PMID:23587127

Aldrich, M. (1997). History of therapeutic cannabis. In: Mathre, M.L. (Ed.), Cannabis in Medical Practice: A Legal, Historical and Pharmacological Overview of the Therapeutic use of Marijuana. McFarland & Co.

Allan, G. M., Finley, C. R., Ton, J., Perry, D., Ramji, J., Crawford, K., Lindblad, A. J., Korownyk, C., & Kolber, M. R. (2018). Systematic review of systematic reviews for medical cannabinoids: Pain, nausea and vomiting, spasticity, and harms. *Canadian Family Physician Medecin de Famille Canadien*, *64*, e78–e94. PMID:29449262

Andries, A., Frystyk, J., Flyvbjerg, A., & Støving, R. K. (2014). Dronabinol in severe, enduringanorexia nervosa: A randomized controlled trial. *International Journal of Eating Disorders*, *47*(1), 18–23. doi:10.1002/eat.22173 PMID:24105610

Babson, K. A., Sottile, J., & Morabito, D. (2017). Cannabis, cannabinoids, and sleep: A review of the literature. *Current Psychiatry Reports*, *19*(4), 23. doi:10.100711920-017-0775-9 PMID:28349316

Badowski, M. E. (2017). A review of oral cannabinoids and medical marijuana for the treatment of chemotherapy-induced nausea and vomiting: A focus on pharmacokinetic variability and pharmacodynamics. *Cancer Chemotherapy and Pharmacology*, *80*(3), 441–449. doi:10.100700280-017-3387-5 PMID:28780725

Barratt, E. S., Beaver, W., & White, R. (1974). The effects of marijuana on human sleep patterns. *Biol. Psychiatry, 8*, 47–54. http://psycnet.apa.org/record/1974-24717001.

Benet, S. (1975). Early diffusion and folk uses of hemp. In: Vera Rubin (Ed.), Cannabis and Culture. Mouton Publishers. doi:10.1515/9783110812060.39

Betthauser, K., Pilz, J., & Vollmer, L. E. (2015). Use and effects of cannabinoids in military veterans with posttraumatic stress disorder. *American Journal of Health-System Pharmacy*, *72*(15), 1279–1284. doi:10.2146/ajhp140523 PMID:26195653

Bonini, S. A., Mastinu, A., Maccarinelli, G., Mitola, S., Premoli, M., La Rosa, L. R., Ferrari Toninelli, G., Grilli, M., & Memo, M. (2016). Cortical structure alterations and social behavior impairment in p50-deðcient mice. *Cerebral Cortex (New York, N.Y.)*, *26*(6), 2832–2849. doi:10.1093/cercor/bhw037 PMID:26946128

Bonnie, R. J., & Whitebread, C. H. (1974). *The Marijuana Conviction: A History of Marijuana Prohibition in the United States*. University Press of Virginia.

Bussmann, R. W., Paniagua Zambrana, N. Y., Sikharulidze, S., Kikvidze, Z., Kikodze, D., Tchelidze, D., Khutsishvili, M., Batsatsashvili, K., & Hart, R. E. (2016). A comparative ethnobotany of Khevsureti, Samtskhe-Javakheti, Tusheti, Svaneti, and RachaLechkhumi, Republic of Georgia (Sakartvelo), Caucasus. *Journal of Ethnobiology and Ethnomedicine*, *12*(1), 43. doi:10.118613002-016-0110-2 PMID:27659258

Butrica, J. L. (2002). The medical use of cannabis among the Greeks and Romans. *Journal of Cannabis Therapeutics*, *2*(2), 51–70. doi:10.1300/J175v02n02_04

Calik, M. W., & Carley, D. W. (2017). Effects of cannabinoid agonists and antagonists on sleep and breathing in Sprague-Dawley rats. *Sleep (Basel)*, *40*(9), zsx112. Advance online publication. doi:10.1093leep/zsx112 PMID:28934522

Carod-Artal, F. J. (2013). Psychoactive plants in ancient Greece. *Neurosci. Hist. 1*, 28–38. áhttp://nah.sen.es/en/130-journals/volume-1/issue-1/241-psychoactive-plants-inancient-greeceñ.

Chait, L. D. (1990). Subjective and behavioral effects of marijuana the morning after smoking. *Psychopharmacology, 100*(3), 328–333. doi:10.1007/BF02244601 PMID:2315429

Couch, D. G., Maudslay, H., Doleman, B., Lund, J. N., & O'Sullivan, S. E. (2018). The use of cannabinoids in colitis: A systematic review and meta-analysis. *Inñamm. Bowel Dis., 24*(4), 680–697. doi:10.1093/ibd/izy014 PMID:29562280

Crippa, J. A., Zuardi, A. W., Martín-Santos, R., Bhattacharyya, S., Atakan, Z., McGuire, P., & Fusar-Poli, P. (2009). Cannabis and anxiety: A critical review of the evidence. *Human Psychopharmacology, 24*(7), 515–523. doi:10.1002/hup.1048 PMID:19693792

Davis, M. P. (2014). Cannabinoids in pain management: CB1, CB2 and non-classic receptor ligands. *Expert Opinion on Investigational Drugs, 23*(8), 1123–1140. doi:10.1517/13543784.2014.918603 PMID:24836296

DiMarzo, V., Fontana, A., Cadas, H., Schinelli, S., Cimino, G., Schwartz, J. C., & Piomelli, D. (1994). Formation and inactivation of endogenous cannabinoid anandamide in central neurons. *Nature, 372*(6507), 686–691. doi:10.1038/372686a0 PMID:7990962

Dragone, D., Prarolo, G., Vanin, P., Zanella, G., (2018). Crime and the legalization of recreational marijuana. *J. Econ. Behav. Organ.* doi:. 02.005. doi:10.1016/j.jebo.2018

Flachenecker, P., Henze, T., & Zettl, U. K. (2014). Spasticity in patients with multiple sclerosis–clinical characteristics, treatment and quality of life. *Acta Neurologica Scandinavica, 129*(3), 154–162. doi:10.1111/ane.12202 PMID:24256407

Fleischhauer, W. (1956). The old man of the mountain: The growth of a legend. Symp. *Q. J. Mod. Lit, 9*(1), 79–90. doi:10.1080/00397709.1956.10113536

Fort, J. (2012). Demic and cultural neolithic diffusion. *Proceedings of the National Academy of Sciences of the United States of America, 109*, 18669–18673. doi:10.1073/pnas.1200662109 PMID:23112147

Freemon, F. R. (1982). The effect of chronically administered delta-9-tetrahydrocannabinol upon the polygraphically monitored sleep of normal volunteers. *Drug and Alcohol Dependence, 10*(4), 345–353. doi:10.1016/0376-8716(82)90036-9 PMID:6299682

Gakuubi, M. M., & Wanzala, W. (2012). A survey of plants and plant products traditionally used in livestock health management in Buuri district, Meru County, Kenya. *Journal of Ethnobiology and Ethnomedicine, 8*(1), 39. doi:10.1186/1746-4269-8-39 PMID:23044218

Gérard, N., Pieters, G., Goffin, K., Bormans, G., & Van Laere, K. (2011). Brain type 1 cannabinoid receptor availability in patients with anorexia and bulimia nervosa. *Biological Psychiatry, 70*(8), 777–784. doi:10.1016/j.biopsych.2011.05.010 PMID:21718968

Giacoppo, S., Mandolino, G., Galuppo, M., Bramanti, P., Mazzon, E., (2014). Cannabinoids: new promising agents in the treatment of neurological diseases. *Molecules.* doi:. doi:10.3390/molecules191118781

Hall, W.D., (2008). The contribution of research to the development of a national cannabis policy in Australia. *Addiction 103*, 712–720. doi:. doi:10.1111/j.1360-0443

Hasenoehrl, C., Storr, M., & Schicho, R. (2017). Cannabinoids for treating inñammatory bowel diseases: Where are we and where do we go? *Expert Review of Gastroenterology & Hepatology*, *11*(4), 329–337. doi:10.1080/17474124.2017.1292851 PMID:28276820

Herzog, S., Shanahan, M., Grimison, P., Tran, A., Wong, N., Lintzeris, N., Simes, J., Stockler, M., & Morton, R. L. (2018). Systematic review of the costs and beneðts of prescribed cannabis-based medicines for the management of chronic illness: Lessons from multiple sclerosis. *PharmacoEconomics*, *36*(1), 67–78. doi:10.100740273-017-0565-6 PMID:28866778

Horn, H., Böhme, B., Dietrich, L., & Koch, M. (2018). Endocannabinoids in body weight control. *Pharmaceuticals*, *11*(2), E55. doi:10.3390/ph11020055 PMID:29849009

Inui, A. (2002). Cancer anorexia-cachexia syndrome: Current issues in research and management. *CA: a Cancer Journal for Clinicians*, *52*(2), 72–91. doi:10.3322/canjclin.52.2.72 PMID:11929007

Jakubovski, E., & Müller-Vahl, K. (2017). Speechlessness in Gilles de la Tourette syndrome: Cannabis-based medicines improve severe vocal blocking tics in two patients. *International Journal of Molecular Sciences*, *18*(8), E1739. doi:10.3390/ijms18081739 PMID:28796166

Jourdan, T., Djaouti, L., Demizieux, L., Gresti, J., Vergès, B., & Degrace, P. (2010). CB1 Antagonism exerts speciðc molecular effects on visceral and subcutaneous fat and reversesliver steatosisindiet-inducedobesemice. *Diabetes*, *59*(4), 926–934. doi:10.2337/db09-1482 PMID:20110567

Keating, G. M. (2017). Delta-9-tetrahydrocannabinol/cannabidiol oromucosal spray (Sativex (®)): A review in multiple sclerosis-related spasticity. *Drugs*, *77*(5), 563–574. doi:10.100740265-017-0720-6 PMID:28293911

Koch, M. (2017). Cannabinoid receptor signaling in central regulation of feeding behavior: A mini review. *Frontiers in Neuroscience*, *11*, 293. doi:10.3389/fnins.2017.00293 PMID:28596721

Koppel, B.S., Brust, J.C., Fife, T., Bronstein, J., Youssof, S., Gronseth, G., Gloss, D., (2014). Systematic review: efficacy and safety of medical marijuana in selected neurologic disorders: report of the Guideline Development Subcommittee of the American Academy of Neurology. *Neurology 82*, 1556–1563. doi:.0000000000000363. doi:10.1212/WNL

Kors, A. C., & Peters, E. (2000). *Witchcraft in Europe, 400–1700: A Documentary History*. University of Pennsylvania Press.

Kowal, M. A., Hazekamp, A., Colzato, L. S., van Steenbergen, H., van der Wee, N. J., Durieux, J., Manai, M., & Hommel, B. (2015). Cannabis and creativity: Highly potent cannabis impairs divergent thinking in regular cannabis users. *Psychopharmacology*, *232*(6), 1123–1134. doi:10.100700213-014-3749-1 PMID:25288512

Kunwar, R.M., Shrestha, K.P., Bussmann, R.W., (2010). Traditional herbal medicine in farwest Nepal: a pharmacological appraisal. J. Ethnobiol. Ethnomed. 6, 35. doi:. doi:10.1186/1746-4269-6-35

Latta, R. P., & Eaton, B. J. (1975).. . *Economic Botany*, *29*, 153. doi:10.1007/BF02863315

Lazzari, P., Sanna, A., Mastinu, A., Cabasino, S., Manca, I., & Pani, L. (2011). Weight loss induced by rimonabant is associated with an altered leptin expression and hypothalamic leptin signaling in diet-induced obese mice. *Behavioural Brain Research, 217*(2), 432–438. doi:10.1016/j.bbr.2010.11.022 PMID:21074566

Lazzari, P., Pau, A., Tambaro, S., Asproni, B., Ruiu, S., Pinna, G., Mastinu, A., Curzu, M. M., Reali, R., Bottazzi, M. E., Pinna, G. A., & Murineddu, G. (2012). Synthesis and pharmacological evaluation of novel 4-alkyl-5-thien-2¢-yl pyrazole carboxamides. *Central Nervous System Agents in Medicinal Chemistry, 12*, 254–276. doi:10.2174/187152412803760636 PMID:22931442

Lazzari, P., Serra, V., Marcello, S., Pira, M., & Mastinu, A. (2017). Metabolic side effects induced by olanzapine treatment are neutralized by CB1 receptor antagonist compounds co-administration in female rats. *European Neuropsychopharmacology, 27*(7), 667–678. doi:10.1016/j.euroneuro.2017.03.010 PMID:28377074

Lee, M. A. (2013). *Smoke Signals: A Social History of Marijuana: Medical, Recreational and Scientiðc.* Scribner Paperback Edition.

Levinthal, C. F. (2012). *Drugs, Behavior, and Modern Society*. Pearson College Div.

Lim, K., See, Y.M., Lee, J., (2017). A systematic review of the effectiveness of medical cannabis for psychiatric, movement and neurodegenerative disorders. *Clin. Psychopharmacol. Neurosci.* 15, 301–312. doi:. 301. doi:10.9758/cpn.2017.15.4

Manca, I., Mastinu, A., Olimpieri, F., Falzoi, M., Sani, M., Ruiu, S., Loriga, G., Volonterio, A., Tambaro, S., Bottazzi, M.E., Zanda, M., Pinna, G.A., Lazzari, P., (2013). Novel pyrazole derivatives as neutral CB_1 antagonists with signiðcant activity towards food intake. *Eur. J. Med. Chem.* 62, 256–269. doi:. 056. doi:10.1016/j.ejmech.2012.12

Mastinu, A., Pira, M., Pani, L., Pinna, G. A., & Lazzari, P. (2012). NESS038C6, a novel selective CB1 antagonist agent with anti-obesity activity and improved molecular proðle. *Behavioural Brain Research, 234*(2), 192–204. doi:10.1016/j.bbr.2012.06.033 PMID:22771813

Mastinu, A., Pira, M., Pinna, G.A., Pisu, C., Casu, M.A., Reali, R., Marcello, S., Murineddu, G., Lazzari, P., (2013). NESS06SM reduces body weight with an improved proðle relative to SR141716A. *Pharmacol. Res.* 74, 94–108. doi:. 2013.06.001. doi:10.1016/j.phrs

Mastinu, A., Premoli, M., Ferrari-Toninelli, G., Tambaro, S., Maccarinelli, G., Memo, M., & Bonini, S. A. (2018). Cannabinoids in health and disease: Pharmacological potential inmetabolic syndrome andneuroinñammation. *Hormone Molecular Biology and Clinical Investigation, 36*(2). Advance online publication. doi:10.1515/hmbci-2018-0013 PMID:29601300

McGinty, E. E., Niederdeppe, J., Heley, K., & Barry, C. L. (2017). Public perceptions of arguments supporting and opposing recreational marijuana legalization. *Preventive Medicine, 99*, 80–86. doi:10.1016/j.ypmed.2017.01.024 PMID:28189806

McKenna, T. (1992). *Food of the Gods: The Search for the Original Tree of Knowledge – A Radical History of Plants, Drugs, and Human Evolution*. Bantam.

McPartland, J., Di Marzo, V., De Petrocellis, L., Mercer, A., & Glass, M. (2001). Cannabinoid receptors are absent in insects. J. *Comp. Neurol.* 436, 423–429. . 1002/cne.1078.

McPartland, J. M. (2004). Phylogenomic and chemotaxonomic analysis of the endocannabinoid system. *Brain Res. Rev.* 45, 18–29. . 1016/j.brainresrev.2003.11.005.

Mechoulam, R., & Gaoni, Y. (1965). A total synthesis of dl-delta-1-tetrahydrocannabinol, the active constituent of hashish. *J. Am. Chem. Soc.* 87, 3273–3275. . 1021/ja01092a065.

Mechoulam, R., Fride, E., & Di Marzo, V. (1998). Endocannabinoids. *European Journal of Pharmacology*, *359*(1), 1–18. doi:10.1016/S0014-2999(98)00649-9 PMID:9831287

Moreau, J. J. (1973). *Hashish and Mental Illness (1845)*. Raven Press.

Mulpuri, Y., Marty, V.N., Munier, J.J., Mackie, K., Schmidt, B.L., Seltzman, H.H., Spigelman, I., (2018). Synthetic peripherally restricted cannabinoid suppresses chemotherapy-induced peripheral neuropathy pain symptoms by CB1 receptor activation. *Neuropharmacology* 139, 85–97. doi:. 07.002. doi:10.1016/j. neuropharm.2018

Naftali, T., Mechulam, R., Lev, L. B., & Konikoff, F. M. (2014). Cannabis for inñammatory bowel disease. *Digestive Diseases (Basel, Switzerland)*, *32*(4), 468–474. doi:10.1159/000358155 PMID:24969296

Nallathambi, R., Mazuz, M., Ion, A., Selvaraj, G., Weininger, S., Fridlender, M., Nasser, A., Sagee, O., Kumari, P., Nemichenizer, D., Mendelovitz, M., Firstein, N., Hanin, O., Konikoff, F., Kapulnik, Y., Naftali, T., & Koltai, H. (2017). Anti-inñammatory activity in colon models is derived from 9-tetrahydrocannabinolic acid that interacts with additional compounds in cannabis extracts. *Cannabis and Cannabinoid Research*, *2*(1), 167–182. doi:10.1089/can.2017.0027 PMID:29082314

Namsa, N. D., Mandal, M., Tangjang, S., & Mandal, S. C. (2011). Ethnobotany of the Monpa ethnic group at Arunachal Pradesh, India. J. Ethnobiol. Ethnomed. 7, 31. . Nichols, D.E., 2016. *Psychedelics. Pharmacol. Rev.* 68 (2), 264–355. doi:1124/pr.115.011478. doi:10.1186/1746-4269-7-31

Nielsen, S., Germanos, R., Weier, M., Pollard, J., Degenhardt, L., Hall, W., Buckley, N., & Farrell, M. (2018). The use of cannabis and cannabinoids in treating symptoms of multiple sclerosis: A systematic review of reviews. *Current Neurology and Neuroscience Reports*, *18*(2), 8. doi:10.100711910-018-0814-x PMID:29442178

O'Shaughnessy, W. B. 1843. On the preparations of the Indian hemp, or Gunjah. Prov. Med. J. *Retrosp. Med. Sci.* 5, 363–369. áhttps://www.ncbi.nlm.nih.gov/pmc/ articles/PMC2490264/ñ.

Panghal, M., Arya, V., Yadav, S., Kumar, S., & Yadav, J. P. (2010). Indigenous knowledge of medicinal plants used by Saperas community of Khetawas, Jhajjar District, Haryana, India. *Journal of Ethnobiology and Ethnomedicine*, *6*(1), 4. doi:10.1186/1746-4269-6-4 PMID:20109179

Pavisian, B., MacIntosh, B. J., Szilagyi, G., Staines, R. W., O'Connor, P., & Feinstein, A. (2014). Effects of cannabis on cognition in patients with MS: A psychometric and MRI study. *Neurology*, *82*(21), 1879–1887. doi:10.1212/WNL.0000000000000446 PMID:24789863

. Pedersen, W., Sandberg, S., (2013). The medicalisation of revolt: a sociological analysis of medical cannabis users. S*ociol. Health Illn.* 35, 17–32. doi:. 1467-9566.2012.01476.x. doi:10.1111/j

Pertwee, R. G. (2006). Cannabinoid pharmacology: The ðrst 66 years. *British Journal of Pharmacology, 147*(S1), S163–S171. doi:10.1038j.bjp.0706406 PMID:16402100

Ramar, K., Rosen, I.M., Kirsch, D.B., Chervin, R.D., Carden, K.A., Aurora, R.N., Kristo, D.A., Malhotra, R.K., Martin, J.L., Olson, E.J., Rosen, C.L., Rowley, J.A., American Academy of Sleep Medicine Board of Directors, (2018). Medical cannabis and the treatment of obstructive sleep apnea: an American academy of sleep medicine position statement. J. *Clin. Sleep. Med.* 14 (4), 679–681. doi:. 7070. doi:10.5664/jcsm

Rampa, A., Bartolini, M., Bisi, A., Belluti, F., Gobbi, S., Andrisano, V., Ligresti, A., & Di Marzo, V. (2012). The ðrst dual ChE/FAAH inhibitors: New perspectives for alzheimer's disease? *ACS Medicinal Chemistry Letters, 3*(3), 182–186. doi:10.1021/ml200313p PMID:24900454

Rice, J., & Cameron, M. (2018). Cannabinoids for treatment of MS symptoms: State of the evidence. *Current Neurology and Neuroscience Reports, 18*(8), 50. doi:10.100711910-018-0859-x PMID:29923025

Riddle, J. M. (2011). *Dioscorides on Pharmacy and Medicine*. University of Texas Press.

Rudroff, T., Honce, J.M., (2017). Cannabis and multiple sclerosis-the way forward. Front. Neurol. 8, 299. . Russo,E. B.,2007.History ofcannabis anditspreparations insaga,science,andsobriquet. *Chem. Biodivers.* 4, 1614–1648. . doi:10.3389/fneur.2017.00299

Ryz, N. R., Remillard, D. J., & Russo, E. B. (2017). Cannabis roots: A traditional therapy with future potential for treating inñammation and pain. *Cannabis and Cannabinoid Research, 2*(1), 210–216. doi:10.1089/can.2017.0028 PMID:29082318

Salzet, M., Breton, C., Bisogno, T., & Di Marzo, V. (2000). Comparative biology of the endocannabinoid system possible role in the immune response. *European Journal of Biochemistry, 267*(16), 4917–4927. doi:10.1046/j.1432-1327.2000.01550.x PMID:10931174

Savonenko, A.V., Melnikova, T., Wang, Y., Ravert, H., Gao, Y., Koppel, J., Lee, D., Pletnikova, O., Cho, E., Sayyida, N., Hiatt, A., Troncoso, J., Davies, P., Dannals, R.F., Pomper, M.G., Horti, A.G., (2015). Cannabinoid CB2 receptors in a mouse model of Aβ amyloidosis: immune histochemical analysis and suitability as a PET biomarker of neuroinñammation. PLoS One 10, e0129618. doi:. 0129618. doi:10.1371/journal.pone

Schenberg, E. E. (2018). Psychedelic-assisted psychotherapy: A paradigm shift in psychiatric research and development. *Frontiers in Pharmacology, 9*, 733. doi:10.3389/fphar.2018.00733 PMID:30026698

Scherma, M., Satta, V., Collu, R., Boi, M. F., Usai, P., Fratta, W., & Fadda, P. (2017). Cannabinoid CB (1)/CB (2) receptor agonists attenuate hyperactivity and body weight loss in a rat model of activity-based anorexia. *British Journal of Pharmacology, 174*(16), 2682–2695. doi:10.1111/bph.13892 PMID:28561272

Schussel, V., Kenzo, L., Santos, A., Bueno, J., Yoshimura, E., de Oliveira Cruz Latorraca, C., Pachito, D. V., & Riera, R. (2018). Cannabinoids for nausea and vomiting related to chemotherapy: Overview of systematic reviews. *Phytotherapy Research, 32*(4), 567–576. doi:10.1002/ptr.5975 PMID:29168289

Sharkey, K. A., Darmani, N. A., & Parker, L. A. (2014). Regulation of nausea and vomiting by cannabinoids and the endocannabinoid system. *European Journal of Pharmacology, 722*, 134–146. doi:10.1016/j.ejphar.2013.09.068 PMID:24184696

Sim, L. J., Hampson, R. E., Deadwyler, S. A., & Childers, S. R. (1996). Effects of chronic treatment with delta9-tetrahydrocannabinol on cannabinoid-stimulated [35S]GTP gamma S autoradiography in rat brain. *The Journal of Neuroscience: The Official Journal of the Society for Neuroscience*, *16*(24), 8057–8066. doi:10.1523/JNEUROSCI.16-24-08057.1996 PMID:8987831

Small, E., & Cronquist, A. (1976). A practical and natural taxonomy for cannabis. *Taxon*, *25*(4), 405–435. doi:10.2307/1220524

Soelberg Sorensen, P. (2017). Safety concerns and risk management of multiple sclerosis therapies. *Acta Neurologica Scandinavica*, *136*(3), 168–186. doi:10.1111/ane.12712 PMID:27891572

Solowij, N., & Battisti, R. (2008). The chronic effects of cannabis on memory in humans: A review. Curr. *Drug Abus. Rev*, *1*(1), 81–98. doi:10.2174/1874473710801010081 PMID:19630708

Starowicz, K., & Finn, D. P. (2017). Cannabinoids and pain: Sites and mechanisms of action. *Advances in Pharmacology (San Diego, Calif.)*, *80*, 437–475. doi:10.1016/bs.apha.2017.05.003 PMID:28826543

Tafelski, S., Häuser, W., & Schäfer, M. (2016). Efficacy, tolerability, and safety of cannabinoids for chemotherapy-induced nausea and vomiting–a systematic review of systematic reviews. *Schmerz (Berlin, Germany)*, *30*(1), 14–24. doi:10.100700482-015-0092-3 PMID:26787227

Tambaro, S., Casu, M. A., Mastinu, A., & Lazzari, P. (2014). Evaluation of selective cannabinoid CB (1) and CB(2) receptor agonists in a mouse model of lipopolysaccharide-induced interstitial cystitis. *European Journal of Pharmacology*, *729*, 67–74. doi:10.1016/j.ejphar.2014.02.013 PMID:24561047

Thompson, S. A., Patterson, K., & Hodges, J. R. (2003). Left/right asymmetry of atrophy in semantic dementia: Behavioral-cognitive implications. *Neurology*, *61*(9), 1196–1203. doi:10.1212/01.WNL.0000091868.28557.B8 PMID:14610120

Tsou, K., Brown, S., Sañudo-Peña, M. C., Mackie, K., & Walker, J. M. (1998). Immuno histochemical distribution of cannabinoid CB1 receptors in the rat central nervous system. *Neuroscience*, *83*(2), 393–411. doi:10.1016/S0306-4522(97)00436-3 PMID:9460749

Zimmer, A., Zimmer, A. M., Hohmann, A. G., Herkenham, M., & Bonner, T. I. (1999). Increased mortality, hypoactivity, and hypoalgesia in cannabinoid CB1receptor knock out mice. *Proceedings of the National Academy of Sciences of the United States of America*, *96*(10), 5780–5785. doi:10.1073/pnas.96.10.5780 PMID:10318961

Whiting, P. F., Wolff, R. F., Deshpande, S., Di Nisio, M., Duffy, S., Hernandez, A. V., Keurentjes, J. C., Lang, S., Misso, K., Ryder, S., Schmidlkofer, S., Westwood, M., & Kleijnen, J. (2015). Cannabinoids for medical use: A systematic review and metaanalysis. *Journal of the American Medical Association*, *313*(24), 2456–2473. doi:10.1001/jama.2015.6358 PMID:26103030

Chapter 2
Historical Evolution of *Cannabis sativa* Transmogrifying Utilizations

Irfan Bashir
University of Kashmir, Srinagar, India

Sameena Bashir
University of Kashmir, Srinagar, India

ABSTRACT

Cannabis sativa is known in India as hemp, ganja, and bhang. Its domestication date is unclear. According to archaeological evidence, hemp was known in the past, with the earliest mentions coming from China and India. Excellent hemp study could help us objectively examine humans' particular interaction with the plant. Different civilizations use the plant in a number of ways. In ancient India, the plant was largely used to make textiles and other therapeutic remedies. Company officials were concerned that its use would lead to insanity during colonial times. According to the 1893-1894 hemp drug committee report, the East India Company officials' perspectives had evolved. They passed a slew of hemp-related legislation and imposed new taxes. According to the commission's findings, Bhang has no biological or societal implications. How did colonial rulers who were against consuming it yet saw it as a good source of fibre change their minds? It is hoped to better understand how perceptions, misperceptions, politics, and rules shape attitudes toward drug use.

INTRODUCTION

Hemp Cultivation in India

With the advent of sedentary life, humans began domesticating many plants and animals. The domestication of a huge number of animals and plants was the most fundamental advancement that influenced the course of human life. Based on archaeological evidence, the earliest domesticated wheat and barley

DOI: 10.4018/978-1-6684-5718-4.ch002

plants are thought to have begun around 7000 BCE. Several locations have revealed a large number of wild precursors of domestic sheep, goats, and cattle that appear to have been domesticated by man between 1000 - 7000 BCE (Chakrabarty, 2009). The domesticated crops that emerged over time were altogether different from the wild ones, and the domesticated ones are morphologically different (Hall, 2008).Sedentarismfavoured man to domesticate, in contrast to hunter-gatherers, as in this stage, they were constantly on the move andalways searching for food. They hardly paid attention to the phenomena of cultivation. Environmental changes prompted him to stay at a particular place to satiate his demands (Blanton, 2002). In the advancing stages of this phase, man developed various skills, such as how plants can be beneficial to them and what their uses and hazards are. Over time, as man's understanding increased, he began employing these plants for therapeutic purposes. This appears to be the case with the cannabissativa, as its transmogrifying use expanded with the advancement of human civilization. To understand the plant, it is necessary to discover when it was first introduced and how its usage has changed over time.

In general, historical academia appears to be less receptive to understanding the relationships that man has built over time with his environment. The reason for this might be traced to several factors, the most significant of which is that history has typically been viewed as the story of great men and important events like battles and other aspects related to war. This led to the fallibility of historians paying less attention to the factors that contributed to the advancement of civilization. However, in recent decades, a considerable transformative shift has occurred in our knowledge of the overall characteristics of human evolution. Historians spent a lot of time figuring out how man interacted with the environment, sustenance, economy, and the interactions of various social units. How society's mechanisms functioned and interacted to explain development over time. How has man's understanding of diverse plants and animals evolved? With the advancement of man's awareness of the various components of the environment and the desire to regulate the various phenomena, human civilization made much progress. However, the topic of how man began to employ these plants for different purposes has always been a mystery. One such explanation may be found in the use of Cannabis Sativa, which has a lengthy history, almost as old as human evolution. Because of the plant's extensive history, we are not sure what it was used for initially and the transmogrifying roles that it assumed in the varied settings. The plant's domestication is traced to the Central Asian and Chinese regions, from where it spread to other parts of the globe (Borougerdi, 2018), (Touw, 1981).

Cannabis sativa is also, in general terms, known as *Ganja,bhang, Charas, and hemp* in the Indian subcontinent. In recent years,the expansion of historical studytouched every aspect of human history, from culinary preferences to agricultural patterns of every known civilization. The history of plants usually forms the dimension of modern research. Still, meagerly full-fledged research is being conducted on herbs and plant-based studies, especially in history discipline. Cannabis is one of the oldest plants,with a long history of being used from the stone Age. It nearly grows in every part of the world. Hemp thrives in almost every climate and improves depleted soil after each crop. Due to hemp's rapid growth in temperate, tropical climes, it has been used for various purposes since ancient times(Singh, Mamania, & Shinde, 2018). Despite the plant's benefits to humanity, little is known about its history due to a dearth of prehistoric and protohistoric literary sources and archaeological evidence. In the absence of records, archaeologists have gathered information about the prehistoric and protohistoric periods by examining remains unearthed from numerous archaeological sites. The archaeological research aided to a considerable extent in assessing the interrelationship between humans and plants during the prehistoric and protohistoric periods.

The earliest traces of Cannabis cultivation come from China, where it comes to the fore from archaeological excavation, which dates back to Neolithic times (Li, 1974). However, in the context of the Indian subcontinent, the earliest traces of it came from the Ellora caves (Singh & Sardesai, 2016). The Ellora caves are located in Maharashtra's Aurangabad district. The caves are dedicated to three major religions predominant in ancient India Buddhism, Hinduism, and Jainism. The evidence of CannabisSativaisreportedly evident in cave 12th of the Ellora, which is dedicated to the Buddhist faith. The hemp employed is blended with other materials in the cave's plaster. The earliest literary reference of hemp is found in the *Atharvaveda* (1500-1000 BCE),one of the important *Ved* among the four Vedas of the Vedicperiod. From the *Atharvaveda*,it is presumed that medicine among the ancient Vedic people began as magical charms and incantations intended to placate, tame, or drive away various types of devils, and demons, that are thought to cause ailments. Thus, the development of medications began with this treatise, and most cures were in the form of amulets and charms. However, enough evidence also makes it implicit that numerous plants and herbs were employed to treat various maladies (Chattopadhyaya, 1978).

Bhang is one of the five sacred plants mentioned in the *Atharvaveda* as a source of anxiety relief. Bhang was initially thought to be a type of wild grass by *Sayana*, but many researchers now associate it with Cannabis (Griffith, 1917). Cannabis is specified as a source of enjoyment, a joy-giver, and a liberator and is considered the most important of the five sacred plants listed in *Atharvaveda*. Numerous allusions imply that cannabis was smoked during daily devotional services in Hinduism. Besides being utilized in religious rites, the herb offers therapeutic properties. Ayurveda has a recorded history of employing plants, animals, metals, and minerals for sustenance and medicine, dating back thousands of years. It has a distinct manner of comprehending plants. The earliest Ayurveda text, Charaka Samhita, offers extensive descriptions of plants and their therapeutic benefits. The information includes nomenclature, identification descriptions, biological properties and actions, habitat, regional specifications for substitutes, collection dates and methods, classification methods, computing and combining plants, processing, application in specific stages of the disease, incompatibility, contraindications, recipes, and poisons, among other things (Verotta, Macchi, & Venkatasubramanian, 2015). Hemp is used as a food ingredient as well as a medicinal herb with therapeutic properties in the Indian subcontinent.

Hemp appears to have a long history of being used to make textiles. Studying the ancient textile industry and the other fabrics used in the process of manufacturing is challenging. The names of many types of clothing are frequently mentioned in literary works, but the source of fabric is rarely mentioned. Hemp is an important source of fibre, and the term hemp was used to denote the numerous parts of the plant. Sana hemp, jute, and true hemp are the three most significant (the dictionaries compiled in mediaeval times unequivocally state that Sana hemp is used for cloth). A weaver wearing a Sana fibre*dhoti*(loincloth) is also mentioned in the Buddhist text Divyadana (Gopal, 1961).This leads us to believe that ordinary people mostly utilise this fibre as fabric.According to the *Colombia History of the world*, the earliest known fabric was likely hemp, which was first processed in the eighth millennium BCE (8000-7000 BCE). Cannabis hemp is the world's strongest, most durable, and most long-lasting natural soft fibre (Herer, 1990).In addition, Pundit Kalhana, a well-known Kashmiri chronicler, penned *Rajatarangini,* a political history of Kashmir in 1049-1050 CE. *Rajatarangini* describes Kashmiri's history from the earliest times up to the author's time. Hemp is listed in this literarywork as a material for manufacturing cloth in Kashmir. However, the references imply that hemp textiles are manufactured for underprivileged segments of society. There is a lack of information on whether the hemp used to manufacture textiles is domesticated or wild-grown (Stein, 1989).

Cannabis sativa's use as a psychoactive substance has a hazy history, as it is not clearly documented or retained in other cultural traits about how the plant came to play the role of intoxicant. It is widely assumed that the plant is utilized both as a psychoactive and medicinal plant in the Indian subcontinent. Its use is widespread and well interwoven not just into people's recreational and sexual lives but also into their religious traditions (Salema et al., 2001).The illustration found from the various sources makes it appear that it was perhaps from the Indian subcontinent that the plant's narcotic and medicinal properties were transmitted to various parts of the globe. The use as mentioned earlier of the plant also implies that hemp is not only being cultivated, but the inhabitants of the land are well-versed in its various applications dating back to ancient times.

The use of cannabis as an intoxicant has a long history in India and Iran. It wasembraced by Muslims in the Middle East two centuries later, following the death of Prophet Mohammad. Cannabis preparations were unknown during his lifetime, so Prophet Mohammad did not specifically condemn cannabis intoxication. Before the 9th century CE, there was a meagre indication of cannabis being used as an intoxicant. The cognizance of cannabis as an intoxicant in other parts of the world appears to have been carried out by traders travelling to Persia from India and Central Asia. Hashish (also known as hash, dried resin of flower tops) is a psychoactive drug created by compressing and processing sections of the cannabis plant. Hashishis conterminous with bhang in Hindu terminology. It was first consumedas an intoxicant by members of religious Persian and Iraqi sects located on the eastern periphery of the Islamic empire. At first, there was some cultural opposition because of the holy Quran, Which, although outlining all of the laws of daily Muslim life, does not explicitly prohibit the eating of Cannabis (Nahas, 1982). The dissemination of hemp to different regions around the world could also be attributed to Muslim traders, as these traders often have served as intermediaries between nations and smoothed the transmission of knowledge from one region to another. Rajan Gurukul has described the phenomenon in his book *History and Theory of Knowledge Production: An Introductory Outline.* The transformation may have occurred due to the overseas trade links between India, Persia, and Europe, which maritime traders facilitated and Jesuit missionaries (Gurukkal, 2018).

However, the usage of cannabis as an intoxicant in India, notably throughout the Middle Ages, appears to be a little hazy from the sources. Cannabis appears to have been grown in all of the Mughal provinces. Its usage seems fashionable among soldiers, and a few emperors appear to have been addicted to it. Although orthodox Islam condemns the use of intoxicants, cannabis seems relatively frequent among Muslims in India during medieval times. The reference, which makes it implicit that it is being used in India, also offers the inference that its use is common among the upper classes of society. *Ma'jun*, a sweat confectionery, was a favourite of Mughal ruler Hamayun. It is thought that the effects of cannabis intake caused his death from a tumble down the stairs. Cannabis is also an addiction of Sikh soldiers who used bhang during combat to help them fight better and dull their pain perceptions; this practice continues to this day in Nihangi's, a Sikh order that consumes intoxicants ritually.

Following the fall of the Mughal Empire, the subcontinent fell into the hands of the East India Company, which came to India for trading objectives but seized control of the country over time. The East India Company ruled India until 1857 when the revolt broke out. In 1858, the British parliament passed the Government of India Act in response to the uprising, transferring the East India Company's authority over India to the British crown. After the uprising of 1857, the British crown assumed the authority to administer India. The firm authorities were taken aback when they learned what had sparked the insurrection in 1857. Over time, much investigation has been done to determine the strengthening forces that led to the event's occurrence. Following a thorough investigation, company officials concluded that the

British meddling in the people's socio-religious structure was the catalyst for the revolt. The inference can be seen in the crown's command to all people of the subcontinent to profess his faith in accordance with his traditions.However, British engagement in Indian affairs persisted, varying in intensity depending on the governor-general in charge and the ideology he supported.

After taking the Diwani rights of Bengal, Bihar, and Orissa with the Treaty of Allahabad on August 12, 1765, the Britishers increasingly began intervening in Indian affairs(Banerjee-Dube, 2014). However, British intervention was always murky and intensified with time. The British administered India under the assumption that Indian society had always been primitive and immobile. They used to attack India's culture, traditions, and faith to demonstrate its underdevelopment. This intervention grew increasingly powerful over time, culminating in the 1857 rebellion. Some scholars have portrayed it as a mutiny, and for others, it was the first war of independence by others (Metcalf & Metcalf, 2006). The revolt was sparked by several factors, the most notable of which was greater British interference in Indian politics, but this did not mean that they avoided intervention totally. Instead, they chose to focus on the Indian people's diverse challenges and customs, in the name of reform. These reforms were not limited to questioning the Indian people's socio-cultural characteristics. The colonialists believe that Indian religions appear to allow them to utilize intoxicants such as cannabis, which they frequently blame for promoting insanity (Mills, 2000).

Despite being aware of the negative consequences of the hemp drug and its derivatives, Company officials did not restrict its usage. This appears to be analogous to the extraction of revenue, which is the company's primary source of income. During this phase, they are more focused on maximising their profits. Subsequently, the efforts of diverse persons contributed to an increase in the colonial authorities' expertise. Important in this regard is the fact that Irish physician William undertook a series of cannabis trials that had no adverse medical effects. In 1842, he wrote about the cannabis sativain his description of the *Bengal Dispensatory and companion to the Pharmacopoeia,* clearing many prior doubts and significantly impacting the next fifty years (Warf, 2014). This work was the basis for all the other volumes of the Pharmacopoeia Indica. For almost a century, O'Shaughnessy's Dispensatory impacted how the British practised medicine and prescribed drugs in India (Salema et al., 2001).It implies that company officials are more interested in profit-making in this phase than in the civilising purpose for which they claim to have arrived.

As early as 1871, the government of India commissioned British civil officers, doctors, and soldiers around south Asia to investigate whether the usage of cannabis was widespread, Resulting in insanity and other harmful repercussions (Mills, 2000). Numerous questions have been raised in the house of commons addressing the ambiguity surrounding the frequency and consumption of hemp by Indians. Some of the individuals who expressed such concerns about banning all intoxicating substances across the British realm believed that cannabis and its allied drugs should be banned as well before the British parliament.The formation of the Hemp Drug Commission in April 1893 was a direct result of the questions raised in the House of Commons by Mark Stewart and William Cain. William Cain's questions led to the establishment of the hemp commissionin 1893 (Commission, 1894).The responses to the enquiries were responded to and sent to Great Britain. The parliamentary commission was tasked with investigating the cultivation of hemp plants in Bengal, the procedure for preparing drugs from it, and the other issues related to trade in this drug. Additionally, the effects of those consuming the drug on the social and moral conditions of the people (Commission, 1894)and the desirability of the people prohibiting the cultivation and sale of Ganja and related drugs.Because the colonial authorities had little knowledge of drugs and their use, they had to rely on the Indians (Borougerdi, 2018). They discovered that hemp leaves are regularly mixed with tobacco and smoked in India to increase their intoxicating properties. In India, hemp is used as an unction for piles by combining it with turmeric, onions, and warm garlic oil.It has led the British to realize that cannabis has a significant therapeutic application, particularly in India. The therapeutic application of the medication began to be prioritized by future companies and crown servants.Hemp is considered a source of potentially valuable medicine. This theme got initially developed through the writings of Irish writers. W. B O'Shaughnessy conducted a number of experiments in Calcutta with hemp derivatives in 1830. He conducted numerous experiments onanimal's reaction to hemp preparations. However, hemp has the potential as medicine in some other effects of stimulating the digestive organ existing cerebral system and relieving pain, which further endorsed him to such extent that he decided to conduct experiments on a human. Rheumatism, hydrophobic cholera, tetanus and infantile convulsions were all treated successfully with various hemp concoctions (Mills, 2000). O'Shaughnessyconcluded that he had gained an anti-conclusion remedy of the greatest value.

The 1893 hemp commission report details several factors that motivated the British government to establish the inquiry. The first appears to be the repeated arguments made by the Britishers to defend their control in India. They saw India as a backward country, believing their western civilization was far superior to the east (Shamir & Hacker, 2001). They thought Indians were unfit to rule themselves and that British authority over India was necessary for the country to progress. The white man's burden theory has similar paradigms, and it seems that theory later got christened after these ideas. The second reason was law and order. People addicted to cannabis frequently resort to violence, which authorities find difficult to control. The plant's commercial importance looks to be the last cause. The plant is illegally utilized or exported to different regions and employed to manufacture several therapeutic medicines. The government began regulating this trafficking to make it more efficient. It is necessary to assess how far the government can reduce the threat of drug consumption and trafficking in the subsequent sections.

Various accounts dealing with the early years of British and company rule imply that British authorities viewed hemp as the root of insanity and other hazardous effects among those addicted to it (Ireland, 1893). However, the evidence supporting such claims appears to be flawed. In the council's inquiry, the governor-general requested that Madras and Bombay explore the effects and abuse of various hemp concoctions. The study should not only focus on hemp's therapeutic benefits but also the alleged role of Ganja and bhang in high-profile violent crimes (Commission, 1894). The investigation's findings revealed various negative consequences for cannabis preparations and users. The enquiry report claimed that hemp drug users were attacking various British officials while under the influence of the substance. The other significant problem that were repeatedly found among the intoxicants are infanticide, immorality, suicide, and the murder of British officers have been linked to cannabis by colonial administrators. Cannabis users were viewed as unpredictable, violent, and deserving of western integrative procedures (Mills, 2000).

Transmuting Role of *Cannabis Sativa*

Even though hemp is cultivated worldwide, the European variety is distinguished from its Asian counterpart since it is mainly valued for its narcotic effects. The distinction throughout time has vanished from literary works. Ganja, Charas, and bhang are the most often utilized forms of cannabis. Ganja consists of a resinous exudate-coated female blooming top and branches. Resinous exudation can be detected on the leaves, young branches, stem bark, and even on the young fruits. Bhang comprises mature leaves and fruits in certain regions of India (Chopra, 1940).

In India, the plant grows in the Himalayan mountains, particularly from Kashmir to the east of Assam. It usually grows up to an altitude of 10,000 meters above sea level (Chopra, 1940). Hemp drug has been utilized in India for a variety of purposes, including overcoming exhaustion and worry, producing Euphoria, and providing relief from worries during times of stress. Drug use can be conveniently classified into three categories: 1) for religious and societal purposes, 2) for therapeutic purposes, and 3) for narcotic and ecstatic pleasure. The hemp commission report demonstrated the disparity in cannabis use in religious and social rituals. The drug's narcotic use appears to be more prevalent in northern India than in southern India, with Bengal dominating consumption, particularly during the Durga Puja (Mills, 2009). This habit is also prevalent during the Holi celebration in numerous places and during Sikh religious rites in Punjab (Warf, 2014). Ganja's ceremonial use is widespread but less prevalent than bhang. It is rarelyconsidered a vital ritual component and is mainly linked with Shiva worship by fakirs, Jogis, Sanyasis, and other ascetics. Where cannabis was more common, the plant was worshipped or, at the very least, venerated (Kalant, 1972).

Secondly, the vast majority of current pharmaceuticals are drawn from natural sources, making natural goods the foundation of traditional treatment and modern medicine. The prevalence of natural items in our culture is staggering. Evidence of India's ancient medical systems dates back to the Indus valley civilization. Archaeological findings from Harappa and Mohanjodaroattestto the existence of a conventional medical system prevalent during the protohistoric times (Borougerdi, 2014). Medicinal plants are supposed to thrive on the slopes of the Himalayas. The notion is echoed in Ramayana, which suggests that the Himalayas are particularly rich in medicinal plants and herbs of therapeutic significance.The hemp plant has been a significant component of traditional medicines throughout history (Borougerdi, 2014). In addition to its usage as an intoxicant, hemp is also an ingredient in a variety of medications. Numerous works from ancient times onwards provide proof of its use. In Hindu medicine, the hemp drug is mentioned in both the classical texts and the medicinal writings. In Sanskrit literature, the hemp plant is referred to as *bhang, indracana,* and *Vijaya or Jaya* (Chopra, 1940). The earliest description of bhang is found in the Atharvaveda, which forms the soma drink along with various other ingredients. Bhang is initially referenced in the *Sushruta Samhita* (6th–7th century CE), which mentions hemp alongside other anti-phlegmatic drugs. It is categorized as an excitant and mentioned alongside opium in the 1500 CE medical text *Sarangadhara Samhita*. Several essential properties of hemp drug are mentioned in the *Bavaprakasha,* compiled in 1600 CE, with particular emphasis on its digestive and stimulant effect on biliary secretion. The texts cited above demonstrate that the hemp plant has a long history of use in India for medicinal purposes. The conventional system of medicine has evolved through time to produce contemporary medications that have the ability to cure a variety of severe ailments.

A British physician introduced the Cannabis plant (Cannabis Sativa and Cannabis Indica) to western medicine in 1839 and discovered that the herb was safe and effective in treating rabies, rheumatism, epilepsy, and tetanus. In 1860, the medication was beneficial for treating stomach pain, birthing psychosis, chronic cough, gonorrhoea, and neuralgia (Heinrich & Mathre, 2001). Cannabinoids and cannabis are used to alleviate cancer-related nausea and vomiting (anti-emetic). HIV patients have traditionally used cannabis, sometimes known as marijuana, as an appetite stimulant and pain reliever (Cinti, 2009). People with multiple sclerosis, a neurological illness, have also utilized cannabinoids to relieve muscle spasms and neuropathic pain(Herer, 1992). One of the most common reasons people use cannabis for therapeutic purposes is chronic pain caused by disease (chronic non-cancer pain). Examples include neuropathic pain, arthritis, back pain, neck and shoulder pain, and headaches. Medical Cannabis and cannabinoids have been pushed for pain relief, appetite stimulation, anxiety reduction, and sleep improvement in terminally sick cancer patients (Mechoulam, 2005).

Additionally, the Indian hemp plant has a history of being used as a home cure for the treatment of minor diseases. It is thought that a moderate beverage produced from bhang leaves stimulates the appetite and aids digestion (Mechoulam, 2005). Indian hemp is most widely smoked and consumed as a beverage due to its purported malaria-preventative properties. The bhang beverage is one of the most popular home treatments for gonorrhoea and dysuria (Brown, 1998; Andrews & Vinkenoog, 1967). Due to their minor diuretic and sedative characteristics, these beverages likely provide some symptomatic relief. Fresh poultices are a typical home cure for severe eye diseases, conjunctivitis, swollen joints, orchitis, and other acute inflammatory disorders.

Moreover, hemp is also used in veterinary medicine. Hemp leaves are mixed with other ingredients such as spices, salt, or sugar candy to cure cattle. Ganja is said to be an effective cure for intestinal worms and footsore illness, while the smoke created by hemp is thought to sterilize sheepfolds. Bhang is used to improve the flow of milk in cows, and bhang, combined with salt, is commonly given to animals as a diarrhoea preventative. Most of these medications are used on the basis of rumour and custom (Chopra, 1940). In addition to the illnesses listed above, cannabis and cannabinoids have been used to treat variousother ailments. Anxiety disorders, such as post-traumatic stress disorder, mood disorders, sleep disorders, such as insomnia, chronic pain, degenerative neurological ailments and inflammatory bowel diseases, such as Crohn's disease, are among these problems.

Cannabis Sativa eventually evolved into a narcotic drug. Cannabis sativa used for psychoactive purposes is generally smoked or consumed orally, depending on the strain, concerning the origin and evolution of hemp's narcotic principle (Brown, 1998). The process is usually linked to and occurs in tandem with several specific morphological changes in plant anatomy. In certain plants, the leaves or primary organs are where narcotic resins are located, whereas, in others, the flowering tops play a key role in storing and secreting the resins. While in the first group, the narcotic qualities are kept on the leaves and produce bhang for commercial use, the fruits and surface of the stem take on themselves and the secretory activities. The second group produces Ganja, while the third group produces Charas. The causes that cause such changes in the physiology of the hemp plant are unknown, as is the resinous material present in the plant. However, the resinous ingredient found in hemp is thought to be the most crucial factor in the drug's physiological effect (Chopra, 1940).

The hemp drug commission of 1893 evaluated the effects of the substance on people with scepticism. Before the panel, the widespread consensus among British government officials seemed to be that the plant has cannabinoid compounds, which is the primary cause of insanity among its addicts. There is no doubt that the plant can impact a person's brain, but it also has many positive properties and should not be overlooked. The commission presented the report of the witnesses with a critical eye, taking the witness's credentials and expertise into account. Some witnesses who are well-versed in the therapeutic application of a substance are surprisingly clueless about its intoxicating properties (Commission, 1894). In determining the adverse effects of cannabis, the quantity and kinds of preparations used, the mode of consumption, and the concurrent use of other medications were crucial considerations.

According to the evidence, Charas and Ganja were more dangerous than bhang, as smoking charas and Ganja was judged more detrimental than drinking bhang. However, excessive usage of the latter might also be harmful. The concept that cannabis use acts as a gateway to more complicated narcotics continues to be supported by data from current studies on cannabis's psychotropic effects (Degenhardt, Hall, & Lynskey, 2001). The frequency with which it is taken, as well as differences in users' neurological sensitivity to the chemical, dictate its effects.The effects are minimal when administered in minute quantities, the patient feels cheery and well-adjusted and becomes more talkative. Consequently, bhang intoxication leads individuals to sing and dance energetically throughout and creates an appetite for their meal intake, which may result in hazardous fights at times. (Poulin & Gram, 2001). Those that consume *Majun* see an increase in both appetite and sexual desire. Happiness is disproportionate to one's situation.

Ganja users experience euphoric reverie while still being able to carry with them their regular responsibilities. On the other hand, the bhang user feels lethargic and weighed down when smoking Ganja. This may be attributed to marijuana's higher THC (Tetrahydrocannabinol) content. Higher doses cause a dreamy, euphoric, altered state of consciousness with feelings of detachment, merriment, and humour. In the presence of others, there is a tendency for uncontrolled, funny laughter and voluble speech. There is a rise in appetite and a heightened appreciation for the flavour of food. The perception of pain and sensitivity to touch are lessened. The hues become more bright, and interest in art and music increases. Concurrent symptoms include a dry mouth, an increased heart rate, and conjunctival suffusion (red eyes). When marijuana is smoked, THC enters the bloodstream and the lungs. The substance enters the brain within minutes. It triggers a variety of brain cell biochemical pathways(Brown, 1998). Although it has been said that cannabis does not induce physical dependence, it does induce substantial psychological dependence. Chronic cannabis use has been linked to dependence and withdrawal symptoms. Symptoms of withdrawal include irritability, melancholy, insomnia, nausea, and tremor. Regular marijuana use may lead to lung problems.Marijuana smoking has been related to lung cancer because it contains four times as much tar and fifty percent more carcinogens than tobacco. Marijuana users had reduced serum testosterone, sperm counts, and sperm motility, which may lead to decreased desire, impotence, and fertility. (Hembree et al., 2001). Additionally, marijuana users tend to be more susceptible to despair and anxiety. The use of marijuana has been related to decreased immunity, greater risk-taking, and an increased risk of myocardial infarction.

Cannabis Sativa: Physical, Mental, and Social Consequences

The hemp drug commission was the first endeavour by the British Indian government to investigate the plant's health effects. Though the commission's recommendations are not founded on modern scientific methodologies, its broad scope makes it essential. The panel determined that modest dosages of cannabis for therapeutic purposes or continuous moderate usage had no appreciable adverse effect save in certain situations and may even be beneficial. Heavy cannabis usage makes users more vulnerable to diseases such as bronchitis caused by smoke inhalation and dysentery caused by direct causes (Commission, 1894). In susceptible individuals, moderate cannabis consumption does not result in mental disease. It also contributes to the development of psychotic disorders by exacerbating mental instability. Though the British Indian administration denies that cannabis usage is the cause of insanity among Indians, it appears to have been exaggerated (Kalant, 1972).

The British Indian government has presumed that those addicted to cannabis sativa are also responsible for disrupting peace and order in the British Indian realm. As is apparent, persistent drug addicts under the substance's effect can produce moral weakness and depravity (Kalant, 1972). Furthermore, frequent heavy drug use may lead to extreme poverty and dishonesty, leading to violent crimes. The hemp drug commission's 1893 assessment of the adverse effects of cannabis Sativa was not based on contemporary scientific standards. It was based solely on the testimony of medical witnesses and centred on the commonly held belief that the medication causes asthma, bronchitis, and dysentery. There was scant evidence of cannabis users being the subject of direct scientific research. In addition, the belief held by authorities at the time that cannabis affects the brain and may lead to insanity is not supported by any firsthand studies of people with mental health condition and their histories.

Cannabis Trade and Narcotics Trafficking

Hemp produced in British Indiaused to be consumed within its domain. The Britishers were less inclined toward the intoxicating aspects of cannabis than hemp fibre, which was widely used in sacks,clothing, and nets. In Europe, Russia was the major hemp supplier,and Britain sought out other sourcesto reduce its reliance on Russia. The demand could be fulfilled in their colonies, that is,India. Bengal produced and consumed the bulk of hemp and its allied preparations. The government initially attempted to control cannabis in this area, and in 1870, Bengal arose as a single province to enforce tight limits on the cultivation, manufacturing, and sale of Ganja. In 1871-1872, most other provinces simply continued to confine their involvement in the cannabis sector to revenue farming and the auctioning of retail or wholesale licences.

The illegal substance of Charas and Ganja was used persistently, and its trafficking increased with time. Charas is an essential commodity traded between Central Asia and India. It is transported from Yarkand in August, when mountain passes are opened, and reaches Leh in Kashmir in September or October. Typically, payment for Charas is paid in kind rather than in cash. All products that are supposedly in high demand in central Asia and India are acceptable for barter. The government of Punjab has regulated Charas trafficking (Chopra, 1940). The bandages of Charas are inspected at Panarmik and Leh in Kashmir to guarantee that any bundle reaching Leh (where the Punjab government erected its storage facilities) is accounted for by the state of Kashmir. Nearly all of India's charas supply passes through Punjab. The Excise Commissioner believes that the overall imports in 1892-93 amounted to 5,000' maunds; nevertheless, this was an extraordinary year, and on average, the imports ranged between 3,000 and 4,000 maunds. The Ganja, Gard, bhang and Churacharas produced in Kashmir are also consumed locally, none is exported to Punjab, according to the Kashmir Governor's Memorandum (Commission, 1894).

The drug trade appears to have benefited the British government. Nevertheless, the appointment of the hemp drug commission for the prohibition of hemp seems to be murky. Although it is a profitable trade, it would be surprising to see authorities intend to impose limitations on it. According to James Mill in *Cannabis Britannica,* the impulse toward prohibition arose from imperialism rather than a scientific, logical assessment of drug use and its effects. Cannabis was the essential source of imperial revenue. The British found themselves in the middle of the world's most significant market for cannabis, which was heavily taxed in India. From 1793 to the 1850s, the British East India Company happily generated a continuous cash stream by taxing cannabis and issuing licences to sellers and distributors. Bengal became a significant exporter throughout India and the Empire during this period. Distributors were required in several provinces to store their crops in government-owned warehouses. When local supplies ran out, the company brought in Charas from Turkestan. Many farmers grew small, distant plots to evade exact counting of their output, and a network of supervisors was created to reduce peasant attempts to avoid taxation. Cannabis taxes in colonial times was increasingly associated with its illegality. Mill contends that colonial officials in India began to associate cannabis with criminality around the same time that they began to tax the trade in Indian hemp products(Warf, 2014).

The Indian hemp drug committee of 1893 ruled that the ban on bhang was completely unjustified since it has been used since antiquity, and its use is firmly rooted in social and religious norms. Moderate usage is safe, and excessive use is not as dangerous as excessive alcohol use. This restriction is impossible to execute due to the plant's uncontrolled proliferation, and even if it were enforced, it would lead to the usage of more dangerous stimulants and widespread unhappiness. Therefore, the government decided to establish more effective control measures. Similarly, the restriction of Charas and Cannabis was deemed unjustified despite the negative consequences of excessive usage having been recognized. The evidence was adequate to establish that Charas was imported from foreign nations such as Turkestan, Yarkand, and other central Asian States (Commission, 1894). Neither their nature nor their scope was sufficient to warrant the prohibition. In 1893, the renowned Indian Hemp Drugs Commission decided in an eight-volume report that bhang was a harmless beverage with no negative biological or social consequences, and the British colonial government decriminalized the narcotic. The cultivation and trade of cannabis appear to have been a flourishing cottage sector on the estate's periphery, where plantation labourers in India learned more specifically about the benefits of Cannabis (Warf, 2014).

CONCLUSION

The cannabis sativa, which is said to have originated in the Central Asian and Himalayan regions, has evidence of use dating back to prehistoric and early mediaeval periods. The herb was first utilised as a ceremonial drink known as soma drink in the Indian subcontinent. Aside from that, the plant has a long history of utilising plaster, evident from the Ellora caves. Additionally, it is used as a fibre material for producing garments, as documented by the Kalhana in his *Rajatarangini.* As the plant interacts with different civilizations, its use appears to have evolved. The plant is used for its medicinal and intoxicating powers, and it was disseminated to other parts of the world from the early mediaeval period onwards, mostly through traders. They are known to have spread its exudations to other parts of the world. The plants' metamorphosis into another region led to its cultivation in numerous locations. However, it is unclear whether the hemp is grown wild or domesticated.

Cannabis plants have different associations in many nations throughout the globe. The plant's socio-religious significance in the Indian subcontinent led to its entrenchment in the Indian social structure. The herb has a therapeutic role, particularly in the ancient and mediaeval Ayurvedic pharmacology system. Nonetheless, it is well-established that the plant is also utilised as an intoxicant, particularly during wartime. However, the usage of cannabis during the medieval era appears to have been restricted to the privileged ones. With the advancement of scientific understanding, the plant has become a vital component of several types of pharmaceuticals that have relieved humankind of numerous chronic conditions. In addition, the plant has a long history of being utilised to treat a variety of veterinary ailments. It is also being used in various homoeopathic preparation for curing minor ailments.

However, with the introduction of British authority in the Indian subcontinent, the conversation around the plant altered completely. Cannabis sativa is supposed to be the cause of insanity, and hemp users have been labelled as lunatics without sufficient scientific study. Despite being well aware of the drug's dangerous consequences, the government's attempts to restrict its utilization appear meagre. Hempdhas been used for a long time. The company authorities did not intervene in advising individuals to avoid hemp usage since they were fully aware of the profits generated by the trade.

Furthermore, Britishers pushed hemp growth for the fibre since they were heavily reliant on importing it from Russia, the world's largest hemp producer.Similarly, to reduce their reliance on Russia, they encouraged the production of hemp throughout their realm. The company officials were well knowledgeable in its psychotropic characteristics but were actively engaged in its commerce, but with the British crown taking control of the subcontinent, the intervention intensified. The likely explanation appears to emphasise the role of the benevolent ruler and the civilised mission that Britishers have taken on to make the people of the subcontinent more civilised.To substantiate their claim of being civilized, they find it plausible to intervene in hemp to assess its adverse effects. In this regard, the British parliament directed its Indian authorities to form the Indian hemp drug commission.

The Indian hemp drug commission of 1893-1894 focused on hemp and related medications. In a well-known eight-volume report published in 1893, the legendary Indian Hemp Drugs Commission ruled that bhang was a safe drink with no harmful biological or social impacts. However, after independence, the Indian government's policies shifted toward development. The Indian government's stance on intoxicant substances is codified in Article 47 of the Indian constitution, which states that the "state should seek to bring about prohibition of the consumption of intoxicating beverages and narcotics that are harmful to health, save for therapeutic purposes." The three international conventions on drug-related issues, namely, the Single Convention on Narcotic Drugs, 1961, the Convention on Psychotropic Substances, 1971, and the UN Convention Against Illicit Traffic in Narcotic Drugs and Psychotropic Substances, 1988, all adopted the same principle of preventing drug use other than for medicinal purposes. These three conventions have been signed and approved by India. The Narcotic Drugs and Psychotropic Substances (NDPS) Act of 1985 forbids the manufacturing, production, trade, and use of narcotic drugs and psychotropic substances except for medicinal or research purposes. The NDPS Act, 1985, section 10, coupled with section 8 of the Act, authorises state governments to licence cannabis cultivation for medicinal and research reasons. Cannabis' medicinal usage has been restricted to complementary medicine such as homoeopathy and Ayurveda. Cannabis cultivation will be authorised for scientific purposes, including trials of various cannabis types. Bhang is a cannabis-based concoction that is drunk during several Indian festivals. The NDPS Act 1985 does not apply to it because it is not derived from cannabis resin or flowering tops. Only the leaves of extensively cultivated cannabis plants will be allowed to be used in the production of Bhang. They are not permitted to utilise the plant's blooming tops or resin. Suppose anybody is caught combining any portion of the flowering tops or the resin generated by cannabis plants with Bhang. In that case, the person will be prosecuted under the relevant sections of the NDPS Act, 1985, and his licence will be revoked. Cannabis plants may be used for industrial purposes as a source of biomass and fibre. Cannabis seeds may be used to make high-value cannabis seed oil. Some nations allow the production of cannabis types with very low levels of tetrahydrocannabinol (THC), the psychoactive element in marijuana. These cannabis types are used to make fibres, which are employed in manufacturing garments and biomass. The government can allow cannabis growing purely for horticultural and industrial uses under Section 14 of the NDPS Act by general or special order. The federal government will support research and trials of cannabis varieties with reduced THC levels. On the other hand, the Central Government will take a careful, evidence-based approach to cannabis growing for horticultural and/or industrial reasons.

REFERENCES

Banerjee-Dube, I. (2014). *A history of modern India*. Cambridge University Press. doi:10.1017/CBO9781107588387

Blanton, R. E. (2002). Empires: Perspectives from Archaeology and History. Latin American Antiquity, 13(2), 237–238.

Borougerdi, B. J. (2014). *Cord of empire, exotic intoxicant: Hemp and culture in the Atlantic world, 1600-1900*. The University of Texas at Arlington.

Borougerdi, B. J. (2018). *Commodifying Cannabis: A Cultural History of a Complex Plant in the Atlantic World*. Rowman & Littlefield.

Brown, D. T. (1998). *Cannabis: The genus cannabis*. CRC Press.

Chakrabarty, D. K. (2009). India: An archaeological history: palaeolithic beginnings to early historic foundations. Oxford University Press. doi:10.1093/acprof:oso/9780198064121.001.0001

Chattopadhyaya, D. (1978). *Science and society in ancient India* (Vol. 22). John Benjamins Publishing.

Chopra, R. N. (1940). Use of hemp drugs in India. *Indian Medical Gazette*, *75*(6), 356. PMID:29013991

Cinti, S. (2009). Medical marijuana in HIV-positive patients: What do we know? *Journal of the International Association of Physicians in AIDS Care*, *8*(6), 342–346. doi:10.1177/1545109709351167 PMID:19952287

Commission, I. H. D. (1894). *Report of the Indian Hemp Drug Commission, 1893-94*. Government Central Printing Office, Simla.

Degenhardt, L., Hall, W., & Lynskey, M. (2001). Alcohol, cannabis and tobacco use among Australians: A comparison of their associations with other drug use and use disorders, affective and anxiety disorders, and psychosis. *Addiction (Abingdon, England)*, *96*(11), 1603–1614. doi:10.1046/j.1360-0443.2001.961116037.x PMID:11784457

Gopal, L. (1961). Textiles in ancient India. *Journal of Economic and Social History of the Orient*, *4*(1), 53–69. doi:10.1163/156852061X00132

Griffith, R. T. H. (1917). *The Hymns of the Atharva-veda* (Vol. 2). EJ Lazarus.

Gurukkal, R. (2018). *History and Theory of Knowledge Production: An Introductory Outline*. Oxford University Press.

Hall, A. (2008). Denis J. Murphy. People, Plants & Genes: The Story of Crops and Humanity. xxiv+ 402 pages, 54 figures, 12 tables. 2007. Oxford: Oxford University Press. *Antiquity*, *82*(316), 505–506. doi:10.1017/S0003598X00097040

Heinrich, J., & Mathre, M. L. (2001). Policy Perspectives: Therapeutic Cannabis. *The American Journal of Nursing*, *101*(4), 61–69. PMID:11301687

Herer, J. (1990). The forgotten history of hemp. *Earth Island Journal*, *5*(4), 35–38.

Herer, J. (1992). *Hemp & the Marijuana Conspiracy: The Emperor Wears No Clothes: the Authoritative Historical Record of the Cannabis Plant, Marijuana Prohibition & how Hemp Can Still Save the World*. Help End Marijuana Prohibition.

Ireland, T. (1893). Indian hemp as a cause of insanity. *British Medical Journal, 2*(1710), 813.

Kalant, O. J. (1972). Report of the Indian Hemp Drugs Commission, 1893-94: A critical review. *The International Journal of the Addictions*, *7*(1), 77–96. doi:10.3109/10826087209026763 PMID:4557840

Mechoulam, R. (2005). *Cannabinoids as therapeutics*. Springer. doi:10.1007/3-7643-7358-X

Metcalf, B. D., & Metcalf, T. R. (2006). *A concise history of modern India*. Cambridge University Press. doi:10.1017/CBO9780511812750

Mills, J. (2000). Madness, Cannabis and Colonialism. *The «Native Only» Lunatic Asylums of British India 1857-1900*.

Mills, J. (2009). Cannabis and the Cultures of Colonialism: Government, medicine, ritual and pleasures in the history of an Asian drug (c. 1800-c. 1895). *Zeitenblicke, 9*(3).

Nahas, G. G. (1982). Hashish in Islam 9th to 18th century. *Bulletin of the New York Academy of Medicine*, *58*(9), 814. PMID:6762898

Salema, A., Valiathan, M. S., Malamound, C., Raghunathan, K., Wujastyk, D., & Walker, T. (2001). *Ayurveda at the crossroads of care and cure*. Indo-European Seminar on Ayurveda Held in Arrabida.

Shamir, R., & Hacker, D. (2001). Colonialism's civilizing mission: The case of the Indian Hemp Drug Commission. *Law & Social Inquiry*, *26*(2), 435–461. doi:10.1111/j.1747-4469.2001.tb00184.x

Singh, M., Mamania, D., & Shinde, V. (2018). *The scope of hemp (Cannabis sativa L.) use in Historical conservation in India*.

Singh, M., & Sardesai, M. M. (2016). Cannabis sativa (Cannabaceae) in ancient clay plaster of Ellora Caves, India. *Current Science*, 884–891.

Stein, M. A. (1989). *Kalhana's Rajatarangini: A Chronicle of the Kings of Kashmir* (Vol. 1 & 2). Motilal Banarsidass Publ.

Touw, M. (1981). The religious and medicinal uses of Cannabis in China, India and Tibet. *Journal of Psychoactive Drugs*, *13*(1), 23–34. doi:10.1080/02791072.1981.10471447 PMID:7024492

Verotta, L., Macchi, M. P., & Venkatasubramanian, P. (2015). *Connecting Indian Wisdom and Western Science: Plant Usage for Nutrition and Health*.

Warf, B. (2014). High points: An historical geography of cannabis. *Geographical Review*, *104*(4), 414–438. doi:10.1111/j.1931-0846.2014.12038.x

Chapter 3
Cultivation of Cannabis:
Medicinal, Social, and Legal Aspects

Khursheed Ahmad Wani
https://orcid.org/0000-0001-5577-3455
Government Degree College Thindim Kreeri, Baramulla, India

Syed Javid Andrabi
SP College, Srinagar, India

Javid Manzoor
https://orcid.org/0000-0002-2821-206X
Government Degree PG College, Bhaderwah, India

Heena Qadir
Government Degree College, Awantipora, India

Kounsar Jan
Government Degree College Thindim Kreeri, Baramulla, India

ABSTRACT

Interest in growing cannabis for medical and recreational purposes is increasing worldwide. This study reviews the cultivation of cannabis, its medicinal significance, and its social impacts. It is believed that cannabis has many medicinal properties that could prove very useful for the managing different disease, and at the same time it has many harmful effects that expose it to many legal and social aspects. Cannabis contains a psychoactive compound called tetrahydrocannabinols (THC) that creates a psychogenic effect. It can be consumed through the respiratory tract and digestive tract through smoking and oral ingesting, respectively. In contrast, cannabidiol (CBD), another component derived from cannabis, is a non-psychoactive cannabinoid that has gained popularity for its medicinal values and as a supplement.

DOI: 10.4018/978-1-6684-5718-4.ch003

INTRODUCTION

It is widely accepted that China is where cannabis was first cultivated, and that it originated in central Asia (Clarke & Merlin 2013; Ranalli 1999; Ren et al. 2019). From Central Asia, it spread to the rest of Asia and eventually Europe (Ranalli 1999). Hemp, one of the plant's many varieties, was put to use for writing materials, textiles, rope, animal feed, edible oil, and even spiritual rituals. Culture, according to Ranalli, plays a role in the cannabis industry (1999). Historically, people in Europe, the northern hemisphere, and East Asia placed a premium on cultivating food sources including fibre and seed. In contrast, societies in the Middle East, Africa, South, and Southern Asia used it first as a hallucinogenic medicine and secondly as a seed plant and a source of fibre.

One interpretation of the current surge in interest in medicinal cannabis is that it represents a return to the drug's traditional medical use. In fact, numerous civilizations across the globe have long recognised the medicinal benefits of cannabis and cannabis-based treatments. Until the 19th century, cannabis had a little part in Western culture, but it gained widespread attention as a popular element in 19th-century European and American medicinal and commercial remedies. In contrast, by the turn of the century, new synthetic medications like aspirin and barbiturates had supplanted cannabis in popularity. Also, in 1961, cannabis was added to the worldwide drugs control system and placed in Schedule I of the Single Convention because to its little therapeutic benefit and considerable misuse potential. This scheduling continues to be the basis for discussions concerning medicinal cannabis (Adu-Gyamfi & Brenya, 2015)

As a matter of fact, the growing interest in medicinal cannabis is contentious. However, additional data is needed before cannabis can be accepted as a medicine by doctors, health officials, and lawmakers. However, state authorities are hesitant to support medical cannabis legalisation for fear that doing so will confuse the public about the distinctions between illicit and legal substances and represent a threat to the ideology of prohibition in drug policy (Adu-Mireku, 2003). Therefore, with the exception of a few U.S. states, most countries that have made medicinal cannabis publicly accessible have done so under a highly controlled system where a patient requires a prescription from a competent doctor and the variety of products available is severely constricted. Medical experts may be sceptical and reluctant to prescribe cannabis treatment to their patients in real practise. The use of tobacco as a delivery mechanism is also problematic. A drug that is smoked is very unlikely to be approved as a therapy in many countries, however other ways of administration, such as vaporisation, remain a possibility (Brown, 1998).

Cannabis is the most widely used illicit drug around the globe and in Europe. Not only are herbal cannabis and cannabis resin now accessible on the black market, but so are a growing number of other, more exotic forms of cannabis. In addition, several businesses in a number of different regions have begun offering items containing trace amounts of THC (the psychoactive component of cannabis) in them. Regulatory reactions are becoming more nuanced and varied as more countries legalise medical cannabis use or are contemplating legalising recreational use under certain circumstances. This is a more nuanced issue, both in terms of description and solution, despite the fact that most health and social problems still revolve around illicit cannabis use. The production, medical value, and societal effects of cannabis are discussed in this article of growing cannabis (Bruce-Amartey et al., 2014).

CANNABIS FOR MEDICINE

The different derivates obtained from cannabis may be used to cure various diseases as shown in Figure 1: However, there is no consistent support to these claims, although trails may prove the fact.

Figure 1. Different types of diseases cured by cannabinoids

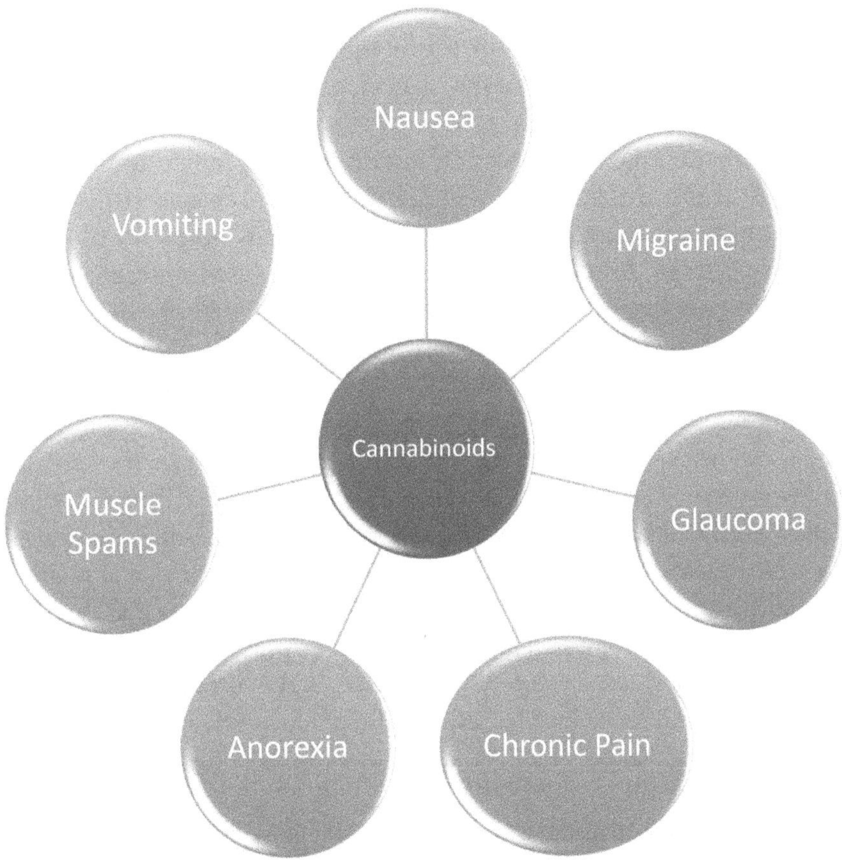

In 2018, the FDA approved Epidiolex as the first CBD-containing prescription medication. Epidiolex is used to treat severe, uncontrollable forms of epilepsy (Holland 2020). CBD has shown to be helpful in mitigating some of chemotherapy's side effects. Patients with cancer who use CBD report less pain, less nausea, and a greater appetite (Davis 2016; Javid et al. 2016). CBD has been shown to inhibit the growth of breast cancer cells and to inhibit the development of prostate cancer in recent research (Sharma et al., 2018). According to the World Health Organization (WHO), there were 912 instances of prostate cancer and 2260 cases of breast cancer in Ghana in 2014.

Cancer rates for both prostate and breast continued to rise in 2020, with respective increases of 2129 and 4482. (GLOBOCAN 2020). Recent increases in the number of reported occurrences of breast and prostate cancer in Ghana have prompted calls for further research on CDB usage. Multiple other pharmacological uses for CBD exist, all of which would be to the advantage of the country. This opens the door for the Ghanaian pharmaceutical sector to study CBD and develop CBD-related medications in light of the recent legalisation and commercialisation. In addition, manufacturers of natural remedies might investigate hemp's therapeutic potential. Nutritional supplements, medicines, and therapeutic goods are among the many uses for hemp.

Plants have been utilised as medicines throughout civilizations for thousands of years. Creating natural substances as single molecules for modern therapeutic usage is time-consuming and costly. Therefore, scientists are focusing on the development of botanical drugs, or entire plant extracts, which are used to treat certain sickness circumstances, drawing cues from traditional medical practises like Ayurveda and Traditional Chinese Medicine (TCM). With this in mind, in 2006 the US Food and Drug Administration (FDA) imposed strict regulations on the manufacture of so-called "Botanical Drugs (Kilmer & Pacula, 2017)

Cannabis varieties vary from one another not only in their chemical composition but also in the proportions of their ingredients, due to differences in their unique botanical characteristics. Different cannabis strains likely have distinct pharmacological effects. Therefore, it is necessary to chemically identify medical cannabis with particular therapeutic action before it may be used in treatment. In terms of R&D, any cannabis preparation (whether it be whole plant or extract) would be classified as a botanical drug and would need complete characterization. As well as defining the product's chemical composition, one would need to demonstrate that it remains constant from batch to batch. In addition, clinical studies are required before botanical medications may be prescribed for certain medical disorders (Kraenzel et al., 1998). Sativex®, also known as nabiximols, was created by G.W. Pharma and is the most well-known botanical medication derived from cannabis. It is an equal mixture of THC and CBD extracts (1:1).

Similarly, "Bedrocan," a cannabis firm located in the Netherlands, sells several cannabis concoctions. The firm provides chemically defined cannabis biomass (buds) to medical marijuana patients in the Netherlands via pharmacies that accept prescriptions. While these items may be purchased without leaving Canada (without prescription). In addition to Bedrocan®, Bedica®, and Bedrobinol®, Bedrocan also offers Bediol®, an intermediate variety (THCCBD), and Bedrolite®, a high CBD variation. In terms of their THC, CBD, and terpene profiles, all of these products are well described. Despite having European certification, the company's goods are not allowed in the United States because to a lack of testing for individual diseases.

However, there are a number of medications, cannabis preparations, and related goods already on the market (in various US states and online) that make unsubstantiated claims of being able to treat a variety of diseases. Patients may be put in risk by receiving a product that does not meet the standards of a legitimate botanical medication, which might lead to a worsening of their health (Kruger et al., 2020).

Many people believe that cannabis plant compositions are more powerful than the individual cannabinoids; they attribute this belief to the "entourage effect". In other words, the action of the primary cannabinoid is amplified by the presence of ancillary cannabinoids, terpenes, and flavonoids present in cannabis. In any case, the clinical evidence supports this claim.

PATTERNS OF CANNABIS USE AND RELATED HARMS

Who is impacted, what drugs are at play, how they are being used, and where the issue is occurring are all crucial pieces of information to have at your disposal when attempting to diagnose and characterise a problem. Drug issues vary over time and between countries, so responses need to be flexible. An extensive number of considerations are discussed at this stage in the Action framework for creating and implementing health and social solutions to drug issues. Cannabinoids and THC are extracted from the Cannabis sativa plant, or the plant itself is used if it is to be smoked. There is a growing selection of cannabis products in Europe, each with its own flavour profile and delivery system (Liao et al, 2020).

Cannabis has the highest prevalence of any illegal substance in Europe and the world. The average age of initial cannabis usage is much younger than that of other illegal substances. There are estimates that between 15 and 20% of Europeans aged 15 to 34 have used cannabis during the last year, with the percentage rising to roughly 16 million among those aged 15 to 24. However, reported levels of usage vary greatly among nations, with prevalence rates often ranging from 3% to roughly 22% among young people. Cannabis usage among young adults is often short-lived and exploratory. However, some people's cannabis usage becomes more chronic and harmful with time; this is especially true of heavy, long-term users.

These issues can range from those related to one's physical health (such as chronic respiratory symptoms) to those related to one's mental health (such as cannabis dependence and psychotic symptoms) to those related to one's social and economic life (such as poor academic performance, dropping out of school, impaired job performance, or involvement with the law) to the potential negative effects on one's unborn child.

Adolescent frequent usage increases the risk of negative mental health, social, and economic effects. Higher potency cannabis products, particularly those with high amounts of tetrahydrocannabinol, the primary psychoactive component of cannabis, may enhance the dangers (THC). Cannabidiol (CBD), another component of cannabis, has shown promise as a potential mediator of the adverse effects of high doses of THC. Furthermore, cannabis usage might result in severe symptoms that need visits to the emergency room. Cannabis is used widely over the globe, but fortunately, it seldom leads to fatalities.

Some nations' criminal penalties for cannabis use and possession are seen with scepticism due to concerns that they may be disproportionate to the damage produced by cannabis usage. As a result, this is one of the reasons why many methods of regulation are being tried out.

Tobacco-infused cannabis smoke is still the norm in Europe. This increases the hazards to health, and the nicotine addiction that often follows increases the difficulty of therapy. It also emphasises the need of looking at cannabis and tobacco policy and reactions in a broader context.

Both the variety of cannabis-based products available and the ways in which they may be used have expanded rapidly in recent years, perhaps in response to the adoption of novel types of cannabis regulation. Vaporizers, concentrates, edibles, and capsules are all becoming more widely accessible. Although these alternatives to combining cannabis with cigarettes may have health benefits, they may also pose new dangers. For instance, young toddlers who are drawn to delicacies like cakes, candies, and chocolate may unintentionally consume too much of the substance and have adverse effects. Dabbing, in which very concentrated extracts are used, also seems to be linked to serious negative health outcomes. Varying vaporizers may provide different dangers depending on the cannabis extract or product being consumed. It seems that an addition or contaminant in illegal vape cartridges is to blame for the 2019-2020 epidemic of serious lung harm in North America linked to the usage of e-cigarettes with cannabis vape liquids (Mensah & Adu-Gyamfi, 2019).

Problems with very strong synthetic cannabinoid receptor agonists, or synthetic cannabinoids, have also been a rising source of concern. Although they share cannabinoid receptors with cannabis, these drugs have quite different effects and may have more serious side effects, including death, when used in excess. The book "New psychoactive substances: health and societal reactions" goes through these topics.

Primary goals of health and social responses to cannabis use and associated problems may include: preventing or delaying use from adolescence until young adulthood; preventing the escalation of use from occasional to regular use; reducing harmful modes of use; providing treatment for people whose cannabis use has become problematic; and reducing the likelihood of people driving after consuming cannabis or engaging in other activities while under the influence of cannabis.

Policymakers should also think about ways to lessen the number of adolescent cannabis users who end up in jail or prison. In addition, the availability of safe products and the enforcement of regulatory measures, such as the prohibition of sales to minors, will be crucial in areas where cannabis is being made legally accessible.

Legal Aspects of Cannabis Cultivation

Producing, harvesting, and processing biomass products, as well as maintaining quality and consistency, are all challenging aspects in the development of plant-based pharmaceuticals. For cannabis in particular, the added complexity stems from the drug's placement in schedule I, where it is subject to strict regulation.

Legalization of cannabis in the United States varies widely from state to state. Some states have legalised cannabis for both medical and recreational use, while many others have done so solely for the former. At the time this article was published, medical cannabis usage was allowed in 33 states in the United States, plus the District of Columbia. Ten states plus the District of Columbia have legalised recreational usage. While growing cannabis is allowed in these states according to state law, it is still against federal law. This makes for an uncommon setting in which to produce a genuine drug. The Food and Medication Administration (FDA) conducts a thorough assessment of each pure/botanical drug manufactured in accordance with federal regulation. There will be no more questions about the product's security or effectiveness. The FDA has several safeguards in place, but drugs and treatments sold under state laws are getting through them.

If you combine Section 8 of the NDPS Act, 1985 with Section 10, the State Governments may issue licences for cannabis growing for medicinal and research reasons. So far, cannabis has only been used in alternative medicine, such as homoeopathy and Ayurveda, for its medicinal properties. The growing of cannabis has not been licenced by state governments. Scientists throughout the world have recently shown a rising interest in investigating the potential medicinal applications of cannabis. Due to the lack of evidence supporting its widespread medicinal use, cannabis cultivation is prohibited. For scientific purposes, including the testing of different cannabis strains, cultivation is allowed.

Bhang, a cannabis leaf mixture, is popular during some Indian celebrations. In accordance with the NDPS Act of 1985, its production is illegal since it does not include the use of cannabis resin or cannabis flowering tops. Many State Governments sanction the cultivation and trade of Bhang. Only those with a legal right to cultivate cannabis in the wild may harvest the leaves needed to make Bhang. They aren't allowed to utilise the plant's resin or blooming tops. Anyone caught adulterating Bhang with cannabis flower tops or resin will face penalties under the NDPS Act, 1985, and if they are a licensee, they will lose their privilege to sell cannabis legally.

The cannabis plant may be used for industrial applications as a source of biomass and fibre. The oil extracted from cannabis seeds is very valuable. There are cannabis strains with relatively little tetrahydrocannabinol (THC), the psychoactive component, that are permitted for growing in certain nations. Fibres extracted from these strains of marijuana are employed in the textile industry for biomass generation. In accordance with Section 14 of the NDPS Act, the Government may, by general or special order, authorise the growing of cannabis for horticultural and industrial uses only. Efforts to discover and test cannabis strains with less psychoactive effects will be supported by the federal government. The federal government, however, must be careful and make judgements based on facts when it comes to allowing cannabis to be grown for horticultural and/or industrial uses.

The NDPS Act makes it illegal to grow opium poppies or cannabis (Cannabis sativa) for recreational purposes. Without a licence, growing opium poppies is illegal and punishable under Section 18, whereas growing cannabis is illegal and punishable under Section 20. All officials of the State and Central governments who are authorised under Section 41, Section 42, or Section 43 shall have the authority of entrance, search, seizure, and arrest in connection to unlawful cultivation offences, as per Section 44. Attach any opium poppy, cannabis, or coca plant which he has reason to believe is being illegally cultivated, and pass such order as he thinks fit, including an order to destroy the crop, if he is a Metropolitan Magistrate, Judicial Magistrate of the first class, or any Magistrate empowered in this behalf by the State Government or any officer of Gazetted rank empowered under section 42. (Section 48).

In spite of these prohibitions, evidence of illicit opium poppy and cannabis growing persists. Such illicit farming is of great concern to the Indian government. The federal and state governments will keep cooperating to address this issue, and they will order all subordinate officials to carry out their duties in accordance with Section 47 of the NDPS Act. Officials who learn of unlawful cultivation are to report it to one or more nodal officers designated by the Central Government and each State Government. Law enforcement at all levels must enforce a zero-tolerance policy against illegal crop production, and the National Crimes Bureau (NCB) and the Central Bank of the United States (CBN) must bring criminal charges against any officials under their jurisdiction who are found to have violated Section 47 of the National Dangerous Plants Act.

In many regions of the United States and the globe, cannabis may be found growing freely. Some of the best conditions for cannabis cultivation include a cold, hilly environment. The NDPS Act requires state government employees to eradicate cannabis plants in the wild to the greatest extent practicable. Except for the leaves, which may be used to make Bhang, wild-grown cannabis is prohibited from being used for any purpose.

Foreign direct investments (FDI) in a nation may increase if industrial hemp is legalised and commercialised. It should be the goal of the Government to help the country wean itself off of international aid and create an economy that is driven by domestic investment. As a result, the government has taken proactive measures and taken pragmatic initiatives, which have been very successful, leading to the establishment of assembly factories in Ghana by automotive giants like Volkswagen and Nissan. There is a lot of money to be made in the cannabis business. Worldwide, there are already over 25,000 items made from industrial hemp. This might include anything from components for automobiles to home furnishings, fabrics, meals, cosmetics, or building materials (Carpenter 2018).

Legal CBD sales in the US, derived from hemp, are projected to reach $20 billion by 2022. (Giammona 2018). According to research conducted by Brightfield Group, the Canadian cannabis market will be worth $5 billion by 2021. By 2025, New Frontier Data estimates, the Canadian cannabis market will be worth $2,000. (Subramaniam 2020). In 2017, the United States imported hemp worth $67.3 million; most of this came from Canada (Johnson 2018). They can't service their domestic cannabis industry without importing either raw ingredients or intermediate goods. The cannabis sector in Lethoso attracted FDI of $13.13m (Prohibition Partners 2019). India's climate and soil are ideal for growing industrial hemp. Despite difficulties with technology, agriculture in India is a major economic and job driver.

CONCLUSION

The new law will likely have beneficial effects on the economy, but it's still vital to examine the entrance criterion for the sector in depth. There is much that India may learn from Africa's existing licencing practises, which seem to unfairly target local farmers and investors. The licencing mechanism should be flexible enough to allow local company owners to enter the hemp sector. In order to boost India's manufacturing sector, the licencing system should favour local investors and farmers in the industrial hemp farming industry. There is a need for more research to be conducted by Indian academics before the country can begin hemp production at large scale keeping its legal approaches in consideration. However, in order for India to effectively control and reap the benefits of hemp cultivation, researchers in India need do many types of study into cannabis importance to society and industry.

REFERENCES

Adu-Gyamfi, S., & Brenya, E. (2015). The marijuana factor in a university in Ghana: A survey. *J Siberian Feder Univ*, *8*(11), 2162–2182. doi:10.17516/1997-1370-2015-8-11-2162-2182

Adu-Mireku, S. (2003). The prevalence of alcohol, cigarette, and marijuana use among Ghanaian senior secondary students in an urban setting. *Journal of Ethnicity in Substance Abuse*, *2*(1), 53–65. doi:10.1300/J233v02n01_05

Brown, D. T. (1998). Non-medical uses of cannabis sativa. In D. T. Brown (Ed.), *Cannabis: the genus cannabis*. Harwood academic publishers.

Bruce-Amartey, E. Jr, Amissah, E. R. K., & Safo-Ankama, K. (2014). The decline of Ghana's textile industry: Its effects on textile education in Ghana. *Arts Design Stud.*, *22*, 36–45.

Carpenter, D. E. (2018). Legal hemp in 2019 may be a boon for stressed out American farmers. *Forbes.* https://www.forbes.com/sites/davidcarpenter/2018/12/20/legal-hemp-in-2019-may-be-a-boon-for-stressed-out-american-farmers/

Clarke, R. C., & Merlin, M. D. (2013). *Cannabis: evolution and ethnobotany*. Univ of California Press. doi:10.1525/9780520954571

Davis, M. P. (2016). Cannabinoids for symptom management and cancer therapy: The evidence. *Journal of the National Comprehensive Cancer Network: JNCCN*, *14*(7), 915–922. doi:10.6004/jnccn.2016.0094 PMID:27407130

Giammona, C. (2018). Trendy hemp compound CBD set for big boost from U.S. *Farm Bill.* https://www.bloomberg.com/news/articles/2018-12-19/trendy-hemp-compound-cbd-set-for-big-boost-from-u-s-farm-bill

GLOBOCAN. (2020). *Cancer today*. GCO. https://gco.iarc.fr/today/home

Holland, K. (2020). CBD vs. THC: properties, benefits, and side effects. *Healthline.* https://www.healthline.com/health/cbd-vs-thc

Javid FA, Phillips RM, Afshinjavid S, Verde R, Ligresti A., (2016). Cannabinoid pharmacology in cancer research: a new hope for cancer patients? *Eur J Pharmacol.* 2775:1–14. doi:. 02.010. doi:10.1016/j.ejphar

Johnson, R. (2018). Hemp as an agricultural commodity (CRS report no. RL32725; p. 48). *Congressional research service.* https://fas.org/sgp/crs/misc/RL32725.pdf

Kilmer, B., & Pacula, R. L. (2017). Understanding and learning from the diversification of cannabis supply laws. *Addiction (Abingdon, England), 112*(7), 1128–1135. doi:10.1111/add.13623 PMID:27891693

Kraenzel, D. G., Petry, T. A., Nelson, B., Anderson, M. J., Mathern, D., & Todd, R. (1998). Industrial hemp as an alternative crop in North Dakota. *Agricultural Economics Report, 402.* doi:10.22004/ag.econ.23264

Kruger, D. J., Moffet, I. M., Seluk, L. C., & Zammit, L. A. (2020). A content analysis of internet information sources on medical cannabis. *J Cannabis Res., 2*(1), 1–6. doi:10.118642238-020-00041-1 PMID:33526127

Liao, J., Zhang, S., & Tang, X. (2020). Sound absorption of hemp fibers (cannabis sativa L.) based nonwoven fabrics and composites: A review. *Journal of Natural Fibers*, 1–13.

Mensah, K.B. & Adu-Gyamfi, P.K.T. (2019). To legalize cannabis in Ghana or not to legalize? Reviewing the pharmacological evidence. *Arch Pharm Pharm Sci.* 3(1):082–8.

Prohibition Partners. (2019). The African cannabis reports. *Prohibition Partners.* https://prohibitionpartners.com/reports/

Ranalli, P. (1999). *Advances in hemp research.* CRC Press. doi:10.1201/9781498705820

Ren, M., Tang, Z., Wu, X., Spengler, R., Jiang, H., Yang, Y., & Boivin, N. (2019). The origins of cannabis smoking: Chemical residue evidence from the first millennium BCE in the Pamirs. *Science Advances, 205*(6), eaaw1391. doi:10.1126ciadv.aaw1391 PMID:31206023

Sharma, D., Kumar, S., & Narasimhan, B. (2018). Estrogen alpha receptor antagonists for the treatment of breast cancer: A review. *Chemistry Central Journal, 12*(1), 107. doi:10.118613065-018-0472-8 PMID:30361894

Subramaniam. (2020). Cannabis industry to be worth just $5 billion by 2021 amid flat rollout, high costs. *Financial Post.* https://financialpost.com/cannabis/cannabis-industry-to-be-worth-just-5-billion-by-2021-amid-flat-rollout-high-costs

World Health Organization (WHO). (2014). *Cancer country profile.* WHO. https://www.who.int/cancer/country-profiles/gha_en.pdf?ua=1

Chapter 4
Medicinal Uses of *Cannabis sativa* and Its Derivatives

Zahid Nabi
Central University of Jammu, India

Javaid Manzoor Lone
https://orcid.org/0000-0002-2821-206X
JJT University, Jhunjhunu, India

Anuradha Sharma
Government Degree College, Bhaderwah, India

ABSTRACT

Cannabis Sativas has found applications in medical industry since time immemorial. With the evolution of time marijuana plant Cannabis sativa, its derivatives, cannabinoids, have grown increasingly popular as a potential treatment for various diseases which include ailments of heart, skin, and other vital organs. Products extracted from Cannabis have found their usage in various stages of medical treatment. Various ailments can be cured by the giving the patient required dose of cannabis or hemp oil. Moreover, Cannabis reduces chronic pain, increases lung capacity, helps lose weight and regulates diabetes.

INTRODUCTION

Cannabis Sativa, usually referred to as marijuana, is an anemophilous herbaceous plant in the Cannabinaceae family. Cannabis plant, which is native to Central or South Asia, has been used for thousands of years in traditional remedies as well as a narcotic for entheogenic and recreational purposes. It is is an herbaceous dioecious annual species that displays considerable variability in phenotypic characteristics (Clarke & Merlin, 2015; Small et al., 2003).

Cannabis is the collective name for all plants that have been included in the Cannabis genus. According to molecular analysis and DNA extraction from modern and archaeobotanical materials, the majority of academics concur that this plant originated in Asia, was transported to Europe, and was farmed as

DOI: 10.4018/978-1-6684-5718-4.ch004

an acrop during the Bronze Age (22nd to the 16th century BC). C. sativa is a plant that is widely grown and produced over the world, including in locations like Africa, Canada, Europe, and the United States in addition to Asian nations (Farinon et al, 2020)

Due to its several uses, this quickly growing plant has recently attracted renewed interest. It is a veritable treasure of phytochemicals and a plentiful supply of both cellulosic and woody fibres. The pharmaceutical and construction industries are both very interested in this plant because its metabolites have powerful biological effects on human health and because its outer and inner stem tissues can be used to produce bioplastics and concrete-like materials, respectively.

Cannabis has been used for food, feed, and therapeutic purposes for a very long time because of its excellent nutritional content. The stem, seeds, roots, and blooms are all a part of this. Hemp seed has been consumed as food from ancient times, especially in Asian cultures, and is important commercially as a source of edible oil. Due to the great nutritional value of the plant, all parts of the cannabis plant, including the stem, seeds, roots, and flowers, have been used for food, feed, and therapeutic purposes for a very long time. Hemp seed has been consumed as food from ancient times, notably in Asian cultures. It is also an economically important source of edible oil (Farinon et al, 2020).

Over 100 chemical components that are active in cannabis are referred to as "cannabinoids". There are an a plenty of cannabinoids in the plant, with delta-9-tetrahydrocannabinol being the most psychotropic (THC). THC is a very promising drug for medical use because it also contains appetite-stimulating, anti-inflammatory, analgesic, and anti-emetic properties..Cannabis contains antioxidants like polyphenols that reduce the risk of chronic illnesses like cancer, neurological disorders, digestive issues, and skin diseases as well as anxiety and oxidative stress. Cannabis has been demonstrated to negatively affect reproductive, driving, and psychomotor processes as well as the respiratory system (De Petrocellis et al, 2011; Sirikantaramas et al., 2005). Nine essential amino acids, including histidine, isoleucine, leucine, lysine, methionine, phenylalanine, threonine, and valine, are present in cannabis sativa (hemp) seeds (Audu, 2015).

Evidence suggests that cannabis and cannabinoids show various medicinal benefits which includes the treatment of adult chronic pain, antiemetics for chemotherapy-induced nausea and vomiting, and a reduction in MS spasticity symptoms as described by patients. Numerous studies have revealed that they have extra health benefits, particularly when used as medicinal agents. The chapter explores various medicinal benefits associated with the use of Cannabis Sativa and products derived from it.

BACKGROUND AND LITERATURE REVIEW

Cannabis sativa is a plant species that has been used for medicinal purposes for centuries. The plant contains compounds called cannabinoids, which have been found to have therapeutic properties. The two main cannabinoids found in the plant are tetrahydrocannabinol (THC) and cannabidiol (CBD).

A literature review published in the journal "Frontiers in Neurology" in 2018, suggests that CBD may have therapeutic potential in treating a wide range of neurological disorders, including epilepsy, multiple sclerosis, and anxiety disorders. CBD has been found to have anti-inflammatory, analgesic, and anti-anxiety properties, which may be useful in treating these conditions (Bitencourt and Takahashi, 2018).

ElSohly et al., 2017 stated that CBD has been found to be effective in treating symptoms of anxiety and PTSD (Post Traumatic Stress Disorder) in human studies. It also reported that CBD has shown promising results in animal studies for treating symptoms of depression.

Sheng et al., 2019, suggested that CBD may have therapeutic potential in treating chronic pain conditions. CBD has been found to have anti-inflammatory and analgesic properties, which may be useful in treating chronic pain conditions such as arthritis, fibromyalgia, and neuropathic pain.

A literature review published in the journal "Cancer Management and Research" in 2017, suggests that CBD may have therapeutic potential in treating cancer symptoms and side effects of cancer treatment. CBD has been found to have anti-inflammatory, analgesic, and anti-anxiety properties, which may be useful in treating cancer symptoms such as pain, nausea, and vomiting.

It is important to note that while these literature reviews suggest the potential therapeutic benefits of CBD, further research is needed to fully understand the medicinal uses of cannabis sativa plant and to establish its safety and efficacy. Moreover, the laws regarding the use of cannabis for medicinal purposes vary depending on the jurisdiction and it is important to be aware of the local laws.

EXPLORING MEDICAL APPLICATIONS OF CANNABIS

The term "medical cannabis," often known as "medical marijuana," refers to the use of cannabis to treat illness or lessen its symptoms, while there is no one definition that is widely accepted (for example, cannabinoids made from cannabis and synthetic cannabinoids are both utilised). Restrictions on production and the fact that many governments consider cannabis to be an illegal narcotic have made it difficult to conduct thorough scientific research into the herb's potential as a therapy.

There is scant evidence to support the use of cannabis to treat chronic pain and muscular spasms, to enhance appetite in HIV/AIDS patients, or to lessen nausea and vomiting associated with chemotherapy. To infer its efficacy or safety from its usage in other medical applications would be inadequate. There is evidence to support the use of cannabis or its derivatives in the treatment of neuropathic pain, multiple sclerosis, and nausea and vomiting brought on by chemotherapy. Its usage for AIDS wasting syndrome, epilepsy, rheumatoid arthritis, and glaucoma is supported by weaker evidence.

Only a small number of countries, including Canada, Belgium, Australia, the Netherlands, and New Zealand, currently permit the use of cannabis for medical purposes. Spain and a number of US states. Typically, a prescription is needed for this usage, and distribution takes place within a framework established by regional regulations.

Due to the abundance of phytochemicals in cannabis Sativa which has been used medicinally since ancient times, scientists are working to maximise the plant's pharmacological potential. The name "cannabis" refers to the produced or obtained goods (drugs and essential oils) made from the annual herb C. sativa and its variations, members of the Cannabacea family.

EXTRACTION OF CANNABINOIDS FROM CANNABIS

Product development and extraction techniques have taken centre stage as the cannabis business moves from an illegal market to a legal market. The dried cannabis flower has historically been a well-liked product for usage in smoking and vaping. However, as the market grows, so does the need for cannabis products, both in terms of variety and potency. Topicals, edibles, drinks, and vaporizer cartridges are some of the goods that are now on the market, whether they be for medical or recreational use. Each product category offers a unique set of benefits and drawbacks, allowing for modification to meet specific needs

(Blake & Nahtigal, 2019). Cannabis is a complex blend of chemicals that is used as a herbal remedy. These chemicals include cannabinoid phenols, non-cannabinoid phenols (such as stilbenes, lignans, spiro-indans, and dihydrophenanthrenes), flavonoids, terpenoids, alcohols, aldehydes, n-alkanes, wax esters, steroids, and alkaloids (Baldino et al., 2020; Lewis., 2017; Jin et al., 2020)

Numerous methods for extracting cannabinoids from Cannabis L. sativa rely on traditional extraction methods like distillation, solvent extraction, Soxhlet, maceration, and sonication; however, these methods take a lot of time and use a significant amount of toxic organic solvents that are harmful to both the environment and human health (Rajaei et al., 2004; Agarwal et al., 2018)

These strategies offer a substantial advantage over traditional ones. Less degradation, the removal of superfluous sample cleaning, lower organic solvent consumption, concentration steps prior to chromatographic analysis, selectivity, improved kinetics, extraction efficiency, and automation ease are some of these benefits (Chemat et al., 2012; Pellati et al., 2018). Pressurized hot water extraction is an alternative to these methods (PHWE). It is viewed as a green extraction technique. Water is employed in its supercritical form as a solvent that has the same solvability characteristics as methanol and ethanol in place of CO2. The recovery of polar and semi-polar bioactive chemicals from plant materials has proven to be a success when using pressurised hot water extraction. The PHWE method relies on using high pressure and temperature to maintain supercritical fluid form of water throughout the extraction process (Bergamashi et al., 2013; Plaza & Turner, 2015; Hawthorne, 1994).

ANTI BACTRIAL PROPERTIES OF CANNABIS

Cannabis has long been thought to have antibacterial properties that can fight off a variety of dangerous bacteria as well as some fungi. Nine-THC and CBD are the key contributors to the antibacterial quality. However, numerous investigations have shown that this action is also present in plant extracts or essential oils. Cannabis leaf extracts made of ethanol and petroleum were tested against several bacteria in 1995 by Wasim and co-workers. According to the findings, both Gram positive (Baccilus subtilus, Baccilus pumilus, Staphlococcus aureus, and Micrococcus flavus) and Gram negative (Proteus vlugaris, Bordetella bronchioseptica) bacteria are strongly inhibited by the extracts. Extracts' antibacterial efficacy was compared to Celphalexin, a widely used antibiotic. In a 2011 study, Ali et al. investigated the effects of Cannabis sativa L. seed oil, petroleum ether, and methanol extracts of the entire plant on two Gram (+) and two Gram (-) organisms, Bacillus subtilis and Staphylococcus aureus (Escherichia coli, Pseudomonas aeruginosa). Strong antibacterial action against Bacillus subtilis and Staphylococcus aureus was shown by the Cannabis sativa seed oil, as well as moderate efficacy (15 mm) against Escherichia coli and Pseudomonas aeruginosa (16 mm). Despite the fact that the extracts were created from various plant sources, these results are comparable to those published by Wasim et al. (1995). The nutritional benefits of cannabis seeds are well recognised, and they are regarded as a fantastic source of fatty acids, however the amount of secondary metabolites is not very high.

ANTIFUNGAL PROPERTIES OF CANNABIS

Few studies have looked into cannabis's and its secondary metabolites' antifungal effects. Some articles claim that plant extracts can be successfully utilised in the management of pathogenic fungus, despite the fact that this impact has not been as thoroughly explored or as strongly demonstrated as in the case of antibacterial properties. The prevalent human pathogenic fungus Candida albicans and Aspergillus niger, which cause black mould in fruits and vegetables, were shown to be efficiently inhibited in their growth and development by Wasim and colleagues (1995) using an ethanol and petroleum extract of cannabis leaves. When compared to an antifungal antibiotic (Nystatin), the zone of inhibition in both cases was significantly higher; however, the concentration of the leaf extract was 10 times higher than that of the antibiotic. A schematic representation of various diseases curable using cannabinoids have been shown below in Figure 1.

Figure 1. List of diseases treatable using cannabinoids

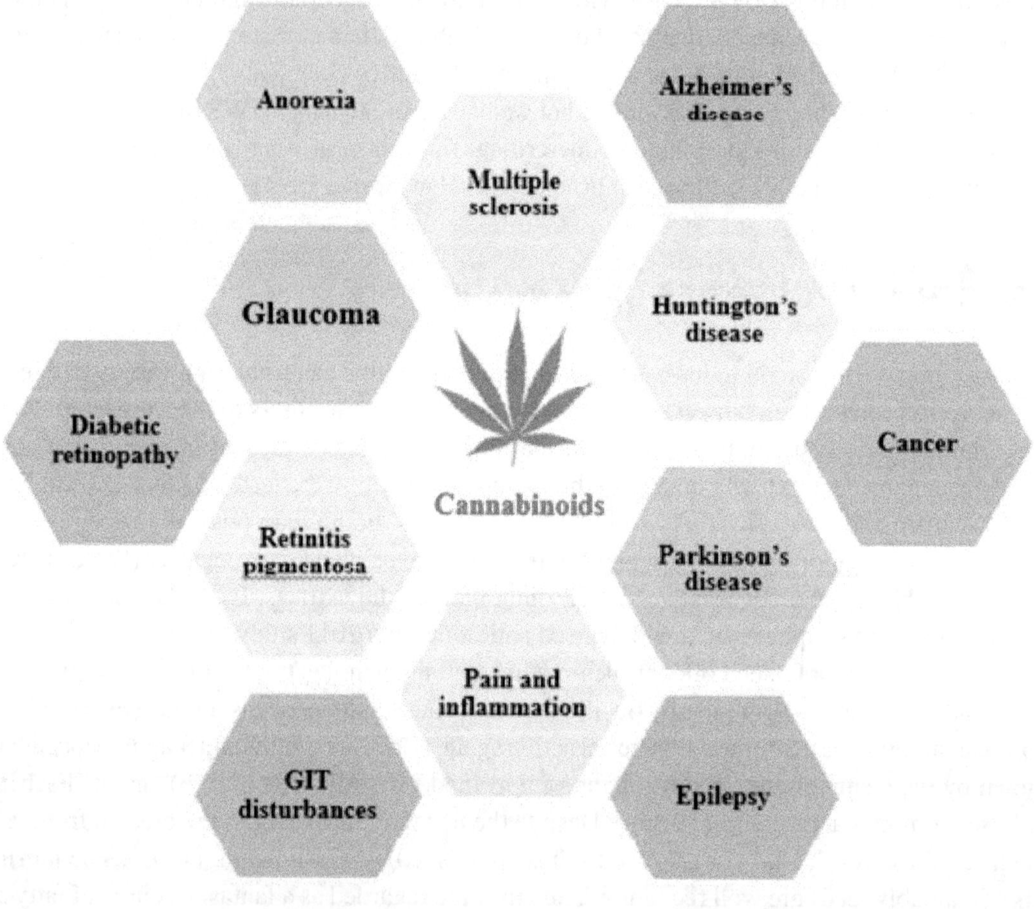

APPLICATION OF CANNABIS SATIVA AND ITS DERIVATIVES IN THE TREATMENT OF VARIOUS AILMENTS

Cancer

According to GHO 2018 projections, cancer was the second leading cause of death worldwide in 2015, accounting for over 8.8 million fatalities—or one in every six fatalities. The starting process of cancer is the development of a paraneoplastic lesion, which progresses into a malignant tumour over time. When the cellular reproduction process degenerates into cancer, it becomes uncontrollable. Uncontrolled, disordered, and undesired cell division characterise this disease. Cancer cells, in contrast to healthy cells, continue to divide and grow throughout their lives, producing dangerous cells (Pellati et al., 2018). It has been demonstrated that cannabinoids can reduce tumour cell proliferation while protecting healthy tissue. For instance, glioma cells exposed to cannabis experience ceramide-induced cell death, but astrocytes are similarly protected from oxidative stress. On glioma cells, cannabidiol makes THC's anti-tumor effects stronger. The expression of CB1 and/or CB2 receptors has also been associated with prognosis in several malignancies. Higher expression of CB2 receptors has been connected to higher tumour grade in gliomas, while higher expression of CB1 and CB2 receptors has been linked to improved prognosis in hepatocellular carcinomas (Flygare & Sander, 2008; Marcu et al., 2010; Xu et al., 2006). In a study, the efficacy and safety of THC were evaluated in individuals with refractory glioblastoma multiform. An infusion catheter was then inserted into the resection cavity after a tumour debulking procedure on nine patients. Every day for 10-64 days, THC was injected into the cavities at doses ranging from 0.80 to 3.29 mg overall. The medication was generally well accepted, with the exception of one patient who experienced a mild psychedelic effect (Bowles et al., 2011).

Skin Disorders

Dermatitis is a term that refers to a group of skin conditions that cause inflammation. These skin ailments include atopic dermatitis (eczema), seborrheic dermatitis (dandruff), and contact dermatitis.

A good source of omega-6 and omega-3 PUFAs is hempseed oil. Dietary hempseed oil and olive oil were contrasted in a 20-week controlled, single-blind, randomised experiment with atopic patients. Fatty acid patterns in plasma triglyceride, cholesteryl, and phospholipid component components were examined in this study. A patient survey was used to gather additional data regarding skin dryness, irritation, and the usage of dermatological medications. On the skin, TEWL (Trans Epidermal Water Loss) was measured.

Skin roughness and itching decreased (p50.027), and the use of topical medications was decreased (p50.024). Consuming hempseed oil significantly changed the plasma lipid composition and reduced the severity of dermatitis symptoms. These benefits are believed to be due to hempseed oil's abundant and well-balanced supply of PUFAs (Callaway et al., 2005). Sleep Related Ailments and Mental Health: Sleep is a crucial physiological activity that aids in the recovery of processes required for regular functioning. Numerous variables, like as duration, timing, effectiveness, and a feeling of restorative sleep that keeps a person aware and productive throughout the day, all have an impact on how well someone sleeps (Buxton et al., 2014; Murawski et al., 2018; Liu et al., 2014). In two studies, cannabinoids (nabilone) were specifically examined for the therapy of sleep issues (5 reports; 54 participants). The first was a parallel-group study with a high risk of bias. In this trial, nabilone was found to be more effective than a placebo at improving the sleep apnea/hypopnea index (mean difference from baseline, 19.64; p value = 0.02). The other was comparing nabilone to amitriptyline in a modest crossover experiment with fibromyalgia patients. This showed that nabilone was associated with improved sleep quality (mean difference from baseline, 0.48) and decreased insomnia (mean difference from baseline, 3.25 (95 percent CI, 5.26 to 1.24) (95 percent CI, 0.01 to 0.95). For extra purposes, sleep was also examined as an outcome in 19 placebo-controlled investigations (chronic pain and MS). Investigations on nabiximols, nabilone, dronabinol, THC/CBD capsules, and smoked THC were all examined in a total of thirteen studies (one at various doses). Oral THC was also examined in two of the nabiximol studies, while oral THC/CBD was examined in the dronabinol trial. Some evidence suggested that cannabinoids might improve these patients' ability to sleep. Cannabinoids, primarily nabiximols, were associated with a larger average improvement in sleep quality and sleep disturbance (WMD, 0.58, 95 percent CI, 0.87 to 0.29; 8 trials) (WMD, 0.26, 95 percent CI, 0.52 to 0.00; 3 trials). While nabiximols were examined in the other experiments while THC/CBD was evaluated in one, the outcomes were comparable for both cannabinoids (Whiting et al., 2015)

Hoch and his colleagues reviewed randomised clinical trials that looked at the efficacy and safety of cannabis-based treatments for mental illnesses. They found some evidence in their systematic review that THC or CBD administered as an additional therapy to other pharmacotherapies and psychotherapy reduced some symptoms of a variety of disorders, including dementia, schizophrenia, cannabis and opioid dependence, generalised social anxiety disorder, post-traumatic stress disorder, anorexia nervosa, attention-deficit/hyperactivity disorder, and Tourette's syndrome. There were some undesirable results described, but they were rarely serious (Hoch et al., 2019).

Inflammatory Bowel Disease (IBD)

Crohn's disease and ulcerative colitis together make up the chronic inflammatory disorder known as inflammatory bowel disease (IBD), which is characterised by relapsing and remitting episodes of inflammation mostly affecting the gastrointestinal tract. Although the pathophysiology of IBD is not yet fully understood, it appears to include an unfavourable inflammatory response and an immunological system that is out of balance in the right environmental and genetic circumstances.

For hundreds of years, anecdotal evidence has shown that cannabis may be beneficial in the management of IBD. In a case report from 1990, patients with IBD were described as using cannabis to keep their condition in remission. 10 Prior to the discovery of the ECS, medical marijuana use was common, which sparked more investigation into cannabis as a potential IBD treatment. There is increasing awareness of the small percentage of IBD patients who use cannabis to treat their IBD symptoms. According to reports, these people successfully manage their gastrointestinal discomfort, joint pain, cramps, diarrhoea, low appetite, weight loss, and nausea (Eisenstein, 2015; Storr et al., 2014).

Treatment of Bowl diseases: Consuming cannabis oil can heal intestinal inflammation in addition to improving digestion. Numerous studies have shown a direct relationship between cannabis oil use and a reduction in inflammation and inflammatory symptoms, including ulcerative colitis and Crohn's disease. THC and CBD, two of the compounds in cannabis oil, interact with cells to strengthen the body's immune system and digestive system. The body creates substances that make the gut wall more susceptible to infections. These toxic substances can be blocked by the cannabinoids in cannabis, which in turn strengthens the intestinal wall. In doing so, it can lessen the likelihood of infections in the gastrointestinal tract.

Alzheimer's Disease

Alzheimer's is one of the brain's most emotionally taxing degenerative diseases. Lack of awareness of one's surroundings and a reversion to one's previous state are some of its symptoms. According to studies, cannabis oil may help this disease progress more slowly.

THC, a cannabis oil component, again decreases the development of amyloid plaque. By preventing the enzyme that produces this plaque, it accomplishes this. Brain cell death caused by amyloid plaque eventually results in Alzheimer's disease. Cannabis oil is undoubtedly useful in maintaining a healthy brain cell count for a longer period of time, despite the fact that there is no known solution for this ailment. Indoor grown, very powerful hemp has a staggering 68 components, of which only 57 could be identified after examination. One and the same, monoterpenes, limonene and myrcene, made up 16% of those that were detected. At a staggering 92%, monoterpenes predominated the chemical composition of cannabis oil. Sesquiterpenes made up 7% of the oil, whereas other substances like esters and ketones made up only approximately 1%.

Cannabis oil made from hemp that was grown outdoors had a monoterpene content of between 47.9 and 92.1%.

CONCLUSION

Despite having some societal taboos attached with its use and applications, Cannabis Sativas has found applications in medical industry since time immemorial. With the evolution of time marijuana plant *Cannabis sativa* and its derivatives, cannabinoids, have grown increasingly popular as a potential treatment for various diseases which include ailments of heart, skin, and other vital organs. Products extracted from Cannabis have found their usage in various stages of medical treatment. Various ailments can be cured by the giving the patient required dose of cannabis or hemp oil. Moreover, Cannabis reduces chronic pain, increases lung capacity, helps lose weight and regulates diabetes. Although use of marijuana has been legalized in many countries; its negative impacts do remain a cause of concern for the society despite having some striking medical benefits.

REFERENCES

Agarwal, C., Máthé, K., Hofmann, T., & Csoka, L. (2018). Ultrasound-Assisted Extraction of Cannabinoids from Cannabis Sativa L. Optimized by Response Surface Methodology. *Journal of Food Science, 83*(3), 700–710. doi:10.1111/1750-3841.14075 PMID:29437231

Ainsworth, C. (2000). Boys and girls come out to play: The molecular biology of dioecious plants. *Annals of Botany, 86*(2), 211–221. doi:10.1006/anbo.2000.1201

Ali EM, Almagboul AZ, Khogali SM, et al. (2012) Antimicrobial Activity of Cannabis sativa L. *Chinese Medicine, 1;3*(1), 61.

Andre, C.M.; Hausman, J.F.; Guerriero, G., (2016). Cannabis sativa: The plant of the thousand and one molecules. *Front Plant Sci. 7*, 19.

Audu, B. S., Ofojekwu, P. C., Ujah, A., & Ajima, M. N. O. (2014). M.N.O. Phytochemical, proximate composition, amino acid profile and characterization of Marijuana (Cannabis sativa L.). *J. Phytopharm*, *3*(1), 35–43. doi:10.31254/phyto.2014.3106

Baldino, L., Scognamiglio, M., & Reverchon, E. (2020). Supercritical fluid technologies applied to the extraction of compounds of industrialinterest fromCannabis sativaL. and to their pharmaceutical formulations: A review. *[PDF] [The Medicinal Natural Products of Cannabis sativa Linn.: A Review.*]. *J. Pharm. Fluids.*, *165*, 104960.

Bergamaschi, M. M., Barnes, A., Queiroz, R. H. C., Hurd, Y. L., & Huestis, M. A. (2013). Impact of enzymatic and alkaline hydrolysis on CBD concentration in urine. *Analytical and Bioanalytical Chemistry*, *405*(14), 4679–4689. doi:10.100700216-013-6837-x PMID:23494274

Bitencourt, R. M., & Takahashi, R. N. (2018). Cannabidiol as a therapeutic alternative for post-traumatic stress disorder: From bench research to confirmation in human trials. *Frontiers in neuroscience*, 502.

Blake, A., & Nahtigal, I. (2019). The evolving landscape of cannabis edibles. *Current Opinion in Food Science*, *28*, 25–31. doi:10.1016/j.cofs.2019.03.009

Bowles, D. W., O'Bryant, C. L., Camidge, D. R., & Jimeno, A. (2012). The intersection between cannabis and cancer in the United States. *Critical Reviews in Oncology/Hematology*, *83*(1), 1–10. doi:10.1016/j.critrevonc.2011.09.008 PMID:22019199

Buxton, O. M., Broussard, J. L., Zahl, A. K., & Hall, M. (2014). Impact of Sleep and Sleep Disturbances on Obesity and Cancer, pp. 25–50. Springer; Berlin/Heidelberg, Germany.

Callaway, J., Schwab, U., Harvima, I., Halonen, P., Mykkänen, O., Hyvönen, P., & Järvinen, T. (2005). Efficacy of dietary hempseed oil in patients with atopic dermatitis. *The Journal of Dermatological Treatment*, *16*(2), 87–94. doi:10.1080/09546630510035832 PMID:16019622

Chemat, F., Vian, M. A., & Cravotto, G. (2012). Green Extraction of Natural Products: Concept and Principles. *International Journal of Molecular Sciences*, *13*(7), 8615–8627. doi:10.3390/ijms13078615 PMID:22942724

Clarke, R. C., & Merlin, M. D. (2015). Letter to the editor: Small, Ernest. 2015. Evolution and Classification of Cannabis sativa (Marijuana, Hemp) in relation to human utilization. Botanical Review 81(3), 189-294.

De Petrocellis, L., Ligresti, A., Moriello, A. S., Allarà, M., Bisogno, T., Petrosino, S., Stott, C. G., & Di Marzo, V. (2011). Effects of cannabinoids and cannabinoid-enriched Cannabis extracts on TRP channels and endocannabinoid metabolic enzymes. *British Journal of Pharmacology*, *163*(7), 1479–1494. doi:10.1111/j.1476-5381.2010.01166.x PMID:21175579

Eisenstein, M. (2015). Medical marijuana: Showdown at the cannabis corral. *Nature*, *525*(7570), S15–S17. doi:10.1038/525S15a PMID:26398734

Elsohly, M. A., Radwan, M. M., Gul, W., Chandra, S., & Galal, A. (2017). Phytochemistry of Cannabis sativa L. *Phytocannabinoids*, *103*, 1–36. doi:10.1007/978-3-319-45541-9_1 PMID:28120229

Farinon, B., Molinari, R., Costantini, L., & Merendino, N. (2020). The seed of industrial hemp (Cannabis sativa L.): Nutritional quality and potential functionality for human health and nutrition. *Nutrients, 12*(7), 1935. doi:10.3390/nu12071935 PMID:32610691

Faux, A. M., Draye, X., Lambert, R., Andrimont, R., Raulier, P., & Bertin, P. (2013). The relationship of stem and seed yields to flowering phenology and sex expression in monoecious hemp (*Cannabis sativa* L.). *European Journal of Agronomy, 47*, 11–22. doi:10.1016/j.eja.2013.01.006

Flygare, J., & Sander, B. (2008). The endocannabinoid system in cancer—Potential therapeutic target? *Seminars in Cancer Biology, 3*(3), 176–189. doi:10.1016/j.semcancer.2007.12.008 PMID:18249558

Hawthorne, S. B., Yang, Y., & Miller, D. J. (1994). Extraction of Organic Pollutants from Environmental Solids with Sub- and Supercritical Water. *Analytical Chemistry, 66*(18), 2912–2920. doi:10.1021/ac00090a019

Hoch, E., Niemann, D., von Keller, R., Schneider, M., Friemel, C. M., Preuss, U. W., Hasan, A., & Pogarell, O. (2019). How effective and safe is medical cannabis as a treatment of mental disorders? A systematic review. *European Archives of Psychiatry and Clinical Neuroscience, 269*(1), 87–105. doi:10.100700406-019-00984-4 PMID:30706168

Jin, D., Dai, K., Xie, Z., & Chen, J. (2020). Secondary metabolites profiled in cannabis inflorescences, leaves, stem barks, and roots formedicinal purposes. *Scientific Reports, 10*, 1–14.

Lewis, M. M., Yang, Y., Wasilewski, E., Clarke, H. A., & Kotra, L. P. (2017). Chemical profiling of medical Cannabis extracts. *ACS Omega, 2*(9), 6091–6103. doi:10.1021/acsomega.7b00996 PMID:30023762

Liu Y., Wheaton A.G., Chapman D.P., Cunningham T.J., Lu H., Croft J.B., (2014). Prevalence of healthy sleep duration among adults—United States. *Morb. Mortal. Wkly.*

Marcu, J. P., Christian, R. T., Lau, D., Zielinski, A. J., Horowitz, M. P., Lee, J., Pakdel, A., Allison, J., Limbad, C., Moore, D. H., Yount, G. L., Desprez, P.-Y., & McAllister, S. D. (2010). Cannabidiol enhances the inhibitory effects of Δ9-tetrahydrocannabinol on human glioblastoma cell proliferation and survival. *Molecular Cancer Therapeutics, 9*(1), 180–189. doi:10.1158/1535-7163.MCT-09-0407 PMID:20053780

Murawski, B., Wade, L., Plotnikoff, R. C., Lubans, D. R., & Duncan, M. J. (2018). A systematic review and meta-analysis of cognitive and behavioral interventions to improve sleep health in adults without sleep disorders. *Sleep Medicine Reviews, 40*, 160–169. doi:10.1016/j.smrv.2017.12.003 PMID:29397329

Pellati, F., Borgonetti, V., Brighenti, V., Biagi, M., Benvenuti, S., & Corsi, L. (2018). Cannabis sativa L. and nonpsychoactive cannabinoids: Their chemistry and role against oxidative stress, inflammation, and cancer. *BioMed Research International, 1691428*, 1–15. doi:10.1155/2018/1691428 PMID:30627539

Pellati, F., Brighenti, V., Sperlea, J., Marchetti, L., Bertelli, D., & Benvenuti, S. (2018). New Methods for the Comprehensive Analysis of Bioactive Compounds in Cannabis sativa L. (hemp). *Molecules (Basel, Switzerland), 23*(10), 2639. doi:10.3390/molecules23102639 PMID:30322208

Plaza, M., & Turner, C. (2015). Pressurized hot water extraction of bioactives. *TrAC* [CrossRef] [Google Scholar]. *Trends in Analytical Chemistry, 71*, 39–54. doi:10.1016/j.trac.2015.02.022

Rajaei, A., Barzegar, M., & Yamini, Y. (2004). Supercritical fluid extraction of tea seed oil and its comparison with solvent extraction. *European Food Research and Technology*, *220*(3-4), 401–405. doi:10.100700217-004-1061-8

Sheng, W. S., Chauhan, P., Hu, S., Prasad, S., & Lokensgard, J. R. (2019). Antiallodynic effects of cannabinoid receptor 2 (CB2R) agonists on retrovirus infection-induced neuropathic pain. *Pain Research and Management*.

Sirikantaramas, S., Taura, F., Tanaka, Y., Ishikawa, Y., Morimoto, S., & Shoyama, Y. (2005). Tetrahydrocannabinolic acid synthase, the enzyme controlling marijuana psychoactivity, is secreted into the storage cavity of the glandular trichomes. *Plant & Cell Physiology*, *46*(9), 1578–1582. doi:10.1093/pcp/pci166 PMID:16024552

Small, E., Pocock, T., & Cavers, P. B. (2003). The biology of Canadian weeds. 119. *Cannabis sativa* L. *Canadian Journal of Plant Science*, *83*(1), 217–237. doi:10.4141/P02-021

Storr, M., Devlin, S., Kaplan, G. G., Panaccione, R., & Andrews, C. N. (2014). Cannabis use provides symptom relief in patients with inflammatory bowel disease but is associated with worse disease prognosis in patients with Crohn's disease. *Inflammatory Bowel Diseases*, *20*(3), 472–480. doi:10.1097/01.MIB.0000440982.79036.d6 PMID:24407485

Wasim, K., Haq, I. U., & Ashraf, M. (1995). Antimicrobial Studies of the Leaf of Cannabis sativa L. *Pakistan Journal of Pharmaceutical Sciences*, *8*, 22–38. PMID:16414764

Whiting, P. F., Wolff, R. F., Deshpande, S., Di Nisio, M., Duffy, S., Hernandez, A. V., Keurentjes, J. C., Lang, S., Misso, K., Ryder, S., Schmidlkofer, S., Westwood, M., & Kleijnen, J. (2015). Cannabinoids for medical use: A systematic review and meta-analysis. *Journal of the American Medical Association*, *313*(24), 2456–2473. doi:10.1001/jama.2015.6358 PMID:26103030

Xu, X., Liu, Y., Huang, S., Liu, G., Xie, C., Zhou, J., Fan, W., Li, Q., Wang, Q., Zhong, D., & Miao, X. (2006). Overexpression of cannabinoid receptors CB1 and CB2 correlates with improved prognosis of patients with hepatocellular carcinoma. *Cancer Genetics and Cytogenetics*, *171*(1), 31–38. doi:10.1016/j.cancergencyto.2006.06.014 PMID:17074588

Chapter 5
Cannabis sativa:
A Versatile Herb - An Overview on Pharmaceutical and Cosmetic Applications

Priyanka Joshi Jain
Principal K.M. Kundnani College of Pharmacy, University of Mumbai, India

Nikhil Prem Rajnani
Principal K.M. Kundnani College of Pharmacy, University of Mumbai, India

Nalini Satish Kurup
Principal K.M. Kundnani College of Pharmacy, University of Mumbai, India

ABSTRACT

Cannabis sativa (Hemp) is an herbaceous species used in foods and beverages, cosmetics, pharmaceuticals, nutraceuticals, etc. It has two active constituents: Tetrahydrocannabinol and Cannabidiol. Cannabinoids suppress uncontrolled growth of cancerous cells, provide pain relief to HIV patients, and help with neurogenic symptoms. Cannabis extracts have exhibited more effectiveness against various bacteria and yeast. Improvement in skin hydration and skin elasticity was observed. Excessive sebum production and proliferation of sebocytes is normalized. Hemp extracts arrest the anagen phase of the hair cycle to cause reversal of the temporal and vertex thinning in Androgenetic alopecia. It has antioxidant potential as well as an anti-ageing effect. Owing to the variability in legislation in different countries, Cannabis sativa poses challenges in research. This chapter discusses the diverse applications of this double-edged herb.

INTRODUCTION

Cannabis, sometimes known as pot, marijuana, weed, or ganja, is the world's most popular illicit recreational drug (Thomas et al., 2014) (Wolff & Jouanjus, 2017). It was initially cultivated in Central Asia, but progressively spread around the world (Singh et al., 2018). Cannabis is typically obtained from one of three cannabis plant strains: *Cannabis sativa*, *Cannabis indica*, or *Cannabis ruderalis*, each of which

DOI: 10.4018/978-1-6684-5718-4.ch005

differs in the composition and quantity of the active chemicals tetrahydrocannabinol (THC) and cannabidiol (CBD) (Singh et al., 2018) (Matsuda et al., 1990) (Figure1).

The THC level is what distinguishes hemp from cannabis. Hemp is merely a term for a plant with lower THC contents (0.3 percent or THC content is lower by dry weight) and greater cannabidiol concentrations (CBD) (Booth et al., 2017).

Thus, the basic materials obtained from the plant are (Peschel, 2016) (Sandle, 2020):

1) Cannabis from the dried flowers of the Cannabis plant, which have medical properties.
2) Hemp fibers derived from the stem are used for making paper, clothes, rope, furnishing fabric and building materials.
3) Cannabis oils are extracted from the plant's flowers. This is used to create high amounts of non-intoxicating and medicinally valuable cannabidiol (CBD).
4) Omega fatty acids are found in hemp seed oil.

Aside from natural sources, the usage of synthetic cannabis (SC), sometimes known as spice, K2 or Kronic, has been more popular over the past decade (Wolff & Jouanjus, 2017).

The use of therapeutic cannabis comes with hazards, which include reduced appetite, dizziness, diarrhea, fatigue, nausea, extreme weakness, hallucinations, mood swings or a shift in conduct, suicidal ideation etc.

Such negative effects do not apply to medicinal cannabis products, which have drug-specific side effects that are detailed in the product information insert. In addition to adverse effects, the mechanisms of action remain unknown (Sandle, 2020).

Cannabis in the form of resins, tinctures, and extracts, has been recognized as a medication in the Pharmacopoeia of the United States (US) since 1851 (Robinson & Adinoff, 2016) (Zuardi, 2006). As per recent legislative developments in the United States and European Union (EU), medicinal cannabis usage is legal in Canada. Scientific studies on the advantages of medicinal cannabis are progressing and there is a surge of interest in cannabinoid (CB) therapy (Bifulco & Pisanti, 2015) (Ko et al., 2016).

This chapter discusses the diverse applications of this double-edged herb with more emphasis on pharmaceutical and cosmetics industry as well as current approved medicinal products to treat various diseases.

Figure 1. Phytocannabinoids (Chemical structures drawn from the ACD/ChemSketch (Freeware)

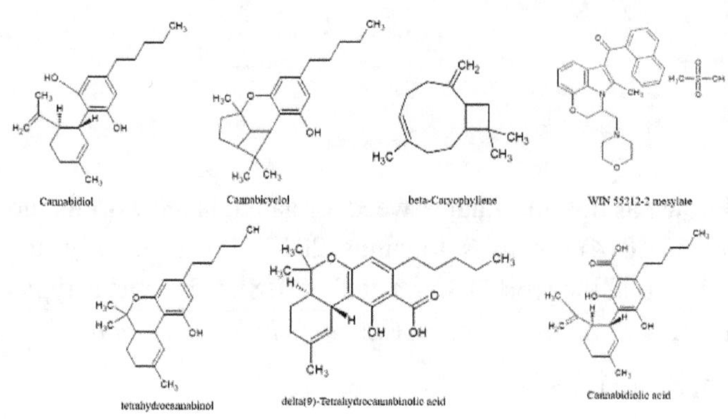

MEDICINAL AND COSMETIC USES

Cancer

In recent years, cannabinoids have been widely studied for their anticancer effects and symptoms in cancer patients (Birdsall et al., 2016) (Davis, 2016) (NCI, 2015). The initial studies demonstrating the anticancer effects of cannabis was published in 1975 (Munson et al., 1975). Current research is focusing on the anticancer action of plant-derived (phytocannabinoids) such as (-)-trans-9-tetrahydrocannabinol (THC), 8-THC, cannabidiol (CBD), cannabinol (CBN), cannabicyclol (CBL), and WIN-55,212-2 (synthetic cannabinoids) (Figure 2) (Birdsall et al., 2016) (Davis, 2016) (Müller et al., 2017). In the 1990s, the endocannabinoid system (ECS) components were discovered as follows: (i) CB1 and CB2 receptors; (ii) two main endogenous ligands also known as endocannabinoids in anandamide / N-arachidonoyl ethanolamine (AEA), mammals, and 2-arachidonoylglycerol (2-AG); and (iii) fatty acid amide hydrolase (FAAH), monoacylglycerol lipase (MAG lipase), and metabolic enzymes of endocannabinoids (Guindon & Hohmann, 2009) (Nadolska & Goś, 2008) (Fogli & Breschi, 2008).

Figure 2. Cannabis phytoconstituents with their therapeutic activity (molecular structures drawn from the ACD/ChemSketch (Freeware)

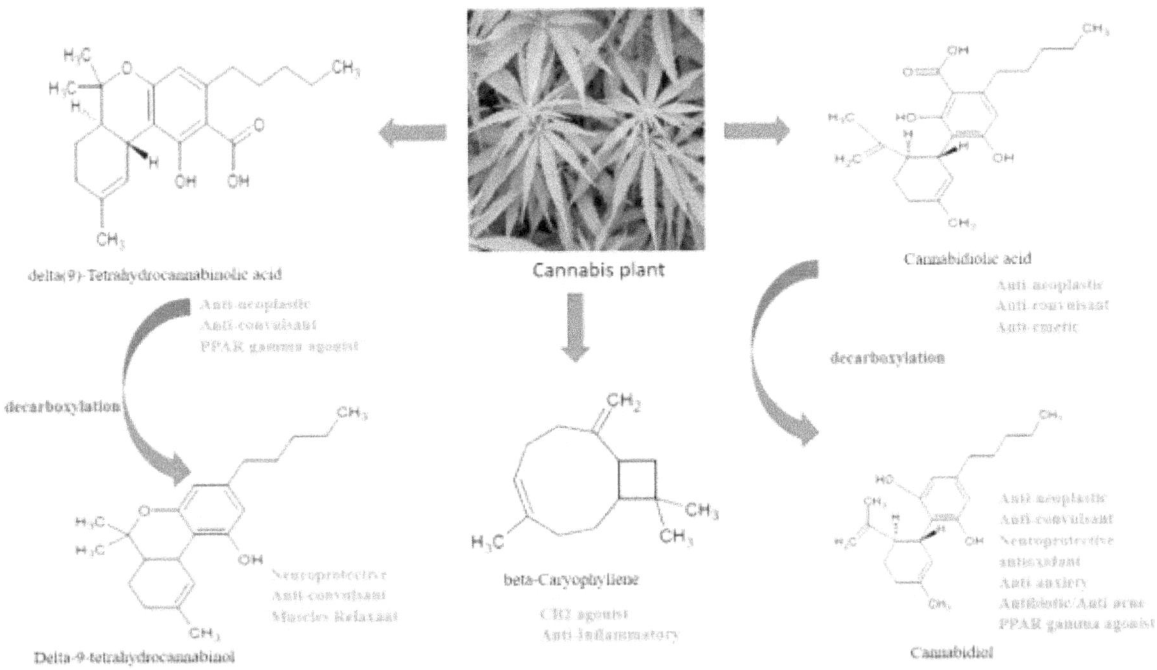

The Endocannabinoid System's Function in Cancer

Endocannabinoids work along with various receptors, including the Gi/o coupled CB1 and CB2 receptors. CB2 receptors are typically present on the immunological cells' surface, whereas CB1 receptors are mostly found in the CNS and, also in some peripheral organs to a lesser extent (Fogli & Breschi, 2008) (Console-Bram et al., 2012). The molecular significance of the ECS in cancer pathophysiology remains unclear, but most studies imply that endogenous ligands for CB receptors are increased in tumor tissue, and overexpression of ligands, receptors, and enzymes which are ECS components is associated with tumor aggressiveness. In cancer cell lines and clinical malignancies, an excess of endocannabinoid-degrading enzymes, have demonstrated that ECS possesses tumor-suppressing properties (Figure 3) (Pérez-Gómez et al., 2015) (Caffarel et al., 2010) (Vercelli et al., 2014) (Chung et al., 2009).

Figure 3. Cannabinoid (CB) receptor expression in a variety of human cancers

Cancer Cell type	Regulation of CB1, CB2	Mechanism and other relevant circumstances
Breast cancer	CB2 receptor expression is increased in HER2-positive breast cancers.	CB2 expression is induced by HER2, which activates ELK1 (MAPK/ERK cascade) and activates pro-oncogenic signaling via the tyrosine kinase c-Src.
	TRPV1 was found in a human breast cancer cell line (MCF-7)	Agonists and antagonists of TRPV1 reduce MCF-7 cell proliferation significantly.
	CB1 receptor expression has increased.	Akt signaling pathway activation has been postulated. CB1 and FAAH levels that are elevated are linked to illness severity.
Prostate cancer	CB1 and CB2 receptors expression is considerably greater in human prostate cancer.	GPR55 has been found to mediate the effects of LPI in DU-145 cell lines and PC-3.
Chemically induced hepatocellular carcinoma	CB1 receptor upregulation	Diethyl nitrosamine was shown to cause liver cancer.
Hepatocellular carcinoma	CB1 and CB2 receptors are overexpressed.	CB1 and CB2 receptor overexpression has been linked to a more favourable outlook (prognosis)
Lung cancer (non-small cell)		MMP9 expression and activity, and Akt signaling pathway activation
Lymphocytic leukemia		The expression of the CB1 receptor was linked to high-risk factors.
Pancreatic cancer	Normal and pancreatic cancer cells express B1 and CB2 receptors (with CB1 expression being greater).	Apoptosis was activated by cannabinoids via the CB2 receptor (ceramide-dependent pathway).

HER2: Human epidermal growth factor receptor 2; c-Src: Tyrosine-protein kinase Src; ELK1: ETS domain-containing protein; TRPV1: Transient receptor potential vanilloid receptor 1, MAPK: Mitogen-activated protein kinase; B; TRPA1: Transient receptor potential ankyrin 1; AR: Androgen receptor; MMP9: Matrix metallopeptidase 9, ERK: Extracellular-signal-regulated kinase, LPI: Lysophosphatidylinositol, Akt: Protein Kinase; and GPR55: Orphan G-protein coupled receptor 55

Cannabinoids influence numerous cellular processes and signaling pathways that are important for tumor growth by concentrating on the ECS. For instance, cause cell cycle halting, increase apoptosis, and reduce the angiogenesis, proliferation, and migration of tumor cells. (Demuth & Molleman, 2006) (Velasco et al., 2016). Cannabis effects appear to be unaffected by CB receptor (e.g., via nicotinic acetylcholine receptor [nAChR] or transient receptor potential V receptor [TRPV1] or 5-hydroxytryptamine [5-HT] among others) in addition to CB1 and CB2 G protein-coupled orphan receptor (Velasco et al., 2016).

HIV

HIV Infection is caused by a virus. It targets the immune system of the body, causing harm to the central nervous system and altering the function of nerve cells (neurons). This can cause inflammation in the spinal cord and brain, as well as impact peripheral sensory nerves (Caffarel et al., 2012). Neuropathic pain is a significant and persistent clinical condition in HIV patients, affecting 30 percent or more of those infected. Despite the fact that antiretroviral (ARV) combination medication has increased HIV immunity and survival, it has had no effect on neuropathic pain. Some HIV reverse transcriptase inhibitors that are nucleoside analogues, include stavudine and didanosine, may play a role in the incidence of painful distal sensory polyneuropathy (DSPN), presumably due to mitochondrial toxicity (Jarai, 2022).

Further research into the potential benefits of cannabis (marijuana) as a medical treatment for a range of illnesses, including neuropathic pain related to HIV DSPN, was recommended by the United States Institute of Medicine in 1999. Tetrahydrocannabinol (THC), the most prevalent element in cannabis, and its synthetic counterparts generate excellent analgesia in the majority of animal pain models (Jarai, 2022) (Ellis et al., 2009) (Watson et al., 2000) (Mao et al., 2000).

THC's antinociceptive properties are mediated by CB1 and CB2 receptors in the central and peripheral nervous systems, which interact with the noradrenergic and k-opioid systems in the spinal cord to block pain perception. Anandamide, CB1's endogenous ligand, is an antinociceptive agent by itself. Medical marijuana has demonstrated tentative benefit towards alleviating neuropathic pain in open-label medical research and one recent controlled experiment (Jarai, 2022) (Martin & Lichtman, 1998) (Calignano et al., 1998).

Benefits of Medicinal Marijuana in HIV

It reduces neuropathic pain: As a result of the infection and certain medications used to treat it, peripheral neuropathic pain is frequent in HIV patients. According to one study, breathing cannabis strains with three times every day for five days with a minimum THC content of 9.4% can help relieve discomfort (Morgan, 2022).

It reduces anxiety: When medical marijuana is used to combat HIV, it produces a 'good drug impact,' which promotes feelings of pleasure as well as confidence while lowering the anxiety and tension that HIV patients experience. Furthermore, the euphoric impact of medicinal marijuana is highly useful in mitigating anxiety and despair linked with HIV/AIDS.

Chronic pain relief: Chronic pain may be relieved with the use of a cannabis strain containing 12.5% THC, which is frequent among HIV patients. A doctor may prescribe medicinal marijuana in the floral, edibles, or concentrates form.

It reduces nausea: As the condition advances, nausea becomes more complicated and noticeable. Using cannabis in conjunction with antiretroviral medication reduces the medicines' negative effects.

It improves appetite: In HIV/AIDS patients, appetite loss and weight loss are prevalent. By improving appetite, medical cannabis works towards reducing weight loss and assists in the treatment of viral symptoms.

NEUROLOGICAL DISORDERS

Cannabidiol has alleged anxiolytic, antipsychotic, and anti-craving properties, with actions that are most certainly tied to the endocannabinoid system, however its exact mode of action is unknown (Abrams et al., 2007) (Batalla et al., 2019). Various receptor types, such as serotonin type 1A (5HT1A), vanilloid receptor 1 (TRPV1), peroxisome proliferator-activated receptor gamma (PPARgamma), GPR55, and GPR18, have also been suggested as molecular targets. CBD has also been observed to increase plasma levels of the cannabinoid anandamide, whose antipsychotic effects have been associated with it (Rohleder et al., 2016) (Jones et al., 2010). It is possible that persons with movement problems, epilepsy, or Alzheimer's disease benefit minimally from marijuana, but it is also possible that very few people with these diseases have tried it (Gururajan & Malone, 2016) (Mack & Joy, 2000).

9-THC is the most researched phytocannabinoid, but it is also the most psychoactive component of Cannabis, severely restricting its medicinal potential as a single agent. As a result, current research has concentrated on non-psychotropic substances, some of which have shown promise as therapeutic agents in preclinical models of CNS disorders (Giacoppo et al., 2014).

Figure 4 gives the overall idea of mode of action and signaling pathway of cannabinoids in the neurological diseases.

Figure 4. Neurological illness and cannabinoid-induced cellular signaling (Giacoppo et al., 2014)

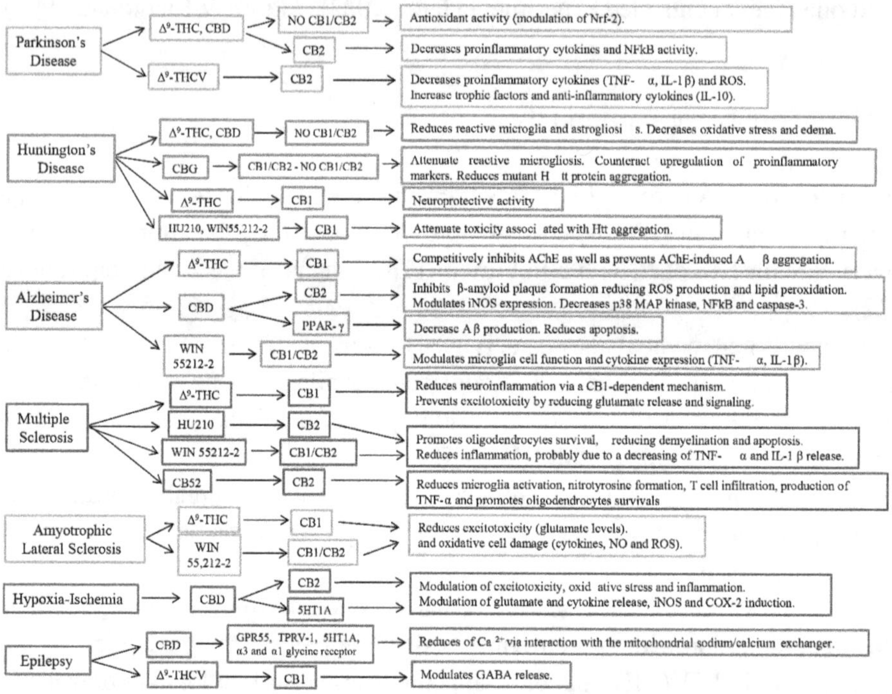

CANNABIS AND INSOMNIA

Cannabis has been used to help people fall asleep for millennia. However, it is only in the last few years that anecdotal evidence has attracted scholarly interest. A growing number of clinical trials exploring the usefulness of cannabis to treat sleep disorders are being done in various nations today. Researchers from the Centre for Sleep Science at the University of Western Australia tested a cannabis-based extract on 23 people with chronic insomnia. Over the course of 14 nights, they were given either the formulation or a placebo. According to the Insomnia Severity Index (ISI), 36 percent of high dose recipients had a significant increase in sleep quality. (Australian Access Clinic, 2021).

CB1 receptors in the body govern sleep patterns biologically. Despite CBD's widespread popularity for its numerous health advantages, research suggests that the THC component of cannabis is what causes sleepiness. THC has an impact on CB1 receptors, which regulate pain alleviation and sleep. A little research suggests that CBD is insufficient to treat insomnia. On the other side, THC-rich strains are understood to promote greater sleep and reduce REM. (rapid eye moment) sleep (which reduces time spent dreaming) (Australian Access Clinic, 2021).

CANNABIS AND DIABETES MELLITUS

According to the American Alliance for Medical Cannabis (AAMC), (Diabetes.co.uk, 2019) cannabis can assist with:

a. Stabilizing blood sugar levels; a growing amount of anecdotal data among diabetics supports this.
b. Reducing part of the arterial inflammation that diabetics typically suffer which could result in cardiovascular disease.
c. Stimulating body and brain receptors that prevent nerve inflammation and relieving the discomfort of neuropathy, the most frequent consequence of diabetes.
d. Over time, lowering blood pressure, thus, helping to minimize heart disease risk and other potential diabetic complications.
e. Improving circulation by keeping blood vessels open.
f. Relieving muscle cramps and gastrointestinal (GI) discomfort.
g. Treating neuropathic pain and tingling in the hands and feet via topical creams.
h. Enhancing metabolism and blood glucose levels along with enhancement in insulin production in human and animal models of diabetes by using tetrahydrocannabivarin (THCV) and CBD according to 2016 research, indicating a “new therapeutic agent for glycemic management.”

CBD therapy decreased inflammation in animal models of diabetes, according to 2017 research from the Medical College of Georgia, which concluded that “the nonpsychotropic CBD is a viable option for anti-inflammatory and neuroprotective therapies.”

ANTIMICROBIAL ACTIVITY

Microorganisms have developed resistance to several antimicrobial agents demanding the need for combination therapies with two or more drugs. Also, the need for newer antimicrobial substances has risen. Cannabis sativa has been investigated as a novel antimicrobial agent. Aqueous, ethanolic and ether extracts of the whole plant have been used to determine their efficacy as also the essential oils and cannabinoids of Cannabis using *in vitro* methods. In conclusion, Cannabis is more effective against Gram positive bacteria as compared to gram negative bacteria. Cannabinoids are capable of inhibiting yeast and multi drug resistant bacteria. Synergistic effects can be achieved if Cannabis extracts are combined with conventional antimicrobial agents (Schofs et al., 2021).

Lorenzo Nissen et al have studied the antimicrobial effects of three different varieties of Cannabis viz. the Italian Carmagnola and Firanova and the French Futura. Gram positive and gram negative bacteria along with some yeast having the ability to cause food spoilage were used in order to test the efficacy of essential oils isolated from these species. These pathogens can cause food poisoning and intestinal syndromes. Amongst the gram positive species that were evaluated were Clostridium, Enterococcus and

Streptococcus while the gram negative ones were Pectobacterium and Pseudomonas species (Nissen et al., 2010).

Johannes Novak et al performed a thin layer chromatographic analysis of the essential oils present in Cannabis from different cultivars. The antimicrobial potential was evaluated on 21 different microbes. A few susceptible ones were *Acinetobacter calcoaceticus, Aeromonas hydrophyla, Bacillus subtilis, Beneckea natriegens, Brevibacterium linens, Brochothrix thermosphacta, Escherichia coli, Flavobacterium suaveolens, Micrococcus luteus, Staphylococcus aureus, Yersinia enterocolitica* (Novak et al., 2001).

Megan Lim and Mark Kirchhoff conducted a survey of data reported by dispensary websites in order to summarize the medicinal and cosmetic applications of cannabis. Dispensaries in Canada, United States and European countries have been included for the same. It can be concluded that although several uses of cannabis have been advertised, most of them are in preliminary testing stages and not approved by medical professionals. Patients have been relying on blogs or the verdict of other patients or salespersons who are not medical professionals (Lim & Kirchhof, 2019).

SKIN DISEASES: PSORIASIS AND PRURITIS

Psoriasis is a chronic inflammatory disorder which was thought to be associated with over activation of T1 helper cells. However, it has been recently discovered that T17 helper cells produce cytokines such as various interleukins which induce keratinocyte proliferation and produce Tumour necrosis factor α in large amounts. TNF-α causes inflammatory cells to migrate from the blood into the skin. This results in inflammation of the skin (Ogawa et al., 2018).

Patients with psoriasis have keratinocytes with oxidative stress and high levels of reactive oxygen species. When such cells are exposed to UV irradiation, this stress is intensified. Treatment with Cannabidiol (CBD) decreases oxidative damage by concentration in the membranes of keratinocytes. It also increases the amount of palmitoylethanolamine, thereby decreasing inflammation. Thus, CBD can help patients with psoriasis especially with UV exposed skin (Jarocka-Karpowicz et al., 2020).

In dermatology patients a common widespread condition is pruritus (itchy skin). Pruritus that lasts longer than six weeks is known as chronic pruritus, and it can be as severe as chronic pain. Currently available therapy are combination of menthol, emollients, topical anaesthetics, glucocorticoids (oral and topical), oral antihistamines, and neuroactive medicines; however, none of these can guarantee constant or complete success. Cannabinoids influence the endogenous endocannabinoid system (ECS) and have showed good activity in the clinical literature for the treatment of itch, which includes clinical research in a variety of conditions, including the management of refractory pruritus.

The central and peripheral actions of the drug are analgesic and antipruritic. CB1 receptors are primarily responsible for analgesic and antipruritic actions in the central nervous system, which is consistent with them being the primary centrally active cannabinoid receptor. TRP ion channels are a family of membrane proteins that conduct sensory responses like nociception and itch in the skin and nervous system. Six TRP channels from three subfamilies are found to interact with endogenous and exogenous cannabinoid receptors, including TRP vanilloid (TRPV1, TRPV2, TRPV3, TRPV4), TRP ankyrin (TRPA1), and TRP melastatin (TRPM1).

Palmitoylethanolamine (PEA), a ligand for TRPV1 channels that has no connection with CB1 and CB2, has been employed for the treatment of pruritus in many of the clinical trials (Avila et al., 2020).

The basal cell layer of the skin is known to rejuvenate every 28 days. In doing so, the older cells get pushed to the surface while the most superficial ones get sloughed off. Cannabinoids have the potential to improve the multiplication and life cycle of these basal cells. This could be associated with their role in anti-ageing and skin repair (Sheriff et al., 2020).

Ligeza et al surveyed 23 healthy volunteers of median 39 years of age for the irritant potential and allergic reaction of hemp oil. A small amount of the oil was applied over blotting paper which was in turn placed on the skin and covered by an occlusive patch. 48 hours later, the irritant potential was evaluated by examining the skin. It was found to be non-irritant and generated no allergic reactions.

An application study was also performed on 80 healthy volunteers of median 41.5 years of age for a period of three days. Hemp oil was evaluated for its appearance, aroma, absorbability, spread ability and consistency. Majority of the participants rated it to have an appealing appearance, good absorbability, spread ability and consistency. However, most rated it to have an unpleasant aroma (Ligęza et al., 2016).

ANTI-ACNE EFFECT

Acne vulgaris is a condition that affects the human skin wherein the sebaceous glands become hyperactive, proliferation of sebocytes occurs accompanied by inflammation possibly when *Propionibacterium acnes* thrive upon the excess sebum. Risk factors include heredity, onset of puberty, insulin resistance and elevated dehydroepiandrosterone in polycystic ovarian syndrome, certain anti-epileptic drugs, anti-cancer drugs and anabolic steroids. Under the influence of androgens, over production of sebum results and defective keratinocyte differentiation causes comedones. The lipids in the sebum get oxidized resulting in inflammatory responses. The comedones provide an anaerobic, lipid rich environment where *P. acnes* thrive and multiply. Acne causes soreness, pain, itching along with the social inhibition associated with it. Conventional drugs include benzoyl peroxide, retinoids, clindamycin, anti-androgens, tetracyclines, erythromycin, isotretinoin etc (Williams et al., 2012).

Attila Olah et al proved that Cannabidiol has a lipostatic and antiproliferative effect on human sebocytes and also an anti-inflammatory effect; hence can prove beneficial in the treatment of acne vulgaris. CBD has the ability to inhibit lipogenic effects of various substances including testosterone and can lower the amount of sebocytes via activation of the transient receptor potential vanilloid 4 ion channels. The anti-inflammatory action is owing to the inhibition of NF-kB signalling which controls the cytokine production and cell survival (Oláh et al., 2014).

Botanix Pharmaceuticals has published promising results exhibiting the anti-acne effects of Cannabidiol in Phase 2 clinical trials. It proved the safety, dosage, efficacy on inflammatory and non-inflammatory skin lesions as well (*Botanix Pharmaceuticals*, n.d.).

A study by Dobrosi N. et al has proved that endocannabinoids have a role in suppressing overproduction of sebum by sebaceous glands, thus useful for treating acne and seborrhea. A cream containing 3% cannabis seed extract was applied to the cheeks of 11 human volunteers for a period of 12 weeks in order to prove significant decrease in sebum produced and erythema of skin. Cannabidiol is known to inhibit the actions of testosterone in an *in-vitro* study on human sebocytes. It also exerts control over the proliferation of sebocytes. (Dobrosi et al., 2008)

ANDROGENETIC ALOPECIA

Androgenetic alopecia is a condition that commonly affects both men and women. Testosterone is metabolized to dihydrotestosterone (DHT) by the enzyme alpha reductase. DHT is responsible for interfering with the hair growth cycle. Typically, the hair follicle has three stages of growth viz. anagen, catagen and telogen. DHT causes a decrease in the anagen: telogen ratio resulting in increased hair loss. It results in decreased hair density in the temporal as well as ventral areas of the scalp. In women, generally, a diffused pattern of baldness is observed. The most conventional synthetic remedies are topical minoxidil and oral finasteride. They have been used in combination as well for synergistic action. However, the benefits are short term and reversible. The most promising results are observed with hair transplant (Amin & Sachdeva, 2013).

The Endocannabinoid system and its association with the hair follicles has been studied. Of the CB1 and CB2 receptors, the former is expressed in large amounts in the hair follicles. The agonism and antagonism at these receptors exhibit decrease and increase in hair shaft elongation respectively.

Tetrahydrocannabinol (THC), a phytocannabinoid, is known to be a partial agonist at the CB1 receptor and hence can be used to get rid of unwanted hair growth. Cannabidiol (CBD) on the other hand is an antagonist at CB1 and hence has a role in promoting hair growth and elongation. This activity is, however, dose dependent; with lower doses exhibiting antagonistic action on the CB1, while higher doses causing premature entry of the follicle into the catagen or the regression phase via a different receptor called the vanilloid receptor.

Gregory Smith and John Satino have conducted a clinical trial on men (aged 28 onwards) and women (aged 46 onwards) for a span of six months in order to prove the efficacy of cannabidiol in androgenetic alopecia. Cannabidiol was extracted from hemp flowers and the content was analyzed. It was then incorporated into a lanolin-based paste in order to yield a 10.8% CBD containing formulation. A $1cm^2$ area was selected in the temporal as well the vertex area of the scalp in order to analyze the performance of the formulation at regular intervals throughout the six-month study. Significant improvement in the hair growth was observed in both men and women. Men showed better results and the hair growth was better in the vertex area as compared to the temporal. Thus, it can be concluded that this therapy should be considered in combination with the existing older therapies in order to yield promising results (Smith & Satino, 2021).

UV PROTECTIVE EFFECTS

The Ultraviolet radiation (UVR) spectrum comprises of three subdivisions viz. UVC (200 to 290nm), UVB (290 to 320nm) and UVA (320 to 400nm). This classification was developed by W.W. Coblentz for the U.S. National Bureau of Standards in the 1930s with the aid of various filters made of barium, pyrex and flint. The ozone layer has the ability to absorb 100% of UVC while the ratio of UVB: UVA that reaches the earth is about 20:1 due to the increasing levels of ozone depletion. The effects of UVR on the body include prolonged pigmentation, sunburn, skin ageing, immunosuppression, precancerous lesions etc. UVA has a negative impact on the number of Langerhans cells while simultaneously increasing the number of inflammatory cells in the dermis. UVB on the other hand is responsible for causing sunburns and also mutations in the DNA linked with skin cancers.

The efficiency of sunscreens can be measured by the sun protection factor (SPF) which can be calculated as follows (Palm & O'Donoghue, 2007):

SPF = Minimal erythema dose (sunscreen protected skin) Minimal erythema dose (unprotected skin)

Photoprotection by the use of sunscreens or sunblock involves reduction in skin damage induced by sun exposure (primarily UVR) by application of an agent that is capable of absorbing the spectrum of UV light or reflecting off the incident light. Chemical sunscreens, owing to their structure, absorbs UV rays and gets excited to higher energy state, which reverts back to low energy upon release of the longer wavelengths. Some chemical sunscreens include aminobenzoates, cinnamates, salicylates, camphor derivatives, benzophenones, anthranilates etc. Physical sunscreens on the other hand do not have the ability to absorb, so they rely solely on their reflective properties in order to scatter the UV light. Hence, a thick coat is essential for greater effectiveness, however, this compromises upon the cosmetic appeal. Physical sunscreen examples are zinc oxide and titanium dioxide (Gabros et al., 2022).

Pranjal Gohad et al studied the UV protective effects of cannabidiol on human primary melanocytes and keratinocytes using cell lines. Both cell lines were treated with different concentrations of cannabidiol followed by increasing exposure time to UV light. MTT assay was carried out in order to determine the cell viability. The efficacy of cannabidiol at preserving cell viability in melanocytes as well as keratinocytes was found to be dose dependent (Gohad et al., 2021).

Young Sun Hwang et al have proved that the CB1 receptors in skin have a vital role in the binding of Cannabidiol administered topically. Once bound it increases the formation of microphthalmia associated transcription factor thus leading to increased levels of tyrosinase enzyme and melanin (Hwang et al., 2017). The role of Cannabidiol in melanogenesis could prove beneficial in the treatment of vitiligo. Axim Biotechnologies, New York has filed a patent with the European Patent Office for developing a topical formulation containing Cannabidiol and Cannabigerol for the treatment of vitiligo (European Patent Office, 2019).

MOISTURIZING POTENTIAL

Factors which contribute to skin hydration include Natural Moisturizing Factor (NMF), increased expression of collagen and decreased expression of metalloproteinases. Loricrin and Filaggrin genes are responsible for skin hydration which leads to increased skin elasticity and anti-wrinkle effects. Mutation of these genes is known to cause Atopic Dermatitis.

Jae-We Cho et al have proved that oral administration of dandelion extract (*Taraxacum platycarpum*) improves skin hydration in NC/Nga mice. The exact mechanism is not known, but it has exhibited significantly increased levels of filaggrin expression. Histopathological analysis showed decreased infiltration of the epidermal tissue by inflammatory mediators when treated with dandelion extract as compared to untreated skin.

The expression of type I collagen protein and metalloproteinases was evaluated in human skin fibroblast cells. Dandelion extract was successful in stimulating the expression of Type I collagen protein and suppressing the expression of Metalloproteinases which are both indicators of improved skin hydration (Cho et al., 2011).

Aquaporin 3 is a protein present in the basal layer of skin keratinocytes encoded by the AQP3 gene. It enables the transport of water when osmotic gradient is present. Mariko Hara et al have used AQP3 null mice which lack these aquaporin 3 channels required for water transport and compared them with wild-type mice. Both species were injected with tritiated water (^3H_2O) intraperitoneally and the stratum corneum was then collected by tape stripping method and incubated in phosphate buffer saline. The radioactivity was measured quantitatively using liquid scintillation spectrometry. It was concluded that AQP3 null mice had reduced water content in their stratum corneum thus confirming the correlation of the Aquaporin protein with water transport (Hara et al., 2002).

Nobutomo Ikarashi et al used HR-1 hairless mice, in order to evaluate the effect of cannabidiol on the skin hydration, transepidermal water loss (TEWL) and the aquaporin 3 levels. The control group was treated with aqueous solution containing propylene glycol and dimethyl sulfoxide, while the test group with aqueous solution containing 1% cannabidiol. The dermal water content was found to be significantly higher in the CBD treated group when measured using a Corneometer, while the TEWL in the CBD treated group was comparable to that of the control when measured using a Tewameter. This proves the improvement in skin hydration and normal barrier function by CBD. Comprehensive analysis of the skin samples using RT-PCR showed significant increase in the expression of Aquaporin 3 protein only amongst other aquaporins (Ikarashi et al., 2021).

Cannabidiol, as well as Cannabis and Cannabis-Derived Products Approved by the FDA

1. Epidiolex, a refined version of the medicinal ingredient cannabidiol (CBD), has been authorized by the FDA for the treatment of seizures associated with Lennox-Gastaut syndrome or Dravet syndrome in kids aged 2 and above. In 2020, FDA also approved Epidiolex to treat tuberous sclerosis complex (FDA Office, 2020). That implies the FDA has determined that it is safe and effective for its intended purpose.
2. In the United States, Marinol and Syndros have been licensed for therapeutic applications, including the treatment of cancer chemotherapy associated nausea and weight loss caused by anorexia in AIDS patients. Their active ingredient dronabinol, is a synthetic delta-9-tetrahydrocannabinol (THC), which is thought to be the psychoactive intoxication component of cannabis (i.e., the component that causes people to get "high" when they use it).
3. Another FDA-approved medicine, Cesamet which has nabilone as the active component is manufactured synthetically and has a molecular structure similar to THC. Like other dronabinol-based medicines Cesamet is used to treat nausea caused by cancer treatment.

Cannabis in Covid-19 Treatment

Small-molecule therapeutic medicines are needed to cure or prevent infections caused by the severe acute respiratory syndrome coronavirus-2 (SARS-CoV-2) and its variations, which cause COVID-19, in addition to vaccinations (van Breeman et al., 2022) (Anil et al., 2021). Botanical ligands to the SARS-CoV-2 spike protein were discovered using affinity selection-mass spectrometry. The anti-inflammatory qualities of C. *sativa* have long been known. COVID-19 causes lung inflammation, which is a serious problem. As a result, the decrease of pulmonary inflammation in mice has been investigated. Cannabinoid isolates like CBD and THC were investigated in humans long before the worldwide pandemic arose as a result of the spread of the severe acute respiratory syndrome coronavirus type 2 (SARS-CoV2) infection. Hemp (Cannabis sativa), Cannabinoid acids were discovered to be allosteric and orthosteric ligands with micromolar affinity for the spike protein. Cannabigerolic acid and cannabidiolic acid blocked infection of human epithelial cells by a pseudovirus producing the SARS-CoV-2 spike protein, as well as the entrance of live SARS-CoV-2 into cells, in follow-up virus neutralization experiments. Cannabigerolic acid and cannabidiolic acid were equally effective against the SARS-CoV-2 alpha variant B.1.1.7 and beta variant B.1.351, which is significant. These cannabinoids, individually or in hemp extracts, are orally accessible and have a long history of safe human usage. They have the potential to prevent and cure SARS-CoV-2 infection.

CONCLUSION

To summarize, while cannabis medications appear to have significant therapeutic promise (medical as well as cosmetic), there is a need for the creation of defined, consistent, and focused solutions. In several countries, regulatory reasons and policies have limited research on the health consequences of cannabis and cannabinoids, leaving patients and health care providers without the data they need to make judgments about cannabis and cannabinoids usage in local settings. CBD has been identified as a possible prophylactic agent for early-stage SARS-CoV-2 infection, and additional clinical investigations are warranted. In a medical setting, marijuana is similar to any other powerful prescription treatment in that it has potentially deadly side effects, and the choice to use it to treat patients must pass the same balancing test as chemotherapy or azidothymidine (AZT): do the drug's therapeutic advantages exceed its negative consequences?

REFERENCES

Abrams, D. I., Jay, C. A., Shade, S. B., Vizoso, H., Reda, H., Press, S., Kelly, M. E., Rowbotham, M. C., & Petersen, K. L. (2007). Cannabis in painful HIV-associated sensory neuropathy: A randomized placebo-controlled trial. *Neurology, 68*(7), 515–521. doi:10.1212/01.wnl.0000253187.66183.9c PMID:17296917

Amin, S. S., & Sachdeva, S. (2013). Alopecia areata: A review. *Journal of the Saudi Society of Dermatology & Dermatologic Surgery, 17*(2), 37–45. doi:10.1016/j.jssdds.2013.05.004

Anil, S. M., Shalev, N., Vinayaka, A. C., Nadarajan, S., Namdar, D., Belausov, E., Shoval, I., Mani, K. A., Mechrez, G., & Koltai, H. (2021). Cannabis compounds exhibit anti-inflammatory activity in vitro in COVID-19-related inflammation in lung epithelial cells and pro-inflammatory activity in macrophages. *Scientific Reports, 11*(1), 1462. doi:10.103841598-021-81049-2 PMID:33446817

Australian Access Clinic. (2021, August 5). *Medical Cannabis for Insomnia: Everything You Need to Know.* Australian Access Clinics. https://www.auscannabisclinics.com.au/medical-cannabis-insomnia/

Avila, C., Massick, S., Kaffenberger, B. H., Kwatra, S. G., & Bechtel, M. (2020). Cannabinoids for the treatment of chronic pruritus: A review. *Journal of the American Academy of Dermatology, 82*(5), 1205–1212. doi:10.1016/j.jaad.2020.01.036 PMID:31987788

Batalla, A., Janssen, H., Gangadin, S. S., & Bossong, M. G. (2019). The Potential of Cannabidiol as a Treatment for Psychosis and Addiction: Who Benefits Most? A Systematic Review. *Journal of Clinical Medicine, 8*(7), E1058. doi:10.3390/jcm8071058 PMID:31330972

Bifulco, M., & Pisanti, S. (2015). Medicinal use of cannabis in Europe: The fact that more countries legalize the medicinal use of cannabis should not become an argument for unfettered and uncontrolled use. *EMBO Reports*, *16*(2), 130–132. doi:10.15252/embr.201439742 PMID:25576303

Birdsall, S. M., Birdsall, T. C., & Tims, L. A. (2016). The Use of Medical Marijuana in Cancer. *Current Oncology Reports*, *18*(7), 40. doi:10.100711912-016-0530-0 PMID:27215434

Booth, J. K., Page, J. E., & Jörg, B. (2017). Terpene synthases from Cannabis sativa. *PLoS One*, *12*(3), e0173911. doi:10.1371/journal.pone.0173911 PMID:28355238

Botanix Pharmaceuticals. (n.d.). *BTX 1503 Acne Phase 2 Study Results Presentation*. ASX. https://www.asx.com.au/asxpdf/20191023/pdf/449s36d2bz6vfr.pdf

Caffarel, M. M., Andradas, C., Mira, E., Pérez-Gómez, E., Cerutti, C., Moreno-Bueno, G., Flores, J. M., García-Real, I., Palacios, J., Mañes, S., Guzmán, M., & Sánchez, C. (2010). Cannabinoids reduce ErbB2-driven breast cancer progression through Akt inhibition. *Molecular Cancer*, *9*(1), 196. doi:10.1186/1476-4598-9-196 PMID:20649976

Caffarel, M. M., Andradas, C., Pérez-Gómez, E., Guzmán, M., & Sánchez, C. (2012). Cannabinoids: A new hope for breast cancer therapy? *Cancer Treatment Reviews*, *38*(7), 911–918. doi:10.1016/j.ctrv.2012.06.005 PMID:22776349

Calignano, A., La Rana, G., Giuffrida, A., & Piomelli, D. (1998). Control of pain initiation by endogenous cannabinoids. *Nature*, *394*(6690), 277–281. doi:10.1038/28393 PMID:9685157

Chung, S. C., Hammarsten, P., Josefsson, A., Stattin, P., Granfors, T., Egevad, L., Mancini, G., Lutz, B., Bergh, A., & Fowler, C. J. (2009). A high cannabinoid CB(1) receptor immunoreactivity is associated with disease severity and outcome in prostate cancer. *European Journal of Cancer (Oxford, England: 1990)*, *45*(1), 174–182. doi:10.1016/j.ejca.2008.10.010

Console-Bram, L., Marcu, J., & Abood, M. E. (2012). Cannabinoid receptors: Nomenclature and pharmacological principles. *Progress in Neuro-Psychopharmacology & Biological Psychiatry*, *38*(1), 4–15. doi:10.1016/j.pnpbp.2012.02.009 PMID:22421596

Davis, M. P. (2016). Cannabinoids for Symptom Management and Cancer Therapy: The Evidence. *Journal of the National Comprehensive Cancer Network: JNCCN*, *14*(7), 915–922. doi:10.6004/jnccn.2016.0094 PMID:27407130

Demuth, D. G., & Molleman, A. (2006). Cannabinoid signalling. *Life Sciences*, *78*(6), 549–563. doi:10.1016/j.lfs.2005.05.055 PMID:16109430

Diabetes.co.uk. (2019, January 15). Cannabis, or marijuana, is a drug derived from the cannabis plant that is used for recreational use, medicinal purposes and religious or spiritual rites. *Diabetes*. https://www.diabetes.co.uk/recreational-drugs/cannabis.html

Dobrosi, N., Tóth, B. I., Nagy, G., Dózsa, A., Géczy, T., Nagy, L., Zouboulis, C. C., Paus, R., Kovács, L., & Bíró, T. (2008). Endocannabinoids enhance lipid synthesis and apoptosis of human sebocytes *via* cannabinoid receptor-2-mediated signaling. *The FASEB Journal*, *22*(10), 3685–3695. doi:10.1096/fj.07-104877 PMID:18596221

Ellis, R. J., Toperoff, W., Vaida, F., van den Brande, G., Gonzales, J., Gouaux, B., Bentley, H., & Atkinson, J. H. (2009). Smoked medicinal cannabis for neuropathic pain in HIV: A randomized, crossover clinical trial. *Neuropsychopharmacology: Official Publication of the American College of Neuropsychopharmacology*, *34*(3), 672–680. doi:10.1038/npp.2008.120 PMID:18688212

European Patent Office. (2019). *European publication server* [European publication server]. Composition Containing Cannabinoids for Use in a Method for the Treatment of Vitiligo. https://data.epo.org/publication-server/document?iDocId=5865308&iFormat=2

FDA. (2020). FDA and Cannabis: Research and Drug Approval Process. *FDA*. https://www.fda.gov/news-events/public-health-focus/fda-and-cannabis-research-and-drug-approval-process

Fogli, S., & Breschi, M. C. (2008). The molecular bases of cannabinoid action in cancer. *Cancer Therapy*, *6*, 103–116.

Gabros, S., Nessel, T. A., & Zito, P. M. (2022). *Sunscreens And Photoprotection*. StatPearls Publishing. https://www.ncbi.nlm.nih.gov/books/NBK537164/

Giacoppo, S., Mandolino, G., Galuppo, M., Bramanti, P., & Mazzon, E. (2014). Cannabinoids: New promising agents in the treatment of neurological diseases. *Molecules (Basel, Switzerland)*, *19*(11), 18781–18816. doi:10.3390/molecules191118781 PMID:25407719

Gohad, P., McCoy, J., Wambier, C., Kovacevic, M., Situm, M., Stanimirovic, A., & Goren, A. (2021). Novel cannabidiol sunscreen protects keratinocytes and melanocytes against ultraviolet B radiation. *Journal of Cosmetic Dermatology*, *20*(4), 1350–1352. doi:10.1111/jocd.13693 PMID:32964699

Guindon, J., & Hohmann, A. G. (2009). The endocannabinoid system and pain. *CNS & Neurological Disorders - Drug Targets*, *8*(6), 403–421. doi:10.2174/187152709789824660 PMID:19839937

Gururajan, A., & Malone, D. T. (2016). Does cannabidiol have a role in the treatment of schizophrenia? *Schizophrenia Research*, *176*(2–3), 281–290. doi:10.1016/j.schres.2016.06.022 PMID:27374322

Hara, M., Ma, T., & Verkman, A. S. (2002). Selectively Reduced Glycerol in Skin of Aquaporin-3-deficient Mice May Account for Impaired Skin Hydration, Elasticity, and Barrier Recovery. *The Journal of Biological Chemistry*, *277*(48), 46616–46621. doi:10.1074/jbc.M209003200 PMID:12270942

Ikarashi, N., Shiseki, M., Yoshida, R., Tabata, K., Kimura, R., Watanabe, T., Kon, R., Sakai, H., & Kamei, J. (2021). Cannabidiol Application Increases Cutaneous Aquaporin-3 and Exerts a Skin Moisturizing Effect. *Pharmaceuticals*, *14*(9), 879. doi:10.3390/ph14090879 PMID:34577578

Jae-We, C., Yeon-Su, J., Ji-Won, H., Young-Jin, C., Hyun-Kyu, K., Min-Young, K., Beom-Joon, K., Ki-Moon, P., Jong-Keun, K., Jae-Hyun, K., & Soo-Muk, C. (2011). Skin Hydration and Collagen Synthesis of AF-343 in HS68 Cell Line and NC/Nga Mice by Filaggrin Expression and Suppression of Matrix Metallopreteinase. *Toxicological Research*, *27*(4), 225–229. doi:10.5487/TR.2011.27.4.225 PMID:24278576

Jarai, M. (2022, March 29). HIV neuropathy: Causes, symptoms, treatment, and more. *Medical News Today*. https://www.medicalnewstoday.com/articles/hiv-neuropathy

Jarocka-Karpowicz, I., Biernacki, M., Wroński, A., Gęgotek, A., & Skrzydlewska, E. (2020). Cannabidiol Effects on Phospholipid Metabolism in Keratinocytes from Patients with Psoriasis Vulgaris. *Biomolecules, 10*(3), 367. doi:10.3390/biom10030367 PMID:32121131

Jones, N. A., Hill, A. J., Smith, I., Bevan, S. A., Williams, C. M., Whalley, B. J., & Stephens, G. J. (2010). Cannabidiol displays antiepileptiform and antiseizure properties in vitro and in vivo. *The Journal of Pharmacology and Experimental Therapeutics, 332*(2), 569–577. doi:10.1124/jpet.109.159145 PMID:19906779

Ko, G. D., Bober, S. L., Mindra, S., & Moreau, J. M. (2016). Medical cannabis—The Canadian perspective. *Journal of Pain Research, 9*, 735–744. doi:10.2147/JPR.S98182 PMID:27757048

Lim, M., & Kirchhof, M. G. (2019). Dermatology-Related Uses of Medical Cannabis Promoted by Dispensaries in Canada, Europe, and the United States. *Journal of Cutaneous Medicine and Surgery, 23*(2), 178–184. doi:10.1177/1203475418808761 PMID:30380925

Mack, A., & Joy, J. (2000). *Marijuana as Medicine? The Science Beyond the Controversy*. National Academies Press (US). https://www.ncbi.nlm.nih.gov/books/NBK224394/

Małgorzata, L., Dominika, W., Aleksandra, T., Kamila, J., & Adam, R. (2016). Natural cold pressed oils as cosmetic products. *Family Medicine and Primary Care Review, 4*, 443–447. doi:10.5114/fmpcr.2016.63699

Mao, J., Price, D. D., Lu, J., Keniston, L., & Mayer, D. J. (2000). Two distinctive antinociceptive systems in rats with pathological pain. *Neuroscience Letters, 280*(1), 13–16. doi:10.1016/S0304-3940(99)00998-2 PMID:10696800

Martin, B. R., & Lichtman, A. H. (1998). Cannabinoid transmission and pain perception. *Neurobiology of Disease, 5*(6, 6 Pt B), 447–461. doi:10.1006/nbdi.1998.0218 PMID:9974177

Matsuda, L. A., Lolait, S. J., Brownstein, M. J., Young, A. C., & Bonner, T. I. (1990). Structure of a cannabinoid receptor and functional expression of the cloned cDNA. *Nature, 346*(6284), 561–564. doi:10.1038/346561a0 PMID:2165569

Morgan, M. (2022, March 11). *Can Medical Marijuana Help With HIV/AIDS?* Medical Marijuana Doctor | West Palm Beach Medical Marijuana. https://mmjhealth.com/can-medical-marijuana-help-with-hiv-aids/

Müller, L., Radtke, A., Decker, J., Koch, M., & Belge, G. (2017). The Synthetic Cannabinoid WIN 55,212-2 Elicits Death in Human Cancer Cell Lines. *Anticancer Research, 37*(11), 6341–6345. doi:10.21873/anticanres.12086 PMID:29061818

Munson, A. E., Harris, L. S., Friedman, M. A., Dewey, W. L., & Carchman, R. A. (1975). Antineoplastic activity of cannabinoids. *Journal of the National Cancer Institute, 55*(3), 597–602. doi:10.1093/jnci/55.3.597 PMID:1159836

Nadolska, K., & Goś, R. (2008). [The role of endocannabinoid system in physiological and pathological processes in the eye]. *Klinika Oczna, 110*(10–12), 392–396. PMID:19195174

NCI. (2015, April 2). *Cancer Statistics*. NCI. https://www.cancer.gov/about-cancer/understanding/statistics

Nissen, L., Zatta, A., Stefanini, I., Grandi, S., Sgorbati, B., Biavati, B., & Monti, A. (2010). Characterization and antimicrobial activity of essential oils of industrial hemp varieties (Cannabis sativa L.). *Fitoterapia, 81*(5), 413–419. doi:10.1016/j.fitote.2009.11.010 PMID:19969046

Novak, J., Zitterl-Eglseer, K., Deans, S. G., & Franz, C. M. (2001). Essential oils of different cultivars ofCannabis sativa L. and their antimicrobial activity. *Flavour and Fragrance Journal, 16*(4), 259–262. doi:10.1002/ffj.993

Ogawa, E., Sato, Y., Minagawa, A., & Okuyama, R. (2018). Pathogenesis of psoriasis and development of treatment. *The Journal ofDermatology, 45*(3), 264–272. doi:10.1111/1346-8138.14139 PMID:29226422

Oláh, A., Tóth, B. I., Borbíró, I., Sugawara, K., Szöllõsi, A. G., Czifra, G., Pál, B., Ambrus, L., Kloepper, J., Camera, E., Ludovici, M., Picardo, M., Voets, T., Zouboulis, C. C., Paus, R., & Bíró, T. (2014). Cannabidiol exerts sebostatic and antiinflammatory effects on human sebocytes. *The Journal of Clinical Investigation, 124*(9), 3713–3724. doi:10.1172/JCI64628 PMID:25061872

Palm, M. D., & O'Donoghue, M. N. (2007). Update on photoprotection: Photoprotection. *Dermatologic Therapy, 20*(5), 360–376. doi:10.1111/j.1529-8019.2007.00150.x PMID:18045361

Pérez-Gómez, E., Andradas, C., Blasco-Benito, S., Caffarel, M. M., García-Taboada, E., Villa-Morales, M., Moreno, E., Hamann, S., Martín-Villar, E., Flores, J. M., Wenners, A., Alkatout, I., Klapper, W., Röcken, C., Bronsert, P., Stickeler, E., Staebler, A., Bauer, M., Arnold, N., & Sánchez, C. (2015). Role of cannabinoid receptor CB2 in HER2 pro-oncogenic signaling in breast cancer. *Journal of the National Cancer Institute, 107*(6), djv077. doi:10.1093/jnci/djv077 PMID:25855725

Peschel, W. (2016). Quality Control of Traditional Cannabis Tinctures: Pattern, Markers, and Stability. *Scientia Pharmaceutica, 84*(3), 567–584. doi:10.3390cipharm84030567 PMID:28117322

Robinson, S. M., & Adinoff, B. (2016). The Classification of Substance Use Disorders: Historical, Contextual, and Conceptual Considerations. *Behavioral Sciences (Basel, Switzerland), 6*(3), E18. doi:10.3390/bs6030018 PMID:27548233

Rohleder, C., Müller, J. K., Lange, B., & Leweke, F. M. (2016). Cannabidiol as a Potential New Type of an Antipsychotic. A Critical Review of the Evidence. *Frontiers in Pharmacology, 7*, 422. doi:10.3389/fphar.2016.00422 PMID:27877130

Sandle, T. (2020, November 24). *Cannabis For Medical And Pharmaceutical Purposes – Part 1: An Overview Of The Development And Application*. IVT Network. https://www.ivtnetwork.com/article/cannabis-medical-and-pharmaceutical-purposes-%E2%80%93-part-1-overview-development-and-application-0

Schofs, L., Sparo, M. D., & Sánchez Bruni, S. F. (2021). The antimicrobial effect behind *Cannabis sativa. Pharmacology Research & Perspectives, 9*(2). Advance online publication. doi:10.1002/prp2.761 PMID:33822478

Sheriff, T., Lin, M. J., Dubin, D., & Khorasani, H. (2020). The potential role of cannabinoids in dermatology. *The Journal of Dermatological Treatment, 31*(8), 839–845. doi:10.1080/09546634.2019.1675854 PMID:31599175

Singh, A., Saluja, S., Kumar, A., Agrawal, S., Thind, M., Nanda, S., & Shirani, J. (2018). Cardiovascular Complications of Marijuana and Related Substances: A Review. *Cardiology and Therapy*, *7*(1), 45–59. doi:10.100740119-017-0102-x PMID:29218644

Smith, G. L., & Satino, J. (2021). Case Study of Hair Regrowth with Topical Cannabidiol (CBD). *International Society of Hair Restoration Surgery*, *31*(4), 140–142. doi:10.33589/31.4.140

Sun, H. Y., Youn-Jung, K., Ok, K. M., Mingyeong, K., & Woong, O. S. (2017). Cannabidiol upregulates melanogenesis through CB1 dependent pathway by activating p38 MAPK and p42/44 MAPK. *Chemico-Biological Interactions*, *273*, 107–114. doi:10.1016/j.cbi.2017.06.005 PMID:28601556

Thomas, G., Kloner, R. A., & Rezkalla, S. (2014). Adverse cardiovascular, cerebrovascular, and peripheral vascular effects of marijuana inhalation: What cardiologists need to know. *The American Journal of Cardiology*, *113*(1), 187–190. doi:10.1016/j.amjcard.2013.09.042 PMID:24176069

van Breemen, R. B., Muchiri, R. N., Bates, T. A., Weinstein, J. B., Leier, H. C., Farley, S., & Tafesse, F. G. (2022). Cannabinoids Block Cellular Entry of SARS-CoV-2 and the Emerging Variants. *Journal of Natural Products*, *85*(1), 176–184. doi:10.1021/acs.jnatprod.1c00946 PMID:35007072

Velasco, G., Sánchez, C., & Guzmán, M. (2016). Anticancer mechanisms of cannabinoids. *Current Oncology (Toronto, Ont.)*, *23*(2), S23–S32. doi:10.3747/co.23.3080 PMID:27022311

Vercelli, C., Barbero, R., Cuniberti, B., Racca, S., Abbadessa, G., Piccione, F., & Re, G. (2014). Transient receptor potential vanilloid 1 expression and functionality in mcf-7 cells: A preliminary investigation. *Journal of Breast Cancer*, *17*(4), 332–338. doi:10.4048/jbc.2014.17.4.332 PMID:25548580

Watson, S. J., Benson, J. A., & Joy, J. E. (2000). Marijuana and medicine: Assessing the science base: a summary of the 1999 Institute of Medicine report. *Archives of General Psychiatry*, *57*(6), 547–552. doi:10.1001/archpsyc.57.6.547 PMID:10839332

Williams, H. C., Dellavalle, R. P., & Garner, S. (2012). Acne vulgaris. *Lancet*, *379*(9813), 361–372. doi:10.1016/S0140-6736(11)60321-8 PMID:21880356

Wolff, V., & Jouanjus, E. (2017). Strokes are possible complications of cannabinoids use. *Epilepsy & Behavior: E&B*, *70*(Pt B), 355–363. doi:10.1016/j.yebeh.2017.01.031

Zuardi, A. W. (2006). History of cannabis as a medicine: A review. *Revista Brasileira De Psiquiatria (Sao Paulo, Brazil: 1999)*, *28*(2), 153–157. doi:10.1590/s1516-44462006000200015

Chapter 6

Role of *Cannabis sativa* L. in the Cosmetic Industry: Opportunities and Challenges

Anup Kumar Sarkar
https://orcid.org/0000-0002-6418-4895
Dukhulal Nibaran Chandra College, India

Sanjoy Sadhukhan
https://orcid.org/0000-0002-2619-8700
Raiganj University, India

ABSTRACT

Cannabis sativa L. is a flowering plant in the family Cannabaceae, and has been cultivated since ancient times for its fibres, oils, resins, dried inflorescences, and leaves. It can be used for a variety of industrial purposes. Over the years, the therapeutic and pharmacological efficacy of its phytoconstituents is shown in a variety of human diseases and health. The use and exploitation of the plant have sparked controversy; however, there are recent legalizations of its use for medical and other purposes in many countries within the corresponding legislative framework. In addition to this legalization, C. sativa is encouraging the very rapid growth of the cannabis oriented pharmaceutical industry. This chapter summarized recent developments in the science of C. sativa and its products about their industrial application, while also addressing gaps in the existing knowledge and future research directions for this high-value multi-use, and potential industrial plant with universal benefits.

INTRODUCTION

Cosmetics are materials used to repair or enhance the appearance of animals and people via care, maintenance, prevention, and therapy (Bijauliya et al., 2017; Lintner, 2009). Technically a cosmetic product is defined as "any ingredient" or "formulation" intended for application to any external area of the human body for the goal of cleansing, perfuming, protecting, and maintaining body parts as well as

DOI: 10.4018/978-1-6684-5718-4.ch006

the entire body. Everyone needs cosmetics to live a happy and healthy life (Devi et al., 2022). Before the discovery of technologies for producing chemicals with similar qualities, plants were the principal source and backbone of all cosmetics. Modern pharmaceutical researchers also use many plant-based bioactive compounds for the improvement of cosmetic products. Since the cosmetics industry is not strictly regulated, cosmetic products do not include monographs controlling their formulation and the chemicals utilized (Gupta et al., 2019). There are only a few criteria that regulate the complete prescription of active substances in cosmetic types (Draelos, 2012). Natural components are ubiquitous and expanding in popularity and the usage of plant extracts in cosmetic composition is increasing day by day. Aromatic herbs and oils have been used as incense, fragrances, perfumes, and for medical and culinary purposes for thousands of years. Many wild and cultivated plants have been used in the pharmaceutical industry for their bioactive compounds. Several researchers have claimed that similar to various herbal formulations and supplements, cultivars of *Cannabis sativa* L. may provide many raw materials for the cosmetics industry and pharmaceutical industry (Vogl et al., 2004). Since then, empirical research has gradually begun to quantify the consequences of cannabis cultivation and, to a lesser extent, consumption. As of early 2020, several nations have established or are in the process of establishing medical access legislation and procedures, and millions of individuals are utilizing cannabis products for medical purposes to treat a variety of medical ailments (Sarma et al., 2020). Historically, cannabis seeds have been gathered for the oil that can be squeezed from them. This oil has found application in a variety of industries, including the food industry as well as manufactures such as soaps, paints, lubricants, and cosmetics (Borhade, 2013; Horne, 2020).

The chemical heterogeneity of cannabis makes pharmaceutical standardisation difficult and needs the employment of complex methodologies to analyse the plant chemotype and the herbal pharmaceutical, as well as extraction processes that are particular to the chemical composition of each substance (Calvi et al., 2018). Due to some uncertain factors, including quantity, dynamics, and mode of administration, the legal medicinal use of cannabis is indeed accompanied by safety concerns (Mead, 2017). Marijuana and hashish are the best-known forms of the *Cannabis* plant. Marijuana is a Mexican phrase that originally referred to cheap tobacco but is now used to denote the dried leaves and blossoms of the cannabis plant, while "Hashish" is an Arabic term for Indian hemp that refers to the plant's resin gum (Amar & Léonard, 2002). Hemp is allowed in much of the area, but marijuana is not (Baral et al., 2020). Cannabinoids are the major chemical components of Cannabis sativa; the principal psychoactive ingredient is -9-tetrahydrocannabinol, while cannabidiol (CBD) is an active nonpsychotic element. Cannabinoids are classified into three types based on their origin: endocannabinoids (ECBs), phytocannabinoids (PCBs), and synthetic cannabinoids (SCs). PCBs are cannabinoids taken from the resin-producing trichomes of the Cannabis sativa L. plant, whereas ECBs are cannabinoids that are naturally created inside the human body. SCs are synthetic cannabinoids created in a lab. The endocannabinoid system (ECS) is a complex intercellular signalling network that plays a crucial role in maintaining human anatomical and physiological homeostasis and through which ECBs exercise their effects (Baswan et al., 2020). Neutral CNBs (like THC and CBD) and Cannabinoid acids may be distinguished from one another by the presence of a carboxyl group (Martins et al., 2022). The resurgence of a historically important plant in modern medicine, cannabis's usage for aesthetic and medicinal reasons has sparked heated debate. Low-THC cannabis is cultivated for commercial purposes, whereas high-THC strains are usually cultivated for medicinal purposes (Zuk-Golaszewska & Golaszewski, 2018).

BOTANICAL AND AGRONOMIC CHARACTERS OF *CANNABIS SATIVA* L

Cannabis sativa L. originated from Eurasia but is now widely dispersed around the world and thrives at varying elevations, habitats, and climate conditions around the globe (Clarke & Merlin, 2016). According to the most widely accepted formal taxonomy, the genus *Cannabis* consists of one species, *C. sativa* L., and three highly polymorphic subspecies – *sativa*, *indica*, and *ruderalis*. The concepts were based on morphological traits as well as chemical profiles of these subspecies (McPartland, 2018; Small, 2015; Zhang et al., 2018). Male flowers are apetalous, with five yellowish sepals and five poricidal stamens. Each female flower consists of a perigonal leaf-like bract, which surrounds the carpel with one single-ovulate ovary (Kuddus et al., 2013). In addition, a growing perianth was observed during the early stages of flower development, which later withered, lost its individuality, and resembled a thin membrane (Spitzer-Rimon et al., 2019). Commercially, the plants are grown for their psychotropic substances, which are synthesized in the trichomes that appear on flower bracts in female inflorescences (Andre et al., 2016). Trichomes are the most significant morphological part of the flower as they have chemotaxonomic and pharmaceutical significance. The plants contain three forms of glandular trichomes which are significantly different from each other-capitate-stalked, capitate-sessile, and bulbous (Aliferis & Bernard-Perron, 2020). In the case of capitate type, the head is composed of eight cells, whereas in bulbous type it is composed of 2-4 cells (Feng et al., 2021; Tian et al., 2017). The fruit is tiny, smooth, light brownish-grey in colour, and loaded with seeds (Kuddus et al., 2013). It is a notoriously resistant plant to transformation, owing to low regeneration efficiency that are depending on cultivar, tissue, plant age, and growth regulator combination (Slusarkiewicz-Jarzina et al., 2005). Cannabis plants have no particular soil specifications; the most essential aspect is the pH of the soil, which should be near neutral or slightly alkaline (Husain et al., 2019; Linger et al., 2005).

BIOACTIVE COMPOUNDS OF *CANNABIS SATIVA* L AND POTENTIAL HEALTH BENEFITS

This plant is responsible for the production of a vast number of secondary metabolites, the vast majority of which are used in various cultures for medicinal reasons. Although it has a very long history of therapeutic use, both its economic and medical value have decreased as a result of the socio-political unrest that has occurred in recent years. In the course of the previous several decades, a significant amount of research has been carried out, which has enabled a clear distinction to be drawn between cannabis in its role as a hazardous drug and its role as a helpful medicinal product. C. sativa is distinguishable from other cannabis species by the complexity of its chemical composition. This composition includes terpenes, carbohydrates, amides, amines, phytosterols, phenolic compounds, fatty acids and their esters, and more (Andre et al., 2016). Cannabinoids, which are classified as terpenophenolics, make up the most common category of bioactive compounds found in cannabis. Cannabinoids make up more than 60 of the plant's compounds, while terpenoids make up more than 140 of the plant's compounds. The plant has more or less 483 distinct components (Rajput & Kumar, 2018). Terpenoids are very potent metabolites, capable of influencing the behaviour of animals and even humans when breathed in very little levels; moreover, some studies have postulated that terpenoids and cannabinoids work synergistically with one another (Russo et al., 2008; Andre et al., 2016; Singh & Sharma, 2015; Tahir et al., 2021). Herbal cannabis includes at least 144 cannabinoids, the most well-known of which are tetrahydrocannabinol (THC), cannabidiol (CBD), cannabinol (CBN), -caryophyllene, Cannabigerol, etc., (Figure 1). This is in contrast to the majority of herbal formulations, which contain only a few pharmacologically active ingredients (Freeman et al., 2019; Rajput & Kumar, 2018). In this respect, the very first problem is to a quality that the overwhelming majority of cannabinoids have in common, namely that they are lipophilic, low melting point semisolids in their physical state (Filer, 2022).

The amount of THC that Is produced by industrial cannabis (hemp) and medicinal cannabis is the key factor that differentiates the two types of cannabis. Cultivation, processing and extraction, manufacturing and packaging, and distribution and sales channels are the four fundamental phases that make up the industrial production of cannabis. Cultivation is the first step in the process. Because the quantity of neutral CNBs in plants is a great deal lower than that of cannabinoid acids, THC and CBD are created by a process that does not include the activity of enzymes called decarboxylation (Tahir et al., 2021). Cannabinoids and non-cannabinoid chemicals, taken as a whole, contribute to an enhancement of *Cannabis sativa* L''s biological activity (Koltai & Namdar, 2020).

Figure 1. Some of the bioactive compounds of cannabis sativa L

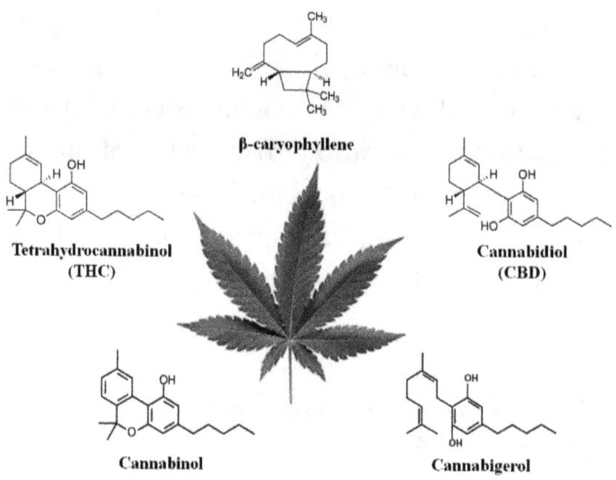

PLANT PHYSIOLOGICAL AND METABOLIC PATHWAYS ASSOCIATED WITH INDUSTRIAL POTENTIAL CONSTITUENTS

The blooms of the plant have a broad range of trichomes, some of which are glandular while others are non-glandular. These trichomes serve as the sites for the synthesis of phytochemicals. The biosynthesis pathways and the storage of cannabinoids and essential oils take place in the glandular trichomes. These trichomes are also responsible for the formation of a resin that is abundant in terpenes (Aliferis & Bernard-Perron, 2020). Several findings reveal variability in trichome size, density, and cannabinoid concentration using metabolic profiling of trichomes. However, the genetic mechanisms driving the alterations in trichome formation and subsequent cannabinoid content remain unexplained (Happyana et al., 2013; Hussain et al., 2021; Small & Naraine, 2016; Richard et al., (2007) discovered that incorporating hemp seed into the rat diet boosted plasma linoleic acid and alpha-linolenic acid levels considerably. These fatty acids regulate fluidity, electrolyte transport, and hormone activity because they are a structural component of phospholipids in cell membranes (Vogl et al., 2004).

UTILIZATION IN COSMETICS INDUSTRY

Nowadays, the global business community and people everywhere regularly refer to cosmetic products as personal care items for both humans and animals. For a few years, cannabis-based products have saturated the market for therapeutic and cosmeceuticals (Bonini et al., 2018). In some countries it is now possible to investigate the medicinal and cosmetic potential of Cannabis derived components, most notably THC and cannabidiol due to the continuousegalizationn trends (Budney & Borodovsky, 2017; Kavousi et al., 2022). *C. sativa* seed oil contains several ingredients like unsaturated fatty acids, vitamins, proteins, phytosterol, and organic compounds that are important in cosmetology. Currently, Cannabis-derived products are used as the common ingredients in skin care products such as body oils, moisturizers, lotions, and lip balms, but scientific research on the topical safety and usefulness of the formulations are scarce (Anwar et al., 2006; Stella et al., 2019). Recently, the endocannabinoid system was found, which comprises receptors, ligands, and enzymes that are broadly expressed in the brain and the periphery, where they operate to achieve stability in many homeostatic processes (Russo & Guy, 2006; Russo, 2017; Vaidya et al., 2022).

Applications in Skin Care

Cannabinoid-rich formulations applied topically to the skin have been proven in a number of trials to significantly enhance patient'' quality of life when used to treat a wide range of skin disorders (Stella et al., 2019). It is also beneficial to use cannabis seed oil as a component in body oils that penetrate the skin and lotions that are rich in lipids (Ali & Akhtar, 2015). As a result of hemp seed oi''s emollient properties, the skin is left feeling smooth and supple, and the oil is thus used in several locations for the purpose of skin care. Cannabis oil is used in the production of a wide variety of skin care products, including but not limited to creams, oils, lotions, moisturisers, ointments, cleansers, exfoliators, gels, lip balms, sunscreen, chemical peel, toner, serums, and so on (Anwar et al., 2006; Bró et al., 2009). These products can be found in the form of creams, oils, lotions, and moisturisers. A number of cannabis-based dermal formulations have shown to be effective in treating a variety of skin conditions, including acne, dermatitis, dry skin, and wrinkled skin. In the skin, the ECS has a role in a variety of processes, including the regulation of cell differentiation, development, and survival; the regulation of inflammatory and immunological responses; nociception; and the growth of hair (Mnekin & Ripoll, 2021). Cannabinoids often perform their functions as exogenous ligands of the ECS, and they have the potential to interact not just with endocannabinoid receptors but also with some membranes and other receptors (Dawidowicz et al., 2021). Both CBN and CBD are drawing attention as potential ingredients for sun protection products (Mnekin & Ripoll, 2021). Hemp seed oil is especially desirable because of the high concentration of flavonoids, terpenes, carotenoids, and phytosterols that it contains. These constituents are responsible for the anti-inflammatory and anti-aging effects of the oil (Mnekin & Ripoll, 2021). It was established by Zagórska-Dziok et al., (2021) that hydrogels based on cannabis extracts may enhance the moisture content of the skin. The findings also indicate that hemp extracts may be a beneficial source of biologically active compounds that may decrease oxidative stress, stop the processes that cause skin to age, and favourably increase the viability of skin cells.

Acne, dark spots, hyperpigmentation, excessive perspiration, fine wrinkles, inflammation, and rashes are some of the skin conditions that may be prevented or treated with the cannabis-based skincare products (Eagleston et al., 2018). Modulating the immune response and lowering the risk of skin inflammation and allergic reactions are both possible benefits of cannabidiol (CBD), which works by acting indirectly on the CB2 receptors. Caspase is an anti-inflammatory enzyme that transmits a signal, which in turn induces death of immune cells. Once CBD attaches to the CB2 receptors on the problematic immune cells, it activates caspase, which in turn activates caspase (Baral et al., 2020). According to Rough (2017), numerous sun protection treatments include sun protection factors (SPF) in addition to cannabis, and these products efficiently prevent skin from sunburn. Interestingly, hemp seed oil deflects specific UV rays without lowering the quantity of vitamin D. It has a high SPF rating and has been found to absorb UV-A, UV-B, and UV-C rays (Atalay et al., 2021; Gogotek et al., 2016; Rodriguez-Morrison et al., 2021). This demonstrates that it has the potential to be utilised as a UV protector at a low level and throughout a wide range. Recent studies suggest that cannabidiol, or CBD, has a protective effect on the survival of keratinocytes and melanocytes after exposure to UV light (Gohad et al., 2021). However, the structure of CBD does not produce a significant amount of UVB absorption; however, because it is an antioxidant, it may be able to defend against the damaging effects of reactive oxygen species (ROS) (Bornheim & Grillo, 1998; Ggotek et al., 2016; Massi et al., 2006). Despite the fact that CBD does not produce substantial UVB absorption, it may be able to protect against the damaging effects of ROS. It is possible that cannabidiol, or CBD, might be a useful component of sunscreens, and it is possible that such products could provide more protection than sunscreen alone. According to Oláh et al. (2014), CBD has a sebostatic effect, which means that it prevents certain molecules, such as arachidonic acid and a mixture of linoleic acid and testosterone, from producing fat.

Hemp contains fatty acids that serve to maintain our skin supple and healthy while also avoiding indications of ageing and sun damage. In addition, hemp oil-based moisturisers and serums can be reported to regenerate healthy skin cells, such as keratinocytes, melanocytes, and Langerhans cells (Sheriff et al., 2020). The phenolic acid, phloroglucinol glucoside found in hemp seed oil is said to fight skin ageing (Hammond & Mahlberg, 1994). Cosmetic preparations containing phenolic extract are marketed with anti-ageing, wound healing, and photoprotection benefits Peyravian et al., 2022. Inhalation, smoking and consumption of medical cannabis can promote the reduction of inflammation and pain as well as the protection of neurons (Xiong et al., 2012). Topical CBD is available in the form of gels, oils, and lotions, and many reputed companies claim that these products are highly successful in eliminating multiple skin-related problems. It might stop the enzyme 5-α reductase from functioning, which would prevent the skin from making too much sebum and make the skin more elastic and moister (Oláh et al., 2014; Vincenzi & Tosti, 2020).

Applications in Oral Care

The cannabinoid-enriched formulation is also used as oral care products in some countries. Many researchers have reported the significant effectiveness of cannabinoids, specifically cannabigerolic acid, cannabinol, cannabigerol, and cannabichromene, to that of conventional dental care products. Cannabinoids may be useful in dentistry for the management of toothaches, microbial infections that cause periodontitis, gingivitis, periodontal disease, tooth decay, salivary gland issues and sores, inflammation-based oral disorders, dental anxiety, and regular oral health maintenance (Lowe et al., 2021). Cannabinoids can effectively reduce the bacterial burden in dental plaque. *C. sativa* seed oil, as well as petroleum-ether extract and methanolic extract of the entire plant, can show antagonistic activity against a variety of bacteria present in dental plaque, such as *Bacillus subtilis*, *Staphylococcus aureus*, *Escherichia coli*, and *Pseudomonas aeruginosa*, and fungi such as *Aspergillus* sp., *Candida albicans*, etc. (Ali et al.,

2012). Mouthwashes infused with cannabinoids have been shown to have the same antibacterial effect on dental plaque samples as chlorhexidine, a commonly used disinfectant and antiseptic (Vasudevan & Stahl, 2020). Cannabinoids were reported to be more effective than well-established conventional dental products like Oral B or Colgate in lowering the colony count of bacterial strains (Stahl & Vasudevan, 2020). Colgate-Palmolive Company (USA) recently filed a patent on personal care compositions including antiperspirant active components and a cannabis-derived natural product in an amount sufficient to create an anti-irritant action on the skin (Bakowska-Barczak et al., 2022; Hernandez et al., 2021).

Hair Care Product

Different products of the *C. sativa* plant have the potential to solve different hair-related issues including hair loss. Currently, several hair-care products contain either CBD or hemp or both and some of the products are CBD scalp calming shampoo, ultra-hydrating herbal conditioner, and CBD anti-dandruff shampoo etc. (Cooper, 2020; Telek et al., 2007). Hemp oil is advertised as an effective cosmetic treatment for hair, with claims that using the oil directly to the hair has hydrating properties, can promote hair growth, may protect the hair and aid in damage healing, and may give shine to the hair (Paul et al., 2019). Cannabis-based hair care products go through a long manufacturing process that starts with the synthesis of the raw materials and ends with cosmeceutical and therapy. The biology of hair follicles is also influenced by cannabinoids and allied compounds. Cannabis-based shampoo offers a variety of benefits that are unavailable elsewhere. This cannabis shampoo contains solely CBD and no THC. The topical application of cannabinoids and hemp oil can potentially improve hair fibres and prevent many issues interlinked with hair follicles (Paul et al., 2019). Almost 69.0 mg/Kg of saponin is present in hemp seed oil, and thus hemp seed oil is recommended for the preparation of shampoo (Cirimele et al., 1999). Recent research by Szabo and colleagues suggests that CBD can be used to treat undesired hair growth and prevent hair loss, depending on the dose of the substance (Szabó et al., 2020). Sub micromolar quantities of CBD have been shown in initial experiments to stimulate hair growth when given at low concentrations. However, greater concentrations inhibit hair growth (Baswan et al., 2020; Wilson, 2021). In a recent investigation, a shampoo containing broad-spectrum CBD was found to be highly efficient in lowering indications of scalp inflammation i.e., arborizing arteries, twisted capillaries, and scales, as well as erythema, scaling, stinging, and burning, after 2 weeks of use (Vincenzi & Tosti, 2020).

Ophthalmic Care Products

Cannabis-based formulations are now widely used in the production of eye care products (Dubald et al., 2018; Lu, 2010; Pacula & Smart, 2017). Mascara is a cosmetic item that is used to improve the eyelashes by making them darker, thicker, lighter, or more defined and they are constructed of a mixture of mineral oils and waxes, with some preservatives added to make them stay longer. Cannabis can be used in place of beeswax, making it a vegan choice. These cannabis-based ophthalmic products have been produced due to their preventive and therapeutic potential, as well as their cosmetic appeal (Punyamurthula et al., 2017; Taskar, 2019). According to Tyrrell, (2019), several cannabis-based compositions lessen dark circles, puffiness, and wrinkles.

Facial Care Products

Different parts of *C. sativa* have been used as raw materials for facial care products like face primer, foundation, glosses, lip balms, lip scrubs, lipsticks, concealer, and many more. CBD-infused chap sticks, glosses, lip balms, lip scrubs, and lipsticks can be found all over the globe. When comes to lip care, CBD is unrivalled. CBD balms for the skin ease tight muscles, stiffness, and give intensive hydration (Stella et al., 2019). Its antimicrobial properties serve to protect, while the antioxidants aid in the restoration of sore and chapped lips. CBD or hemp-based exfoliating cleansers have been reported to wash and softened the skin (Zagórska-Dziok et al., 2021). These cannabis-based products not only have a pleasing appearance and fragrance but also aid to reduce the visibility of scar tissue and have a strong anti-ageing impact (Nadar et al., 2022). CBD can also help to reduce inflammation and discomfort caused by cold sores.

Pain Relieving Product

Painful joints or muscles can get quick relief from the CBD-infused lotion or cream (Miller & Miller, 2017). The therapeutic use of *C. sativa* and its products for chronic pain is gaining popularity around the world, and the percentage of patients who take it either by prescription or as self-medication is constantly increasing (Compton et al., 2017; Han et al., 2018). Vulfsons et al., (2020) reviewed the therapeutic effects of cannabis compounds for the management of pain, and reported that they do not appear to be useful in the control of acute pain, but have mild therapeutic benefits for the treatment of neuropathic pain and may be effective in the management of core orthopaedic musculoskeletal pain. Sativex or Nabiximols, which contain the 1:1 ratio of THC and CBD, are now employed as medications to treat spasticity in individuals with multiple sclerosis (Devinsky et al., 2016; Pertwee, 2008).

Other Uses

C. sativa includes a large number of extremely volatile terpenoids which act as insect repellent and are regularly used in insect repellent cream (Booth et al., 2017). When THC is added to cannabis oil, neurobehavioral symptoms like delusions, agitation, irritability, apathy, lack of sleep, and caregiver stress go down by a massive proportion (Verma et al., 2021). *C. sativa* seeds are also processed to produce natural colour and dye (Vogl et al., 2004). Some researchers claimed that THC can lessen the risk of nausea and vomiting by activating the CB1 receptor and thus can be utilized in the preparation of anti-vomiting formulation (Badowski, 2017).

IMPROVEMENT OF INDUSTRIAL POTENTIAL THROUGH BIOTECHNOLOGY

C. sativa is a perfect example of a versatile crop owing to its large potential for usage in numerous industrial sectors, such as textile, paper, construction materials, bioenergy, bioplastics, pharmaceutical industry, vegetable oil, animal products, cosmetics, etc. Researchers claim to have produced cosmetic formulations containing a CBD source and several other components (Bakowska-Barczak et al., 2022). Due to its high lipophilicity, CBD can easily pass through biological barriers and is swiftly absorbed (Brunetti et al., 2020). Because of the growing importance of cannabinoids as industrial raw materials along with the increasing number of novel applications of medicinal cannabis, seed firms must use

Figure 2. Various applications of Cannabis sativa l., in cosmetics Industry

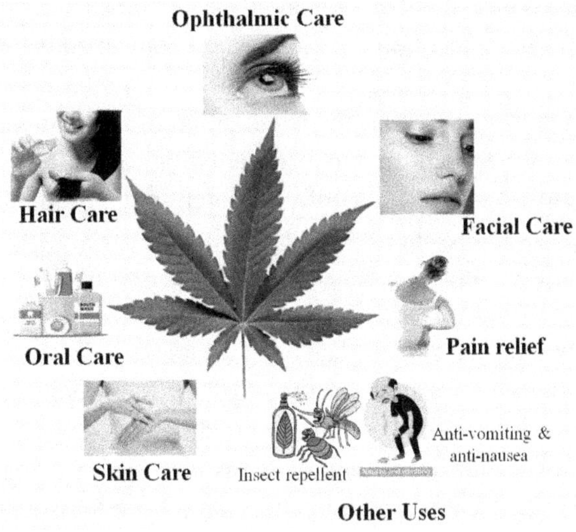

both traditional and novel breeding approaches to create new *C. sativa* genotypes (Chandra et al., 2017; Grof, 2018; Naim-Feil et al., 2021). Cannabis research in recent years has mostly focused on the genetic control of cannabinoid production and the relationship between environmental conditions, physiological features, and the secondary metabolite profile of the plant (Allen et al., 2019; Braich et al., 2019; Grassa et al., 2018; Van Bakel et al., 2011). Phytocannabinoid concentration is mostly determined by genetic variables that are inheritable and differ in expression depending on variety, tissue type, tissue position, and growth stage.

RESEARCH TRENDS, CHALLENGES AND NEW-AGE PERSPECTIVES AS INDUSTRIAL CROP

The plant is widely characterised as a potent hallucinogenic narcotic, however, there are various indications that it is also utilized as an industrial plant. Some products of the plant have unbelievable efficacy as cosmetics. Despite multitudinous use in the cosmetic industry comparatively little study has been conducted on its improvement and many studies have demonstrated the relative safety of cannabis-based cosmetics. To validate their positive and detrimental effects for aesthetic, cosmeceutical, diagnostic, preventive, and therapeutic usage, these formulations must be extensively studied using appropriate *in vitro* and *in vivo* models (Nadar et al., 2022). The ongoing controversy over the legality issue of the plant has impeded progress in the field of cannabis research. Despite there is the tremendous therapeutic potential of cannabis there are still certain chemical issues. To better comprehend the pharmaceutical implications and applications of active cannabinoids in the cosmetic industry, additional chemical and toxicological research is required. Since *C. sativa* contains a huge number of bioactive cannabinoid compounds and as cannabinoid receptors are found throughout the human body, every consideration of medical cannabis will necessarily require a simplification of a very complicated system including multivariate interactions. Although human studies with *C. sativa*-derived pharmaceuticals are essential to verify their effectiveness and tolerability in various clinical settings. A cosmetic product is not designated as a "Drug" since a drug is typically a natural product or chemically synthesized substance that influences the structural and/or functional attributes of humans or any animals when consumed or otherwise delivered into the body (Pandey et al., 2021).

Another big issue is the controversy about the legalization of the plant and its products. The prohibition on the production and utilization of cannabis plants for recreational, medical, pharmaceutical, and industrial purposes severely restricted scientific research in the field. Several studies have already identified some distinct barriers to the approval of new clinical trials using cannabis-based drugs that are raising concerns, particularly among ethics and governance committees, and consequently putting up barriers that are impeding the advancement of their use as a medicine as well as cosmetics (Martin et al., 2020). Over the last two decades, there has been an increase in the legalisation of medical and recreational cannabis cultivation and consumption around the world (Bahji & Stephenson, 2019; Chouvy, 2019). While marijuana is prohibited at the federal level in the USA, several states are decriminalising it and making it legal to sell it to consumers at retail and this is one of the biggest challenges in the USA. Researchers studying cannabis and chemical compounds have faced logistical and regulatory challenges due to its quasi-legal status in many places and persisting societal prejudice. Workers in both cannabis extraction and edible marijuana production may be exposed to various chemicals, particularly in the later sector, as edible products are typically prepared in hygienic conditions. Skin rashes and burns, frostbite, and the risk of fires or explosions are a few of the associated health hazards for the employees.

The social acceptability of cannabis and its cosmetic benefits are critical factors for industrial hemp to gain attention. The advantages and practical applications of cannabis have stimulated study on its cultivation, quality characteristics, and use in novel products. Existing knowledge concerning industrial cannabis cultivation is fragmented and mostly based on junk science and/or indoor and outdoor growth approaches, but the agronomic demands of industrial cannabis cultivated under field settings in most developed countries have never been investigated.

FUTURE PROSPECTS AND CONCLUSIONS

There has been a substantial increase in the demand for cosmetics during the past few decades as a result of the growth of the third-world economy, the improvement in living standards, and the spread of specialty stores (Gupta et al., 2019). Companies that produce cosmetics are employing a variety of strategies for identifying biologically derived products to maintain and strengthen their market position. There is no doubt that Cannabis derived natural products have gained a lot of attention as the raw material of the cosmetic industry. Despite the contentious discussions surrounding the legalisation of cannabis for use in pharmaceuticals, cosmetics, and other products, the plant's extraordinary bioactive compounds and the appropriate regulatory environment indicate an imperative need for additional research and development in a variety of fields. Fueled by recent prospects afforded by shifting legislation as well as the latest scientific developments, Cannabis product market potential has increased by up to tenfold within a decade (Valizadehderakhshan et al., 2021). As the cannabis industry transforms from the black market to the legal market, product design and extraction techniques have come to the forefront. Comprehensive research on chemical components has uncovered an abundance of terpenes and flavonoids, which may also contribute to its cosmetic properties. Furthermore, while improvements in science and technology have enhanced many essential crops in the past few decades, cannabis has not been appraised using modern technologies and accurate scientific procedures due to its illicit status.

REFERENCES

Aldrich, M. (1997). History of Therapeutic Cannabis. In M. L. Mathre (Ed.), *Cannabis in Medical Practice: a Legal, Historical and Pharmacological Overview of the Therapeutic use of Marijuana* (pp. 35–55). McFarland & Co.

Ali, A., & Akhtar, N. (2015). The safety and efficacy of 3% *Cannabis* seeds extract cream for reduction of human cheek skin sebum and erythema content. *Pakistan Journal of Pharmaceutical Sciences*, *28*(4), 1389–1395. PMID:26142529

Ali, E. M., Almagboul, A. Z., Khogali, S. M., & Gergeir, U. M. (2012). Antimicrobial Activity of *Cannabis sativa* L. *Chinese Medicine*, *3*(1), 61–64. doi:10.4236/cm.2012.31010

Aliferis, K. A., & Bernard-Perron, D. (2020). Cannabinomics: Application of Metabolomics in Cannabis (*Cannabis sativa* L.) Research and Development. *Frontiers in Plant Science*, *11*, 554. doi:10.3389/fpls.2020.00554 PMID:32457786

Allen, K. D., McKernan, K., Pauli, C., Roe, J., Torres, A., & Gaudino, R. (2019). Genomic characterization of the complete terpene synthase gene family from *Cannabis sativa*. *PLoS One*, *14*(9), e0222363. doi:10.1371/journal.pone.0222363 PMID:31513654

Amar, M. B., & Léonard, L. (2002). Cannabis. In L. Léonard & M. B. Amar (Eds.), Les psychotropes: pharmacologie et toxicomania [Psychotropics: Pharmacology and Addiction] (pp. 571–627). Les Presses del'Université de Montréal.

Andre, C. M., Hausman, J.-F., & Guerriero, G. (2016). *Cannabis sativa*: The Plant of the Thousand and One Molecules. *Frontiers in Plant Science*, *7*, 19. doi:10.3389/fpls.2016.00019 PMID:26870049

Anwar, F., Latif, S., & Ashraf, M. (2006). Analytical characterization of hemp (*Cannabis sativa*) seed oil from different agro-ecological zones of Pakistan. *Journal of the American Oil Chemists' Society*, *83*(4), 323–329. doi:10.100711746-006-1207-x

Atalay, S., Gęgotek, A., Wroński, A., Domigues, P., & Skrzydlewska, E. (2021). Therapeutic application of cannabidiol on UVA and UVB irradiated rat skin. A proteomic study. *Journal of Pharmaceutical and Biomedical Analysis*, *192*, 113656. doi:10.1016/j.jpba.2020.113656 PMID:33086172

Badowski, M. E. (2017). A review of oral cannabinoids and medical marijuana for the treatment of chemotherapy-induced nausea and vomiting: A focus on pharmacokinetic variability and pharmacodynamics. *Cancer Chemotherapy and Pharmacology*, *80*(3), 441–449. doi:10.100700280-017-3387-5 PMID:28780725

Bahji, A., & Stephenson, C. (2019). International Perspectives on the Implications of Cannabis Legalization: A Systematic Review & Thematic Analysis. *International Journal of Environmental Research and Public Health*, *16*(17), 3095. doi:10.3390/ijerph16173095 PMID:31454942

Bakowska-Barczak, A., Esparza, Y., Kaur, H., & Popek, T. (2022). Industrial hemp-based dietary supplements and cosmetic products. In M. Pojić & B. K. Tiwari (Eds.), *Industrial Hemp: Food and Nutraceutical Applications* (pp. 247–299). Academic Press. doi:10.1016/B978-0-323-90910-5.00010-5

Baral, P., Bagul, V., & Gajbhiye, S. (2020). Hemp seed oil for skin care (non-drug *Cannabis sativa* L.): A review. *World Journal of Pharmaceutical Research*, *9*(8), 2534–2556.

Baswan, S. M., Klosner, A. E., Glynn, K., Rajgopal, A., Malik, K., Yim, S., & Stern, N. (2020). Therapeutic Potential of Cannabidiol (CBD) for Skin Health and Disorders. *Clinical, Cosmetic and Investigational Dermatology*, *13*, 927–942. doi:10.2147/CCID.S286411 PMID:33335413

Bijauliya, R. K., Alok, S., Kumar, M., Chanchal, D. K., & Yadav, S. (2017). A comprehensive review on herbal cosmetics. *International Journal of Pharmaceutical Sciences and Research*, *8*(12), 4930–4949. doi:10.13040/IJPSR.0975-8232.8(12).4930-49

Bonini, S. A., Premoli, M., Tambaro, S., Kumar, A., Maccarinelli, G., Memo, M., & Mastinu, A. (2018). *Cannabis sativa*: A comprehensive ethnopharmacological review of a medicinal plant with a long history. *Journal of Ethnopharmacology*, *227*, 300–315. doi:10.1016/j.jep.2018.09.004 PMID:30205181

Booth, J. K., Page, J. E., & Bohlmann, J. (2017). Terpene synthases from *Cannabis sativa. PLoS One*, *12*(3), e0173911. doi:10.1371/journal.pone.0173911 PMID:28355238

Borhade, S. S. (2013). Chemical Composition and Characterization of Hemp (*Cannabis sativa*) Seed oil and essential fatty acids by HPLC Method. *Archives of Applied Science Research*, *5*(1), 5–8.

Bornheim, L. M., & Grillo, M. P. (1998). Characterization of Cytochrome P450 3A Inactivation by Cannabidiol: Possible Involvement of Cannabidiol-Hydroxyquinone as a P450 Inactivator. *Chemical Research in Toxicology*, *11*(10), 1209–1216. doi:10.1021/tx9800598 PMID:9778318

Braich, S., Baillie, R. C., Jewell, L. S., Spangenberg, G. C., & Cogan, N. O. (2019). Generation of a Comprehensive Transcriptome Atlas and Transcriptome Dynamics in Medicinal Cannabis. *Scientific Reports*, *9*(1), 1–12. doi:10.103841598-019-53023-6 PMID:31719627

Brunetti, P., Faro, A. F. L., Pirani, F., Berretta, P., Pacifici, R., Pichini, S., & Busardò, F. P. (2020). Pharmacology and legal status of cannabidiol. *Annali dell'Istituto Superiore di Sanita*, *56*(3), 285–291. doi:10.4415/ANN_20_03_06 PMID:32959794

Budney, A. J., & Borodovsky, J. T. (2017). The potential impact of cannabis legalization on the development of cannabis use disorders. *Preventive Medicine*, *104*, 31–36. doi:10.1016/j.ypmed.2017.06.034 PMID:28668544

Bíró, T., Tóth, B. I., Haskó, G., Paus, R., & Pacher, P. (2009). The endocannabinoid system of the skin in health and disease: Novel perspectives and therapeutic opportunities. *Trends in Pharmacological Sciences*, *30*(8), 411–420. doi:10.1016/j.tips.2009.05.004 PMID:19608284

Calvi, L., Pavlovic, R., Panseri, S., Giupponi, L., Leoni, V., & Giorgi, A. (2018). Quality Traits of Medical *Cannabis sativa* L. Inflorescences and Derived Products Based on Comprehensive Mass-Spectrometry Analytical Investigation. In W. J. Costain & R. B. Laprairie (Eds.), *Recent Advances in Cannabinoid Research* (pp. 55–78). IntechOpen. doi:10.5772/intechopen.79539

Cassano, T., Villani, R., Pace, L., Carbone, A., Bukke, V. N., Orkisz, S., Avolio, C., & Serviddio, G. (2020). From *Cannabis sativa* to Cannabidiol: Promising Therapeutic Candidate for the Treatment of Neurodegenerative Diseases. *Frontiers in Pharmacology*, *11*, 124. doi:10.3389/fphar.2020.00124 PMID:32210795

Chandra, S., Lata, H., Khan, I. A., & ElSohly, M. A. (2017). *Cannabis sativa* L.: Botany and Horticulture. In S. Chandra, H. Lata, & M. ElSohly (Eds.), *Cannabis sativa L. - Botany and Biotechnology* (pp. 79–100). Springer. doi:10.1007/978-3-319-54564-6_3

Chouvy, P.-A. (2019). Cannabis cultivation in the world: Heritages, trends and challenges. *EchoGéo*, (48). doi:10.4000/echogeo.17591

Cirimele, V., Kintz, P., Jamey, C., & Ludes, B. (1999). Are Cannabinoids Detected in Hair After Washing With Cannabio® Shampoo? *Journal of Analytical Toxicology*, *23*(5), 349–351. doi:10.1093/jat/23.5.349 PMID:10488922

Clarke, R. C., & Merlin, M. D. (2016). *Cannabis* Domestication, Breeding History, Present-day Genetic Diversity, and Future Prospects. *Critical Reviews in Plant Sciences*, *35*(5-6), 293–327. doi:10.1080/07352689.2016.1267498

Compton, W. M., Han, B., Hughes, A., Jones, C. M., & Blanco, C. (2017). Use of Marijuana for Medical Purposes Among Adults in the United States. *Journal of the American Medical Association*, *317*(2), 209–211. doi:10.1001/jama.2016.18900 PMID:27992636

Cooper, S. (2020). *4 Reasons to use CBD oil for healthy hair*. American Spa. https://www.americanspa.com/cbd/4-reasons-use-cbd-oil-healthy-hair

Dawidowicz, A. L., Olszowy-Tomczyk, M., & Typek, R. (2021). CBG, CBD, Δ9-THC, CBN, CBGA, CBDA and Δ9-THCA as antioxidant agents and their intervention abilities in antioxidant action. *Fitoterapia*, *152*, 104915. doi:10.1016/j.fitote.2021.104915 PMID:33964342

Degenhardt, F., Stehle, F., & Kayser, O. (2017). The Biosynthesis of Cannabinoids. In V. R. Preedy (Ed.), *Handbook of Cannabis and Related Pathologies: Biology, Pharmacology, Diagnosis, and Treatment* (pp. 13–23). Elsevier. doi:10.1016/B978-0-12-800756-3.00002-8

del Río, C., Millán, E., García, V., Appendino, G., DeMesa, J., & Muñoz, E. (2018). The endocannabinoid system of the skin. A potential approach for the treatment of skin disorders. *Biochemical Pharmacology*, *157*, 122–133. doi:10.1016/j.bcp.2018.08.022 PMID:30138623

Devi, M., Thalkari, A. B., & Thorat, V. M. (2022). Overview of Herbal Cosmetics. *Research Journal of Topical and Cosmetic Sciences*, *13*(1), 27–34. doi:10.52711/2321-5844.2022.00005

Devinsky, O., Marsh, E., Friedman, D., Thiele, E., Laux, L., Sullivan, J, & Filloux, F. (2016). Cannabidiol in patients with treatment-resistant epilepsy: An open-label interventional trial. *Lancet Neurology*, *15*(3), 270–278. doi:10.1016/S1474-4422(15)00379-8 PMID:26724101

Draelos, Z. D. (2012). Cosmetics, categories, and the future. *Dermatologic Therapy*, *25*(3), 223–228. doi:10.1111/j.1529-8019.2012.01498.x PMID:22913438

Dubald, M., Bourgeois, S., Andrieu, V., & Fessi, H. (2018). Ophthalmic Drug Delivery Systems for Antibiotherapy—A Review. *Pharmaceutics*, *10*(1), 10. doi:10.3390/pharmaceutics10010010 PMID:29342879

Eagleston, L. R., Kalani, N. K., Patel, R. R., Flaten, H. K., Dunnick, C. A., & Dellavalle, R. P. (2018). Cannabinoids in dermatology: A scoping review. *Dermatology Online Journal*, *24*(6), 1–17. doi:10.5070/D3246040706 PMID:30142706

Feng, Z., Bartholomew, E. S., Liu, Z., Cui, Y., Dong, Y., Li, S., Wu, H., Ren, H., & Liu, X. (2021). Glandular trichomes: New focus on horticultural crops. *Horticulture Research*, *8*(1), 158. doi:10.103841438-021-00592-1 PMID:34193839

Filer, C. N. (2022). Cannabinoids as Cocrystals. *Medical Cannabis and Cannabinoids*, *5*(1), 7–8. doi:10.1159/000521137 PMID:35224435

Freeman, T. P., Hindocha, C., Green, S. F., & Bloomfield, M. A. P. (2019). Medicinal use of cannabis based products and cannabinoids. *BMJ (Clinical Research Ed.)*, *365*, l1141. doi:10.1136/bmj.l1141 PMID:30948383

Gagne, S. J., Stout, J. M., Liu, E., Boubakir, Z., Clark, S. M., & Page, J. E. (2012). Identification of olivetolic acid cyclase from *Cannabis sativa* reveals a unique catalytic route to plant polyketides. *Proceedings of the National Academy of Sciences of the United States of America*, *109*(31), 12811–12816. doi:10.1073/pnas.1200330109 PMID:22802619

Gohad, P., McCoy, J., Wambier, C., Kovacevic, M., Situm, M., Stanimirovic, A., & Goren, A. (2021). Novel cannabidiol sunscreen protects keratinocytes and melanocytes against ultraviolet B radiation. *Journal of Cosmetic Dermatology*, *20*(4), 1350–1352. doi:10.1111/jocd.13693 PMID:32964699

Grassa, C. J., Wenger, J. P., Dabney, C., Poplawski, S. G., Motley, S. T., Michael, T. P., & Weiblen, G. D. (2018). A complete *Cannabis* chromosome assembly and adaptive admixture for elevated cannabidiol (CBD) content. *bioRxiv*, *458083*. doi:10.1101/458083

Grof, C. P. (2018). Cannabis, from plant to pill. *British Journal of Clinical Pharmacology*, *84*(11), 2463–2467. doi:10.1111/bcp.13618 PMID:29701252

Gupta, P. L., Rajput, M., Oza, T., Trivedi, U., & Sanghvi, G. (2019). Eminence of Microbial Products in Cosmetic Industry. *Natural Products and Bioprospecting*, *9*(4), 267–278. doi:10.100713659-019-0215-0 PMID:31214881

Gęgotek, A., Biernacki, M., Ambrożewicz, E., Surażyński, A., Wroński, A., & Skrzydlewska, E. (2016). The cross-talk between electrophiles, antioxidant defence and the endocannabinoid system in fibroblasts and keratinocytes after UVA and UVB irradiation. *Journal of Dermatological Science*, *81*(2), 107–117. doi:10.1016/j.jdermsci.2015.11.005 PMID:26674123

Hammond, C. T., & Mahlberg, P. G. (1994). Phloroglucinol glucoside as a natural constituent of *Cannabis sativa*. *Phytochemistry*, *37*(3), 755–756. doi:10.1016/S0031-9422(00)90352-2

Han, B., Compton, W. M., Blanco, C., & Jones, C. M. (2018). Trends in and correlates of medical marijuana use among adults in the United States. *Drug and Alcohol Dependence*, *186*, 120–129. doi:10.1016/j.drugalcdep.2018.01.022 PMID:29567626

Happyana, N., Agnolet, S., Muntendam, R., Van Dam, A., Schneider, B., & Kayser, O. (2013). Analysis of cannabinoids in laser-microdissected trichomes of medicinal Cannabis sativa using LCMS and cryogenic NMR. *Phytochemistry, 87*, 51–59. doi:10.1016/j.phytochem.2012.11.001 PMID:23280038

Hernandez, C. M., Orsini, C. A., Blaes, S. L., Bizon, J. L., Febo, M., Bruijnzeel, A. W., & Setlow, B. (2021). Effects of repeated adolescent exposure to cannabis smoke on cognitive outcomes in adulthood. *Journal of Psychopharmacology (Oxford, England), 35*(7), 848–863. doi:10.1177/0269881120965931 PMID:33295231

Horne, M. R. (2020). Bast fibres: hemp cultivation and production. In R. M. Kozłowski & M. Mackiewicz-Talarczyk (Eds.), *Handbook of Natural Fibres* (2nd ed., Vol. 1, pp. 163–196). Woodhead Publishing., doi:10.1016/B978-0-12-818398-4.00007-4

Husain, R., Weeden, H., Bogush, D., Deguchi, M., Soliman, M., Potlakayala, S., Katam, R., Goldman, S., & Rudrabhatla, S. (2019). Enhanced tolerance of industrial hemp (*Cannabis sativa* L.) plants on abandoned mine land soil leads to overexpression of cannabinoids. *PLoS One, 14*(8), e0221570. doi:10.1371/journal.pone.0221570 PMID:31465423

Hussain, T., Jeena, G., Pitakbut, T., Vasilev, N., & Kayser, O. (2021). *Cannabis sativa* research trends, challenges, and new-age perspectives. *iScience, 24*(12), 103391. doi:10.1016/j.isci.2021.103391

Kavousi, P., Giamo, T., Arnold, G., Alliende, M., Huynh, E., Lea, J., & Yee, A. (2022). What do we know about opportunities and challenges for localities from Cannabis legalization? *The Review of Policy Research, 39*(2), 143–169. doi:10.1111/ropr.12460

Koltai, H., & Namdar, D. (2020). Cannabis Phytomolecule 'Entourage': From Domestication to Medical Use. *Trends in Plant Science, 25*(10), 976–984. doi:10.1016/j.tplants.2020.04.007 PMID:32417167

Kuddus, M., Ginawi, I. A., & Al-Hazimi, A. (2013). *Cannabis sativa*: An ancient wild edible plant of India. *Emirates Journal of Food and Agriculture, 25*(10), 736–745. doi:10.9755/ejfa.v25i10.16400

Linger, P., Ostwald, A., & Haensler, J. (2005). *Cannabis sativa* L. growing on heavy metal contaminated soil: Growth, cadmium uptake and photosynthesis. *Biologia Plantarum, 49*(4), 567–576. doi:10.100710535-005-0051-4

Lintner, K. (2009). Cosmetic ingredients: Definitions, legal requirements, and an attempt to harmonize (global?) characterization. In K. Lintner (Ed.), *Global Regulatory Issues for the Cosmetics Industry* (pp. 31–53). Elsevier. doi:10.1016/B978-0-8155-1569-2.50009-9

Lowe, H., Toyang, N., Steele, B., Bryant, J., Ngwa, W., & Nedamat, K. (2021). The Current and Potential Application of Medicinal Cannabis Products in Dentistry. *Dentistry Journal, 9*(9), 106. doi:10.3390/dj9090106 PMID:34562980

Lu, G. W. (2010). Recent Advances in Developing Ophthalmic Formulations: A Patent Review. *Recent Patents on Drug Delivery & Formulation, 4*(1), 49–57. doi:10.2174/187221110789957246 PMID:19807679

Machado Bergamaschi, M., Helena Costa Queiroz, R., Waldo Zuardi, A., & Crippa, A. S. (2011). Safety and Side Effects of Cannabidiol, a *Cannabis sativa* Constituent. *Current Drug Safety, 6*(4), 237–249. doi:10.2174/157488611798280924 PMID:22129319

Marks, M. D., Tian, L., Wenger, J. P., Omburo, S. N., Soto-Fuentes, W., He, J., Gang, D. R., Weiblen, G. D., & Dixon, R. A. (2009). Identification of candidate genes affecting Δ^9-tetrahydrocannabinol biosynthesis in *Cannabis sativa. Journal of Experimental Botany*, *60*(13), 3715–3726. doi:10.1093/jxb/erp210 PMID:19581347

Martin, J. H., Hill, C., Walsh, A., Efron, D., Taylor, K., Kennedy, M., & Irving, H. (2020). Clinical trials with cannabis medicines—guidance for ethics committees, governance officers and researchers to streamline ethics applications and ensuring patient safety: Considerations from the Australian experience. *Trials*, *21*(1), 1–7. doi:10.118613063-020-04862-6 PMID:33203469

Martins, A. M., Gomes, A. L., Vilas Boas, I., Marto, J., & Ribeiro, H. M. (2022). Cannabis-Based Products for the Treatment of Skin Inflammatory Diseases: A Timely Review. *Pharmaceuticals*, *15*(2), 210. doi:10.3390/ph15020210 PMID:35215320

Massi, P., Vaccani, A., Bianchessi, S., Costa, B., Macchi, P., & Parolaro, D. (2006). The non-psychoactive cannabidiol triggers caspase activation and oxidative stress in human glioma cells. *Cellular and Molecular Life Sciences CMLS*, *63*(17), 2057–2066. doi:10.100700018-006-6156-x PMID:16909207

McPartland, J. M. (2018). *Cannabis* Systematics at the Levels of Family, Genus, and Species. *Cannabis and Cannabinoid Research*, *3*(1), 203–212. doi:10.1089/can.2018.0039 PMID:30426073

Mead, A. (2017). The legal status of cannabis (marijuana) and cannabidiol (CBD) under US law. *Epilepsy & Behavior*, *70*, 288–291. doi:10.1016/j.yebeh.2016.11.021 PMID:28169144

Miller, R. J., & Miller, R. E. (2017). Is cannabis an effective treatment for joint pain? *Clinical and Experimental Rheumatology*, *35*(5), 59–67. PMID:28967368

Mnekin, L., & Ripoll, L. (2021). Topical Use of Cannabis sativa L. Biochemicals. *Cosmetics*, *8*(3), 85. doi:10.3390/cosmetics8030085

Nadar, R. M., Pathak, S., Ramesh, S., Govindarajulu, M., Moore, T., Agrawal, D. C., & Dhanasekaran, M. (2022). Cannabis-Based Cosmetic Products and Their Uses. In D. C. Agrawal, R. Kumar, & M. Dhanasekaran (Eds.), *Cannabis/Marijuana for Healthcare* (pp. 253–269). Springer., doi:10.1007/978-981-16-8822-5_13

Naim-Feil, E., Pembleton, L. W., Spooner, L. E., Malthouse, A. L., Miner, A., Quinn, M., Polotnianka, R. M., Baillie, R. C., Spangenberg, G. C., & Cogan, N. O. (2021). The characterization of key physiological traits of medicinal cannabis (*Cannabis sativa* L.) as a tool for precision breeding. *BMC Plant Biology*, *21*(1), 1–15. doi:10.118612870-021-03079-2 PMID:34174826

Napimoga, M. H., Benatti, B. B., Lima, F. O., Alves, P. M., Campos, A. C., Pena-dos-Santos, D. R., Severino, F. P., Cunha, F. Q., & Guimarães, F. S. (2009). Cannabidiol decreases bone resorption by inhibiting RANK/RANKL expression and pro-inflammatory cytokines during experimental periodontitis in rats. *International Immunopharmacology*, *9*(2), 216–222. doi:10.1016/j.intimp.2008.11.010 PMID:19070683

Oláh, A., Tóth, B. I., Borbíró, I., Sugawara, K., Szöllõsi, A. G., Czifra, G., & Camera, E. (2014). Cannabidiol exerts sebostatic and antiinflammatory effects on human sebocytes. *The Journal of Clinical Investigation*, *124*(9), 3713–3724. doi:10.1172/JCI64628 PMID:25061872

Pacula, R. L., & Smart, R. (2017). Medical Marijuana and Marijuana Legalization. *Annual Review of Clinical Psychology, 13*(1), 397–419. doi:10.1146/annurev-clinpsy-032816-045128 PMID:28482686

Pandey, A., Jatana, G. K., & Sonthalia, S. (2021). Cosmeceuticals. In *StatPearls*. StatPearls Publishing.

Paul, R., Williams, R., Hodson, V., & Peake, C. (2019). Detection of cannabinoids in hair after cosmetic application of hemp oil. *Scientific Reports, 9*(1), 1–6. doi:10.103841598-019-39609-0 PMID:30796346

Pertwee, R. (2008). The diverse CB_1 and CB_2 receptor pharmacology of three plant cannabinoids: Δ^9-tetrahydrocannabinol, cannabidiol and Δ^9-tetrahydrocannabivarin. *British Journal of Pharmacology, 153*(2), 199–215. doi:10.1038j.bjp.0707442 PMID:17828291

Peyravian, N., Deo, S., Daunert, S., & Jimenez, J. J. (2022). The Anti-Inflammatory Effects of Cannabidiol (CBD) on Acne. *Journal of Inflammation Research, 15*, 2795–2801. doi:10.2147/JIR.S355489 PMID:35535052

Punyamurthula, N. S., Adelli, G. R., Gul, W., Repka, M. A., ElSohly, M. A., & Majumdar, S. (2017). Ocular Disposition of Δ^8-Tetrahydrocannabinol from Various Topical Ophthalmic Formulations. *AAPS PharmSciTech, 18*(6), 1936–1945. doi:10.120812249-016-0672-2 PMID:27905004

Raharjo, T. J., Chang, W.-T., Choi, Y. H., Peltenburg-Looman, A. M., & Verpoorte, R. (2004). Olivetol as product of a polyketide synthase in *Cannabis sativa* L. *Plant Science, 166*(2), 381–385. doi:10.1016/j.plantsci.2003.09.027

Rajput, R., & Kumar, K. (2018). A Review on *Cannabis sativa*: Its Compounds and Their Effects. *International Journal of Pharmaceutical Sciences Review and Research, 53*(2), 59–63.

Richard, M., Ganguly, R., Steigerwald, S., Al-Khalifa, A., & Pierce, G. (2007). Dietary hempseed reduces platelet aggregation. *Journal of Thrombosis and Haemostasis, 5*(2), 424–425. doi:10.1111/j.1538-7836.2007.02327.x PMID:17155962

Rodriguez-Morrison, V., Llewellyn, D., & Zheng, Y. (2021). Cannabis Inflorescence Yield and Cannabinoid Concentration Are Not Increased With Exposure to Short-Wavelength Ultraviolet-B Radiation. *Frontiers in Plant Science, 12*, 725078. doi:10.3389/fpls.2021.725078 PMID:34795683

Rough, L. (2017). 7 Must-Try Cannabis Topicals for Those Scorching Summer Days. *Leafly*. https://www.leafly.com/news/strains-products/cannabis-topicals-for-summer

Russo, E., & Guy, G. W. (2006). A tale of two cannabinoids: The therapeutic rationale for combining tetrahydrocannabinol and cannabidiol. *Medical Hypotheses, 66*(2), 234–246. doi:10.1016/j.mehy.2005.08.026 PMID:16209908

Russo, E. B. (2017). Cannabidiol Claims and Misconceptions. *Trends in Pharmacological Sciences, 38*(3), 198–201. doi:10.1016/j.tips.2016.12.004 PMID:28089139

Russo, E. B., Jiang, H.-E., Li, X., Sutton, A., Carboni, A., Del Bianco, F., & Bera, S. (2008). Phytochemical and genetic analyses of ancient cannabis from Central Asia. *Journal of Experimental Botany, 59*(15), 4171–4182. doi:10.1093/jxb/ern260 PMID:19036842

Sarma, N. D., Waye, A., ElSohly, M. A., Brown, P. N., Elzinga, S., Johnson, H. E., & Deyton, L. (2020). Cannabis Inflorescence for Medical Purposes: USP Considerations for Quality Attributes. *Journal of Natural Products*, *83*(4), 1334–1351. doi:10.1021/acs.jnatprod.9b01200 PMID:32281793

Sheriff, T., Lin, M. J., Dubin, D., & Khorasani, H. (2020). The potential role of cannabinoids in dermatology. *The Journal of Dermatological Treatment*, *31*(8), 839–845. doi:10.1080/09546634.2019.1675854 PMID:31599175

Singh, B., & Sharma, R. A. (2015). Plant terpenes: defense responses, phylogenetic analysis, regulation and clinical applications. *3 Biotech*, *5*(2), 129-151. doi:10.1007/s13205-014-0220-2

Slusarkiewicz-Jarzina, A., Ponitka, A., & Kaczmarek, Z. (2005). Influence of cultivar, explant source and plant growth regulator on callus induction and plant regeneration of *Cannabis sativa* L. *Acta Biologica Cracoviensia. Series; Botanica*, *47*(2), 145–151.

Small, E. (2015). Classification of *Cannabis sativa* (Marijuana, Hemp) in Relation to Human Utilization. *Botanical Review*, *81*(3), 189–294. doi:10.100712229-015-9157-3

Small, E., & Naraine, S. G. (2016). Size matters: Evolution of large drug-secreting resin glands in elite pharmaceutical strains of *Cannabis sativa* (marijuana). *Genetic Resources and Crop Evolution*, *63*(2), 349–359. doi:10.100710722-015-0254-2

Spindle, T. R., Bonn-Miller, M. O., & Vandrey, R. (2019). Changing landscape of cannabis: Novel products, formulations, and methods of administration. *Current Opinion in Psychology*, *30*, 98–102. doi:10.1016/j.copsyc.2019.04.002 PMID:31071592

Spitzer-Rimon, B., Duchin, S., Bernstein, N., & Kamenetsky, R. (2019). Architecture and Florogenesis in Female *Cannabis sativa* Plants. *Frontiers in Plant Science*, *10*, 350. doi:10.3389/fpls.2019.00350 PMID:31001293

Stahl, V., & Vasudevan, K. (2020). Comparison of Efficacy of Cannabinoids versus Commercial Oral Care Products in Reducing Bacterial Content from Dental Plaque: A Preliminary Observation. *Cureus*, *12*(1), e6809. doi:10.7759/cureus.6809 PMID:32038896

Stella, A., Palmieri, B., Laurino, C., & Vadalà, M. (2019). A therapeutic effect of cbd-enriched ointment in inflammatory skin diseases and cutaneous scars. *La Clinica Terapeutica*, *170*(2), e93–e99. doi:10.7417/CT.2019.2116 PMID:30993303

Stout, J. M., Boubakir, Z., Ambrose, S. J., Purves, R. W., & Page, J. E. (2012). The hexanoyl-CoA precursor for cannabinoid biosynthesis is formed by an acyl-activating enzyme in *Cannabis sativa* trichomes. *The Plant Journal*, *71*(3), 353–365. doi:10.1111/j.1365-313X.2012.04949.x PMID:22353623

Suryavanshi, S. V., Kovalchuk, I., & Kovalchuk, O. (2020). Cannabinoids as Key Regulators of Inflammasome Signaling: A Current Perspective. *Frontiers in Immunology*, *11*, 613613. doi:10.3389/fimmu.2020.613613 PMID:33584697

Szabó, I. L., Lisztes, E., Béke, G., Tóth, K. F., Paus, R., Oláh, A., & Bíró, T. (2020). The Phytocannabinoid (–)-Cannabidiol Operates as a Complex, Differential Modulator of Human Hair Growth: Anti-Inflammatory Submicromolar versus Hair Growth Inhibitory Micromolar Effects. *The Journal of Investigative Dermatology*, *140*(2), 484–488. doi:10.1016/j.jid.2019.07.690 PMID:31369737

Tahir, M. N., Shahbazi, F., Rondeau-Gagné, S., & Trant, J. F. (2021). The biosynthesis of the cannabinoids. *Journal of Cannabis Research*, *3*(1), 1–12. doi:10.118642238-021-00062-4 PMID:33722296

Taskar, P. (2019). *Formulation development, preclinical testing, and primary packaging optimization for cannabinoids and other therapeutics*. University of Mississippi.

Telek, A., Bíró, T., Bodó, E., Tóth, B. I., Borbíró, I., Kunos, G., & Paus, R. (2007). Inhibition of human hair follicle growth by endo-and exocannabinoids. *The FASEB Journal*, *21*(13), 3534–3541. doi:10.1096/fj.06-7689com PMID:17567570

Tian, N., Liu, F., Wang, P., Zhang, X., Li, X., & Wu, G. (2017). The molecular basis of glandular trichome development and secondary metabolism in plants. *Plant Gene*, *12*, 1–12. doi:10.1016/j.plgene.2017.05.010

Tyrrell, S. (2019). *How Cannabis Eye Creams Can Help With Puffy-Looking Eyes*. Cannabis MD. https://cannabismd.com/beauty/skin-care/how-cannabis-eye-creams-can-help-with-puffy-looking-eyes/

Vaidya, M., Choudhury, A., Brumlik, C., Agrawal, D. C., & Kumar, R. (2022). A Complete Patent Analysis of Cannabis/Marijuana in Drug Delivery and Disease Conditions. In D. C. Agrawal, R. Kumar, & M. Dhanasekaran (Eds.), *Cannabis/Marijuana for Healthcare* (pp. 1–34). Springer. doi:10.1007/978-981-16-8822-5_1

Valizadehderakhshan, M., Shahbazi, A., Kazem-Rostami, M., Todd, M. S., Bhowmik, A., & Wang, L. (2021). Extraction of Cannabinoids from *Cannabis sativa* L. (Hemp)—. *Revista de Agricultura (Piracicaba)*, *11*(5), 384. doi:10.3390/agriculture11050384

Van Bakel, H., Stout, J. M., Cote, A. G., Tallon, C. M., Sharpe, A. G., Hughes, T. R., & Page, J. E. (2011). The draft genome and transcriptome of *Cannabis sativa. Genome Biology*, *12*(10), 1–18. doi:10.1186/gb-2011-12-10-r102 PMID:22014239

Vasudevan, K., & Stahl, V. (2020). Cannabinoids infused mouthwash products are as effective as chlorhexidine on inhibition of total-culturable bacterial content in dental plaque samples. *Journal of Cannabis Research*, *2*(1), 1–9. doi:10.118642238-020-00027-z PMID:33526124

Verma, R., Hoda, F., Arshad, M., Iqubal, A., Siddiqui, A. N., Khan, M. A., Haque, S. E., Akhtar, M., & Najmi, A. K. (2021). Cannabis, a Miracle Drug with Polyvalent Therapeutic Utility: Preclinical and Clinical-Based Evidence. *Medical Cannabis and Cannabinoids*, *4*(1), 43–60. doi:10.1159/000515042 PMID:34676349

Vincenzi, C., & Tosti, A. (2020). Efficacy and Tolerability of a Shampoo Containing Broad-Spectrum Cannabidiol in the Treatment of Scalp Inflammation in Patients with Mild to Moderate Scalp Psoriasis or Seborrheic Dermatitis. *Skin Appendage Disorders*, *6*(6), 355–361. doi:10.1159/000510896 PMID:33313051

Vogl, C. R., Mölleken, H., Lissek-Wolf, G., Surböck, A., & Kobert, J. (2004). Hemp (*Cannabis sativa* L.) as a resource for green cosmetics: Yield of seed and fatty acid compositions of 20 varieties under the growing conditions of organic farming in Austria. *Journal of Industrial Hemp*, *9*(1), 51–68. doi:10.1300/J237v09n01_06

Vulfsons, S., Minerbi, A., & Sahar, T. (2020). Cannabis and Pain Treatment—A Review of the Clinical Utility and a Practical Approach in Light of Uncertainty. *Rambam Maimonides Medical Journal*, *11*(1), e0002. doi:10.5041/RMMJ.10385 PMID:32017678

Wilson, D. (2021). *Cannabidiol (CBD) in Hair Oil*. Science Senior Seminar.

Xiong, W., Cui, T., Cheng, K., Yang, F., Chen, S.-R., Willenbring, D., & Xu, Y. (2012). Cannabinoids suppress inflammatory and neuropathic pain by targeting α3 glycine receptors. *The Journal of Experimental Medicine*, *209*(6), 1121–1134. doi:10.1084/jem.20120242

Zagórska-Dziok, M., Bujak, T., Ziemlewska, A., & Nizioł-Łukaszewska, Z. (2021). Positive Effect of *Cannabis sativa* L. Herb Extracts on Skin Cells and Assessment of Cannabinoid-Based Hydrogels Properties. *Molecules (Basel, Switzerland)*, *26*(4), 802. doi:10.3390/molecules26040802 PMID:33557174

Zhang, Q., Chen, X., Guo, H., Trindade, L. M., Salentijn, E. M., Guo, R., Guo, M., Xu, Y., & Yang, M. (2018). Latitudinal Adaptation and Genetic Insights Into the Origins of *Cannabis sativa* L. *Frontiers in Plant Science*, *9*, 1876. doi:10.3389/fpls.2018.01876 PMID:30627133

Zuk-Golaszewska, K., & Golaszewski, J. (2018). *Cannabis sativa* L.–cultivation and quality of raw material. *Journal of Elementology*, *23*(3), 971–984. doi:10.5601/jelem.2017.22.3.1500

Chapter 7
Bioactive Properties and Food Applications of *Cannabis sativa* and Applications of Its Molecular Modeling

Sefa Celik
https://orcid.org/0000-0001-6216-1297
Istanbul University, Turkey

Elif Cakir
Istanbul Aydin University, Turkey

Alev Er
Istanbul University, Turkey

ABSTRACT

In addition to being the oldest cultivated plant from past to present as a raw material source, Cannabis sativa L. is a strategically characteristic plant used for food, medicine, cosmetics, and pharmacological purposes. Molecular modeling is an important means for elucidating molecular structures and plays an important role in the design and development of new pharmaceuticals. This chapter includes the beneficial properties of the primary and secondary metabolites contained in cannabis such as foaming, emulsifying, gelling, film formation; antioxidant, antimicrobial activities and bakery products by means of their superior nutritional values, snack products, dairy products, processed meat products, in beverages such as coffees, teas, soda and functional food ingredients in many other areas of the food industry, nutritional supplements, usability in the development of new food formulations on hemp and molecular modeling studies on constituents of cannabis sativa.

DOI: 10.4018/978-1-6684-5718-4.ch007

INTRODUCTION

Cannabis, named *Cannabis sativa* L., belongs to the Cannabaceae family and is among the herbal raw material sources, except pleasurable strain (medical cannabis); food, textile, paper, building materials (Schluttenhofer & Yuan, 2017; Zhang et al., 2016), medicine (Andre et al., 2016), is an industrial plant for nutraceutical and cosmetic purposes (Liu et al., 2022) with multifunctional economic benefits in different industries (Lu & Clarke, 1995; Zhang et al., 2016). Cannabis was initially known as a pleasure ingredient, but after research, it was classified according to its psychoactive properties according to the amount of tetra-hydrocannabinol (THC) it contains. While Cannabis sativa subsp. indica species which contains more than 0.3% THC (Chen & Pan, 2021; Guo et al., 2018; Liu et al., 2022) is classified as pleasurable, the specie contains less than 0.3% THC (Guo et al., 2018) is classified as Cannabis sativa subsp. sativa characterized as a specie used in the pharmaceutical industry (Andre et al., 2016; Small & Cronquist, 1976).

Most European countries allow the cultivation of hemp containing the upper legal limit of 0.2% THC for fiber and seed production (Petrović et al., 2015; Russo & Marcu, 2017). For these reasons, it has been a forbidden plant to be grown, kept and used in most countries. Thanks to increasing scientific research in recent years, it is a strategic plant that has been determined to have functional product development potential thanks to bioactive compounds such as protein, amino acids, cannabinoids and terpenes obtained from cannabis plants (Andre et al., 2016; Pap et al., 2020). It is among the plants cultivated from the past to the present (Pellati et al., 2018; Xu et al., 2021) and has been the focus of attention of investors with its ability to keep up with variable agro-climatic conditions. Hemp is harvested for its fibers and seeds. Hemp plants harvested for their fiber are taller and have a very low cannabinoid content. The cannabis plant harvested for cannabinoids is shorter and rich in cannabinoid content (Chen & Pan, 2021). The fact that hemp is rich in fiber contributes to the development of the textile industry, while increasing its popularity in the food industry thanks to the amino acids, essential oils and bioactive components it contains (Christinat et al., 2020).

NUTRITIONAL PROPERTIES OF CANNABIS

In particular, hemp proteins have high nutritional value quality with their essential amino acid content (Callaway, 2004; Shen et al., 2021). It has been determined that hemp seeds contain 25-35% fatty acids, 20-25% protein, 20-30% carbohydrates, 10-15% fiber and trace amounts of minerals, amino acids containing good amount of sulphur in terms of protein structure with high nutritional value and all nine essential amino acids in an appropriate ratio with very high arginine and glutamic acid (Callaway, 2004).

Hemp seeds have legumin and albumin two main proteins and are especially rich in arginine and glutamic acid amino acids and are easily digestible (Callaway et al., 2004; Dunford, 2015; Odani & Odani, 1998). While in studies on the digestibility of hemp proteins, the digestibility of peeled off hemp seeds was found as 90.8%-97.5%, this value was comparable to casein (97.6%), it was stated that the digestibility of hemp seeds increased as peel off and it was emphasized that it was an efficient protein source for human consumption (House et al., 2010; Xian-Sheng, 2007). Stearidonic acid (C18:4 omega-3), obtained from hemp seed is considered very valuable for its content (Callaway et al., 2004; Iványi, 2006). These seeds are also seen as a source of dietary fiber. The thiamine content of hemp is competitive with cereals such as oats, wheat, and rye (Murkovic et al., 1997). In addition, the seeds are often marketed with glume or without glume hemp seeds, and oil is produced by extraction and cold pressing (Ferrante et al., 2019).

Common *Cannavis sativa* L varieties have 20–36% ratio of oil content, with the main fatty acid being linoleic acid. Apart from this, linolenic and stearidonic acid are found in remarkable proportions. Research has shown that the seed oil's 6:3 fatty acid composition sets it apart from more conventional seed oils and presents new possibilities for the creation of innovative dietary supplements (Dunford, 2015).

It has been reported that approximately 200 cannabinoids obtained from the leaves of *C. sativa* have been identified (Baldino et al., 2020). One of its important secondary metabolites is alkaloids, and about 70 alkaloids (Janeczek et al., 2018) have been identified, of which D9-THC is the most psychoactive substance. *C. sativa* is rich in terpenoids, as the primary source of aroma (Booth & Bohlmann, 2019).

USE OF HEMP IN FOOD PRODUCTION

Hemp is used as an effective strategy in bioactive compounds that increase nutritional value in human nutrition and provide protective properties and in the production of new or developed high-quality food products that increase the functional properties of food products. Studies report that the global market for edible hemp products for 2017 is \$8.4 billion, and the market share will reach an estimated \$25.7 billion after 2022 (King, 2019). The fact that the cholesterol-free seeds of hemp (*Cannabis sativa L.*) are rich in protein, vitamins and minerals, contain plenty of dietary fiber and bioactive are seen as a raw material source in the food industry (Chen & Pan, 2021). Studies have shown that the protein solubility of hemp seed cake through enzymatic processes will directly affect its applicability in food products and play an important role in the functional character of the product (Wang et al., 2019).

The hemp plant is seen as a very valuable fiber and oil plant. While fiber is obtained from the stems of the plant, oil is obtained from the seed of the plant. Hemp (*Cannabis sativa L.*), grown for industrial use and harvested for fiber, seeds, oil, flour, is gaining great interest as a sustainable crop that does not require fertilizers, herbicides, and pesticides (Ferrante et al., 2019; Vonapartis et al., 2015). In a study on seed oil (Borhade, 2013), it was determined that hemp seed oil extracted with hexane is liquid at room temperature, has a yellow color and a soft taste, depending on its full maturity it can have strong and sharp taste (Blade et al., 2006). Since hemp oils used in food products are bitter, have tar-like properties on the consistency, and because of their viscosity, they pose a challenge in the formulation of their final products.

Working on constitute to standard procedure and addition to aroma-bearing components for these kind of final product formulations appealing to consumers (Kladar et al., 2021). De-oiled and ground seed pulp is considered as protein-rich flour (Callaway et al., 2004).

Hemp seeds are used extensively in the food industry, and improved products such as powders, concentrates, hemp cake, isolates of hemp produced with different technologies; it has been evaluated in bakery products, snack products, beverages, dairy products, processed meat products and in many more areas. It is especially used in salad souce, crackers, chips, bread, macaroni cookies, ice cream production (Apostol et al., 2015; Dabija et al., 2018) and in the food industry as a stand-alone snack (Lachenmeier, 2004). It is also included in Europe in breakfast cereals, coffees, teas, carbonated beverages to which cannabinoid extracts are added, health-beneficial honeys and formulations of fortified sports products (Doğan & Doğan, 2021; King, 2019) and in different kinds of food products.

Although bread has been included in the diet of human beings from past to present, today's view of bread has changed as a result of consumers demand for healthy and nutritious products. Grinding the seed plays a role in turning it into fine flour with a grain-like composition (Perlín, 2002). Flour obtained from hemp has antiallergic, antiatherogenic, anti-inflammatory, antimicrobial, antiviral, anticancer and cardioprotective effects thanks to the bioactive compounds it contains (Callaway, 2004; Manach et al., 2005). After the extraction for the production of hemp seed oil, a cake with is obtained seed pulp is obtained together with the residual oil with high nutritional value containing hemp protein (Callaway, 2004; Mattila et al., 2018; Pap et al., 2020) and these obtained products can be used as a replacement agent instead of some components in foods or by adding to the formulation (Ferrante et al., 2019). In addition, the essential amino acids contained in hemp are rich in sulfur (Wang et al., 2008), hemp proteins are generally well tolerated and show very rare or mild allergic reactions were determined by the work done. For this reason, bakery products are at the forefront of the sectors in which hemp use is the most researched subject and in particular, research has been carried out on functional components to improvement of bread in terms of nutrition and health.

In a study, they examined effects on the rheological properties of the dough which they produce by used hemp flour and hemp protein concentrate instead of 10% or 20% starch and the quality of the bread crumb and the staling rate in gluten-free breads made of cornstarch and potato starch. While the addition of hemp flour causes the dough structure to weaken and become more susceptible to deformation, 20% of the hemp protein concentrate strengthens the structure of the dough tested. In addition, it has been determined that it increases the fiber content and bread volume, and the color of the bread crumb and the taste of the bread are accepted sensory (Korus et al., 2017).

In another study on bakery, they examined the effects of breads made by replacing 550 types of wheat flour (PZZ Krakow, Poland) with degreased hemp flour at certain rates on chemical, texture, organoleptic properties, and furan derivatives. The addition of hemp flour increased the protein content and polyphenol content of the breads and used hemp flour causes the formation of furan derivatives were determined. It has been stated that industrial production should be below this value as a result of the fact that hemp flour exceeding 30% did not receive a positive score in the sensory evaluation (Mikulec et al., 2019).

Another study on hemp is the effect of hemp by-products on lactic acid bacteria in fermented foods. One of the studies conducted for this purpose is on the prebiotic potential activity of seed bran fermented by Lactobacilli. It has been shown that hemp seed bran can be considered as a product with prebiotic activity with organic acids that support the growth of probiotics and bioactive compounds in its content. As a result of the study, it was seen that hemp seed bran is the source of life for starter lactobacilli in fermentation. Fermentation improved the prebiotic potential of hemp seed bran (Nissen et al., 2021).

In another study (Nionelli et al., 2018), Lactobacillus plantarum, *Pediococcus acidilactici* and *Leuconostoc mesenteroides* lactic acid bacteria isolated and identified from type I sourdough produced from hemp (Cannabis sativa L.) flour is used as starter culture in wheat sourdough production. These sourdoughs were included in the formulation of 5% - 15% wheat bread and they produced wheat bread with hemp sour yeast. It has been determined that breads enriched with hemp sourdoughs increase protein digestibility, significantly reduce the predicted glycemic index and improve texture compared to wheat bread (Nionelli et al., 2018).

In a study on gluten-free bread, acceptability potential and quality of gluten-free corn/rice bread of sourdough which produced using chia, quinoa, hemp flour and *Lactobacillus sanfranciscensis* lactic acid bacteria were investigated.

Studies was done conducted on biscuits and gluten-free cracker containing hemp flour, hemp seeds, hemp fiber. In one of these studies, biscuits based on corn- hemp flour (80/20, 40/60 and 60/40) blends (Korus et al., 2017; Xu et al., 2020) were developed. However, the protein and total polyphenol content of the biscuits were shown to rise with the addition of hemp flour, offsetting the biscuits' decreased volume and increased hardness. Further, it was found that the biscuits had a greater propensity toward a deeper hue as the proportion of hemp flour rose (Korus et al., 2017).

Hemp and decaf green tea leaves have been shown to enhance the level of protein, fibre, antioxidants, minerals, and fatty acids relative to the control (Radočaj et al., 2014; Xu et al., 2020). It has also been developed as gluten-free crackers in by-products like 4-14% seeds and fewer than 9% seed pods, and favourable improvements in protein, fibre, and antioxidant activities of crackers have been discovered. The research in this area has been promising (Martin-Diana et al., 2017; Xu et al., 2020).

Hemp cake, a by-product of cold pressing hemp seeds to extract oil, was added to potato chips in various concentrations to examine its influence on the chips' physicochemical and antioxidant qualities. Protein, total dietary fibre, and phenolic content were all shown to be considerably higher with the addition of 20% hemp seed cake. Unsaturated fatty acid residues in the hemp seed cake were said to hasten lipid oxidation in the sample, suggesting the necessity for more research on chips (Feng et al., 2022). With regards to edibles, it has been observed that the cannabinoids found in hemp are mostly used in tea and tea mixes. To make hemp tea or a tea mix based on hemp, the cannabinoids-rich hemp leaves are employed in several countries (Ferrante et al., 2019; Kladar et al., 2021). It is well knowledge that the inflorescences (or "flowers") of the hemp plant contain the highest concentrations of cannabinoids. These inflorescences are made up of glandular structures called trichomes (Glivar et al., 2020). Hemp inflorescences are a good source of cannabinoids, hence teas (or tea blends) containing them are preferable. (King, 2019). Hemp milk, made from hemp seeds that have been roasted and shelled, is hypoallergenic because it retains most of its natural nutrients and is lactose-free. Hemp seeds have been linked to a drop in blood cholesterol, triacylglycerol, and thyroid hormones. That's why many people are switching to hemp milk from other options like almond, soy, and even hazelnut (Wang et al., 2018).

Milk alternatives like soy and rice drinks are the subject of much research. Researchers fermented commercial hemp seed with *Lactobacillus fermentum, Lactobacillus plantarum*, and *Bifidobacterium bifidum* to create a novel beverage recipe. The bioactive chemicals in hemp seeds have been studied, and it has been shown that they promote the health and viability of probiotic strains and activate prebiotics (Nissen et al., 2020).

Nanoemulsions are also included in studies on hemp. Nanoemulsions have a wide range of uses in the food industry to increase the shelf life and improve the quality of foods. In a study done it was used to form a stable nanoemulsion of hemp seed (*Cannabis sativa*) oil as emulsifier with lecithin as co-surfactant. It has been found to be important in terms of showing good stability property, not having a negative effect on taste in terms of sensory and offering potential usage opportunities in biomedical and cosmetic applications (Jarzębski et al., 2019).

Molecular Modeling Applications on Constituents of *Cannabis sativa* and Its Derivatives

Numerous theoretical and computational approaches are at the heart of molecular modelling, which is then utilised to illustrate molecular, ionic, or particle structures (Barbosa et al., 2017). When John Dalton proposed that atoms are the fundamental building blocks of matter, it was the early 1800s (Dalton, 1808).

Given that he included sketches of atoms and compounds in his writings, his sketches may be considered the earliest visual depiction of molecules. Edward Frankland introduced the concept of atomic bonding in 1852 (Frankland, 1852). In 1858, Archibald Couper added to this hypothesis by demonstrating that carbon is tetravalent and may be linked together to create lengthy chains (Couper, 1858). In his essay, Couper demonstrated the links between atoms by the use of dashed lines. Later on, it was developed by Alexander Crum Brown, who portrayed each atom as a letter inside of a circle and linked it to its neighbours using straight lines (Crum Brown, 1864; 1867). With only minor modifications, these structural formulas are still used today (Perkins, 2005).

The structure-activity correlations of medications and their mechanisms of action may be better understood with the use of an essential technique known as molecular modelling. Molecular modelling tools allow for the electrical and steric molecular features of the interaction between pharmaceuticals and macromolecules to be shown in three dimensions. This allows for a more accurate understanding of the interaction. (Santos et al., 2014). Thanks to the significant advances in molecular modeling techniques in recent years, molecular modeling has become fundamental components of chemical, physical and biological studies (Saxena et al., 2009).

Below are the researches of molecular modeling applications in the subject area:

In a study conducted in 2017, molecular docking studies were done with the Arachidonate 5-lypoxygenase enzyme of some fundamental cannabinoids included in Cannabis sativa. As a result of this analysis, it was found that the docking between the 5-LO enzyme and Cannabigerol was more stable compared to the other molecules used in the study. Cannabinoids obtained from the Cannabis sativa L. plant and the seized cannabis resin were found to inhibit the Arachidonate 5-lipoxygenase enzyme better than the drug Zileuton. When molecular docking results were compared, cannabigerol was found to be the best inhibitor (Bouchentouf et al., 2017). Medical cannabis contains many chemical molecules such as cannabigerol, cannabidol, cannabichromene, tetrahydrocannabivarin, cannabigerovarinic acid and cannabidiolic acid. Calculations were done in the 2020 research to compare the chemical and biological functions of these six compounds. These compounds' quantum chemical properties were computed using the DFT/B3LYP approach and several basis sets. Additionally, these compounds' biological activity against Liver Cancer 1 were investigated. Investigations were done on interactions impacting the cannabichromene molecule's biological activity. Gaussian and docking calculations showed that the Cannabichromene molecule has the highest biological and chemical activity (Tuzun, 2020). In the study conducted on the derivatives of cannabinoids in 2018, the optimized molecular structures of 5 different cannabinoid derivatives containing indole-3-carboxylate and indazole-3-carboxylate were determined by DFT/B3LYP/6-311G** level of theory. As a result of the calculations, it was found that the energy band gap of the Naphthalene-1-yl 1-(5-fluoropentyl)-1H-indazole-3-carboxylate molecule has the lowest band gap energy indicating the effect on intramolecular charge transfer (Abdulsalami et al., 2018). In the study conducted by Silva and co-workers in 2008, 30 cannabinoid metabolites were investigated using electronic and chemometric methods. Optimized geometries and energies were calculated using density functional calculations (Silva et al., 2008). In the study conducted in 2021, strong interactions were found between the β2 adrenergic receptor of the adrenergic system and the Cannabidiol (CBD) and Δ-9-tetrahydrocannabinol (Δ-9-THC) molecules with molecular docking studies. As a result of the calculation, it was found that the Δ-9-THC molecule had the best binding affinity with -9 kcal/mol. The interaction of the human β2 adrenergic receptor with amino acid TYR316 caused it to have a strong binding potential. It has been calculated that the CBD molecule interacts with the amino acids TYR308 and THR110 of the human β2 adrenergic receptor and has a binding energy of -8.7 kcal/mol (Erukainure et al., 2021[a]). In 2021, the Gaussian09 software was used to optimise the chemical structure of compounds including tetrahydrocannabivarin, cannabispiran, cannabidiol tetrahydrocannabinol, cannabigerol, and cannabinol. These compounds' structures, together with their interactions and binding energies, were determined by docking them into the active conformation of the chosen receptors. Hydrogen bonds, hydrophobic contacts, and others not often seen in nature are all examples of these interactions (Erukainure et al., 2021[b]).

Geometry optimization of 1-Pentyl-3-(4-methoxy-1-naphthoyl) indole and 2-(2-methoxy-phenyl)-1-(1-pentyl-1H-indol-3-yl)-ethanone molecules were done by DFT/B3LYP/6-31G** level of theory and their electronic structures were determined. It has been found that intramolecular and intermolecular hydrogen bonds contribute to the conformation of both molecules (Nycz et al., 2010).

In a study conducted in 2018, theoretical and experimental studies were done on the molecule 5F-PB-22 (1-(5-fluoropentyl)-8-quinolinyl ester-1H-indole-3-carboxylic acid), which is a synthetic cannabinoid. The optimized geometry of this molecule was determined by using DFT/B3LYP/3-21 level of theory (Alkaseem et al., 2018).

In the study conducted in 2021, (-)-trans-Δ^9- tetrahydrocannabinol and (-)-cannabidiol molecules, which are natural cannabinoids found in the cannabis plant, were investigated. These compounds also interact with cannabinoid receptors in the human body. The structural calculations of the conformers of these compounds were made by using B3LYP-D3BJ/6-31+G(d,p) level of theory. Conformational flexibility was investigated depends on the alkyl side chain (Baranović, 2021).

In the study conducted by Bindesri, tetrahydrocannabinol and carboxy-tetrahydrocannabinol molecules were optimized by various methods and checked the z matrix coordinates by using vibrational frequencies (Bindesri et al., 2020).

The antioxidant mechanism of tetrahydrocannabinol and cannabidiol molecules was interpreted in 2013 by comparing them to -tocopherol, butylhydroxytoluene, and hydroxytoluene using the DFT approach. The electronic characteristics were studied, including the kind of frontier orbitals present, the ionisation potential, the dissociation energy of O-H bonds, the stabilisation energy, and the distribution of spin densities. Based on calculated HOMO and ionisation potential values, it was determined that the tetrahydrocannabinol molecule has a greater antioxidant potential than the phenol, ether, and alkyl molecules (Borges et al., 2013).

In the study by Crocioni, Δ^9-Tetrahydrocannabinolic acid, cannabidiolic acid, cannabigerolic acid, Δ^9-tetrahydrocannabinol, cannabidiol and cannabigerol molecules, which are the most relevant in terms of concentration and properties, were optimized with the MMFF94 force field using the Avagadro program. Then, the equilibrium structure was determined with the DFT/B3LYP/6-31G(d,p) level of theory. Molecular geometries obtained by using DFT were compared with the initial geometry (Crocioni, 2021).

Kazami and co-workers performed molecular docking analysis between P-glycoprotein (P-gp) and lignanamides which were obtained from cannabis sativa. Tariquidar and zosuquidar molecules, which are P-gp inhibitors, were chosen as control ligands in this study. Therefore, a comparison was made between the binding affinities discovered using molecular docking research. Findings showed that both cannabisin M and cannabisin N molecules had greater binding affinities than the control ligands. The findings suggest that cannabisins M and N are promising therapeutic options for treating P-gp receptor dysfunction (Kazemi et al., 2021).

To aid in the fight against malaria, scientists in 2021 performed in-depth computational analyses of 125 chemicals isolated from cannabis sativa L. to determine their potential to block the enzyme plasmodium falciparum dihydrofolate reductase-thymidinesynthase. The molecules of cycloguanil and

WR99210 were used as a reference in the molecular docking study. The highest docking score among the compounds was achieved by compound 9 (Quan et al., 2021).

CONCLUSION

Hemp (*Cannabis sativa* subsp. sativa) has been accepted as an important symbol of sustainability in the food industry and an alternative food source. Trends towards the consumption of functional foods indicate that hemp and its by-products can play an important role in the development of special and new foods. More work is needed on the development of efficient extraction, separation, purification and identification technologies for bioactive compounds in hemp. Hemp products show that it will increase its share in the global market with its consumer potential targeting diet and nutrition. The overall increasing popularity and availability of hemp-based foods has led to the need to control of products on the market.

REFERENCES

Abdulsalami, I. O., Adeoye, M. D., Alabi, K. A., Abdulsalami, B. A., & Abolurin, N. O. (2018). Comparative Analysis of Theoretical and Empirical Data of Synthetic Cannabinoids. *Fountain Journal of National Ad Applied Sciences*, *7*(1), 29–41. doi:10.53704/fujnas.v7i1.247

Alkaseem, M., & Baron, M. (2018). SERS and DFT study of 5F-PB-22. *Journal of Raman Spectroscopy: JRS*, *49*(10), 1594–1606. doi:10.1002/jrs.5444

Andre, C. M., Hausman, J.-F., & Guerriero, G. (2016). Cannabis sativa: The plant of the thousand and one molecules. *Frontiers in Plant Science*, *7*, 19. doi:10.3389/fpls.2016.00019 PMID:26870049

Apostol, L., Popa, M., & Mustatea, G. (2015). Cannabis sativa L partially skimmed flour as source of bio-compounds in the bakery industry. *Romanian Biotechnological Letters*, *20*(5), 10835–10844.

Baldino, L., Scognamiglio, M., & Reverchon, E. (2020). Supercritical fluid technologies applied to the extraction of compounds of industrial interest from Cannabis sativa L. and to their pharmaceutical formulations: A review. *The Journal of Supercritical Fluids*, *165*, 104960. doi:10.1016/j.supflu.2020.104960

Baranović, G. (2021). Understanding the conformational, electronic and vibrational properties of Tetrahydrocannabinol (THC) and Cannabidiol (CBD). Pharmacophoric similarities and differences. *Journal of Molecular Structure*, *1244*, 130945. doi:10.1016/j.molstruc.2021.130945

Barbosa, N. S. V., de Almeida Lima, E. R., & Tavares, F. W. (2017). *Molecular modeling in chemical engineering*.

Bindesri, S. D., Jebailey, R., Albarghouthi, N., Pye, C. C., & Brosseau, C. L. (2020). Spectroelectrochemical and computational studies of tetrahydrocannabinol (THC) and carboxy-tetrahydrocannabinol (THC-COOH). *Analyst (London)*, *145*(5), 1849–1857. doi:10.1039/C9AN02173F PMID:31967120

Blade, S. F., Ampong-Nyarko, K., & Przybylski, R. (2006). Fatty acid and tocopherol profiles of industrial hemp cultivars grown in the high latitude prairie region of Canada. *Journal of Industrial Hemp*, *10*(2), 33–43. doi:10.1300/J237v10n02_04

Booth, J. K., & Bohlmann, J. (2019). Terpenes in Cannabis sativa–From plant genome to humans. *Plant Science, 284*, 67–72. doi:10.1016/j.plantsci.2019.03.022 PMID:31084880

Borges, R. S., Batista, J. Jr, Viana, R. B., Baetas, A. C., Orestes, E., Andrade, M. A., Honório, K., & Da Silva, A. B. (2013). Understanding the molecular aspects of tetrahydrocannabinol and cannabidiol as antioxidants. *Molecules (Basel, Switzerland), 18*(10), 12663–12674. doi:10.3390/molecules181012663 PMID:24129275

Borhade, S. S. (2013). Chemical Composition and Characterization of Hemp (Cannabis sativa) Seed oil and essential fatty acids by HPLC Method. *Archives of Applied Science Research, 5*(1), 5–8.

Bouchentouf, S., Ghalem, S., Allali, H., & Missoum, N. (2017). Investigating the Inhibition of 5-LO Enzyme by Main Cannabinoids Contained in Cannabis safiva and Seized Resin Cannabis by Using Molecular Modeling. *Insights Enzyme Res, 1*(1), 10.

Callaway, J., Schwab, U., Harvima, I., Halonen, P., Mykkänen, O., Hyvönen, P., & Järvinen, T. (2004). Efficacy of dietary hempseed oil on plasma lipids and skin quality in patients with atopic dermatitis. *The Journal of Dermatological Treatment.*

Callaway, J. C. (2004). Hempseed as a nutritional resource: An overview. *Euphytica, 140*(1), 65–72. doi:10.100710681-004-4811-6

Chen, C., & Pan, Z. (2021). Cannabidiol and terpenes from hemp–ingredients for future foods and processing technologies. *Journal of Future Foods, 1*(2), 113–127. doi:10.1016/j.jfutfo.2022.01.001

Christinat, N., Savoy, M.-C., & Mottier, P. (2020). Development, validation, and application of a LC-MS/MS method for quantification of 15 cannabinoids in food. *Food Chemistry, 318*, 126469. doi:10.1016/j.foodchem.2020.126469 PMID:32143130

Couper, A. S. (1858). On a new chemical theory. *Philosophical Magazine, 4*(16), 104–116.

Crocioni, E. (2021). *Raman spectroscopy of Cannabis Sativa trichomes and selected cannabinoids.* Politecnico Milano1863.

Crum Brown, A. (1864). On the theory of isomeric compounds. *Transactions of the Royal Society of Edinburgh, 23*, 234.

Crum Brown, A. (1867). On the Classification of chemical substances, by means of generic radicals. *Transactions of the Royal Society of Edinburgh, 24*(2), 331–339. doi:10.1017/S0080456800018597

Dabija, A., Codină, G. G., Gâtlan, A.-M., Sănduleac, E. T., & Rusu, L. (2018). Effects of some vegetable proteins addition on yogurt quality. *Scientific Study & Research. Chemistry & Chemical Engineering, Biotechnology. Food Industries, 19*(2), 181–192.

Dalton, J. C. (1808). *A New System of Chemical Philosophy.* doi:10.5479il.324338.39088000885681

Doğan, N., & Doğan, C. (2021). Mucizevi Bitki Kenevir'in (Cannabis sativa L.) Gıda Endüstrisinde Kullanımı. *Bozok Veterinary Sciences, 2*(2), 47–56.

Dunford, N. (2015). Hemp and flaxseed oil: properties and applications for use in food. In *Specialty oils and fats in food and nutrition* (pp. 39–63). Elsevier. doi:10.1016/B978-1-78242-376-8.00002-8

Erukainure, O., Matsabisa, M., Salau, V., Oyedemi, S., Oyenihi, O., Ibeji, C., & Islam, M. (2021). [a]). Cannabis sativa L.(var. indica) Exhibits Hepatoprotective Effects by Modulating Hepatic Lipid Profile and Mitigating Gluconeogenesis and Cholinergic Dysfunction in Oxidative Hepatic Injury. *Frontiers in Pharmacology*, *12*, 12. doi:10.3389/fphar.2021.705402 PMID:34992528

Erukainure, O. L., Matsabisa, M. G., Muhammad, A., Abarshi, M. M., Amaku, J. F., Katsayal, S. B., & Nde, A. L. (2021). [b]). Targeting of Protein's Messenger RNA for Viral Replication, Assembly and Release in SARS-CoV-2 Using Whole Genomic Data From South Africa: Therapeutic Potentials of Cannabis Sativa L. *Frontiers in Pharmacology*, *12*, 2314. doi:10.3389/fphar.2021.736511

Feng, X., Sun, G., & Fang, Z. (2022). Effect of Hempseed Cake (Cannabis sativa L.) Incorporation on the Physicochemical and Antioxidant Properties of Reconstructed Potato Chips. *Foods*, *11*(2), 211. doi:10.3390/foods11020211 PMID:35053943

Ferrante, C., Recinella, L., Ronci, M., Menghini, L., Brunetti, L., Chiavaroli, A., Leone, S., Di Iorio, L., Carradori, S., Tirillini, B., Angelini, P., Covino, S., Venanzoni, R., & Orlando, G. (2019). Multiple pharmacognostic characterization on hemp commercial cultivars: Focus on inflorescence water extract activity. *Food and Chemical Toxicology*, *125*, 452–461. doi:10.1016/j.fct.2019.01.035 PMID:30711720

Frankland, E. (1852). On a New Series of Organic Bodies Containing Metals. *Philosophical Transactions of the Royal Society.*, *142*, 417–444. doi:10.1098/rstl.1852.0020

Glivar, T., Eržen, J., Kreft, S., Zagožen, M., Čerenak, A., Čeh, B., & Benković, E. T. (2020). Cannabinoid content in industrial hemp (Cannabis sativa L.) varieties grown in Slovenia. *Industrial Crops and Products*, *145*, 112082. doi:10.1016/j.indcrop.2019.112082

Guo, T., Liu, Q., Hou, P., Li, F., Guo, S., Song, W., Zhang, H., Liu, X., Zhang, S., Zhang, J., Ho, C.-T., & Bai, N. (2018). Stilbenoids and cannabinoids from the leaves of Cannabis sativa f. sativa with potential reverse cholesterol transport activity. *Food & Function*, *9*(12), 6608–6617. doi:10.1039/C8FO01896K PMID:30500001

House, J. D., Neufeld, J., & Leson, G. (2010). Evaluating the quality of protein from hemp seed (Cannabis sativa L.) products through the use of the protein digestibility-corrected amino acid score method. *Journal of Agricultural and Food Chemistry*, *58*(22), 11801–11807. doi:10.1021/jf102636b PMID:20977230

Iványi, I. (2006). Effect of genotype and environmental on the oil content and fatty acid composition of hempseed. *Cereal Research Communications*, *34*(1), 493–496. doi:10.1556/CRC.34.2006.1.123

Janeczek, A., Zawadzki, M., Szpot, P., & Niedzwiedz, A. (2018). Marijuana intoxication in a cat. *Acta Veterinaria Scandinavica*, *60*(1), 1–4. doi:10.118613028-018-0398-0 PMID:29996908

Jarzębski, M., Fathordoobady, F., Guo, Y., Xu, M., Singh, A., Kitts, D. D., Kowalczewski, P. Ł., Jeżowski, P., & Pratap Singh, A. (2019). Pea protein for hempseed oil nanoemulsion stabilization. *Molecules (Basel, Switzerland)*, *24*(23), 4288. doi:10.3390/molecules24234288 PMID:31775277

Kazemi, F., Karimi, I., & Yousofvand, N. (2021). Molecular docking study of lignanamides from Cannabis sativa against P-glycoprotein. *In Silico Pharmacology*, *9*(1), 1–7. doi:10.100740203-020-00066-7 PMID:33442533

King, J. W. (2019). The relationship between cannabis/hemp use in foods and processing methodology. *Current Opinion in Food Science*, *28*, 32–40. doi:10.1016/j.cofs.2019.04.007

Kladar, N., Čonić, B. S., Božin, B., & Torović, L. (2021). European hemp-based food products–Health concerning cannabinoids exposure assessment. *Food Control*, *129*, 108233. doi:10.1016/j.foodcont.2021.108233

Korus, A., Gumul, D., Krystyjan, M., Juszczak, L., & Korus, J. (2017). Evaluation of the quality, nutritional value and antioxidant activity of gluten-free biscuits made from corn-acorn flour or corn-hemp flour composites. *European Food Research and Technology*, *243*(8), 1429–1438. doi:10.100700217-017-2853-y

Korus, J., Witczak, M., Ziobro, R., & Juszczak, L. (2017). Hemp (Cannabis sativa subsp. sativa) flour and protein preparation as natural nutrients and structure forming agents in starch based gluten-free bread. *Lebensmittel-Wissenschaft + Technologie*, *84*, 143–150. doi:10.1016/j.lwt.2017.05.046

Lachenmeier, D. (2004). Hemp food products-A problem? *Deutsche Lebensmittel-Rundschau*, *100*(12), 481–490.

Liu, Y., Liu, H.-Y., Li, S.-H., Ma, W., Wu, D.-T., Li, H.-B., Xiao, A.-P., Liu, L.-L., Zhu, F., & Gan, R.-Y. (2022). Cannabis sativa bioactive compounds and their extraction, separation, purification, and identification technologies: An updated review. *Trends in Analytical Chemistry*, *149*, 116554. doi:10.1016/j.trac.2022.116554

Lu, X., & Clarke, R. C. (1995). The cultivation and use of hemp (Cannabis sativa L.) in ancient China. *Journal of the International Hemp Association*, *2*(1), 26–30.

Manach, C., Mazur, A., & Scalbert, A. (2005). Polyphenols and prevention of cardiovascular diseases. *Current Opinion in Lipidology*, *16*(1), 77–84. doi:10.1097/00041433-200502000-00013 PMID:15650567

Martin-Diana, A. B., Izquierdo, N., Albertos, I., Sanchez, M. S., Herrero, A., Sanz, M. A., & Rico, D. (2017). Valorization of carob's germ and seed peel as natural antioxidant ingredients in gluten-free crackers. *Journal of Food Processing and Preservation*, *41*(2), e12770. doi:10.1111/jfpp.12770

Mattila, P. H., Pihlava, J.-M., Hellström, J., Nurmi, M., Eurola, M., Mäkinen, S., Jalava, T., & Pihlanto, A. (2018). Contents of phytochemicals and antinutritional factors in commercial protein-rich plant products. *Food Quality and Safety*, *2*(4), 213–219. doi:10.1093/fqsafe/fyy021

Mikulec, A., Kowalski, S., Sabat, R., Skoczylas, Ł., Tabaszewska, M., & Wywrocka-Gurgul, A. (2019). Hemp flour as a valuable component for enriching physicochemical and antioxidant properties of wheat bread. *Lebensmittel-Wissenschaft + Technologie*, *102*, 164–172. doi:10.1016/j.lwt.2018.12.028

Murkovic, M., Draxl, S., & Pfannhaeser, W. (1997). Vitamin B1 in Austrian cereals. *Ernaehrung*, *21*, 263–265.

Nionelli, L., Montemurro, M., Pontonio, E., Verni, M., Gobbetti, M., & Rizzello, C. G. (2018). Pro-technological and functional characterization of lactic acid bacteria to be used as starters for hemp (Cannabis sativa L.) sourdough fermentation and wheat bread fortification. *International Journal of Food Microbiology*, *279*, 14–25. doi:10.1016/j.ijfoodmicro.2018.04.036 PMID:29715603

Nissen, L., Casciano, F., Babini, E., & Gianotti, A. (2021). Prebiotic potential and bioactive volatiles of hemp byproduct fermented by lactobacilli. *Lebensmittel-Wissenschaft + Technologie, 151*, 112201. doi:10.1016/j.lwt.2021.112201

Nissen, L., di Carlo, E., & Gianotti, A. (2020). Prebiotic potential of hemp blended drinks fermented by probiotics. *Food Research International, 131*, 109029. doi:10.1016/j.foodres.2020.109029 PMID:32247454

Nycz, J. E., Malecki, G., Zawiazalec, M., Pazdziorek, T., & Skop, P. (2010). 1-Pentyl-3-(4-methoxy-1-naphthoyl) indole and 2-(2-methoxy-phenyl)-1-(1-pentyl-1H-indol-3-yl)-ethanone: X-ray structures and computational studies. *Journal of Molecular Structure, 984*(1-3), 125–130. doi:10.1016/j.molstruc.2010.09.016

Odani, S., & Odani, S. (1998). Isolation and primary structure of a methionine-and cystine-rich seed protein of Cannabis sativa. *Bioscience, Biotechnology, and Biochemistry, 62*(4), 650–654. doi:10.1271/bbb.62.650 PMID:9614695

Pap, N., Hamberg, L., Pihlava, J.-M., Hellström, J., Mattila, P., Eurola, M., & Pihlanto, A. (2020). Impact of enzymatic hydrolysis on the nutrients, phytochemicals and sensory properties of oil hemp seed cake (Cannabis sativa L. FINOLA variety). *Food Chemistry, 320*, 126530. doi:10.1016/j.foodchem.2020.126530 PMID:32222655

Pellati, F., Borgonetti, V., Brighenti, V., Biagi, M., Benvenuti, S., & Corsi, L. (2018). Cannabis sativa L. and nonpsychoactive cannabinoids: Their chemistry and role against oxidative stress, inflammation, and cancer. *BioMed Research International, 2018*, 2018. doi:10.1155/2018/1691428 PMID:30627539

Perkins, J. A. (2005). A history of molecular representation. Part one: 1800 to the 1960s. *The Journal of Biocommunication, 31*(1), 1.

Perlín, C. (2002). Hemp as food. *Výživa a potraviny, 61*, 121-122.

Petrović, M., Debeljak, Ž., Kezić, N., & Džidara, P. (2015). Relationship between cannabinoids content and composition of fatty acids in hempseed oils. *Food Chemistry, 170*, 218–225. doi:10.1016/j.foodchem.2014.08.039 PMID:25306338

Quan, P. M., Toan, T. Q., Hung, N. P., Nam, P. H., Kiet, N. T., Ha, N. X., & Thi, H. H. P. (2021). Cannabis sativa L. chemical compositions as potential plasmodium falciparum dihydrofolate reductase-thymidinesynthase enzyme inhibitors: An in silico study for drug development. *Open Chemistry, 19*(1), 1244–1250. doi:10.1515/chem-2021-0102

Radočaj, O., Dimić, E., & Tsao, R. (2014). Effects of hemp (Cannabis sativa L.) seed oil press-cake and decaffeinated green tea leaves (Camellia sinensis) on functional characteristics of gluten-free crackers. *Journal of Food Science, 79*(3), C318–C325. doi:10.1111/1750-3841.12370 PMID:24527987

Russo, E. B., & Marcu, J. (2017). Cannabis pharmacology: The usual suspects and a few promising leads. *Advances in Pharmacology, 80*, 67–134. doi:10.1016/bs.apha.2017.03.004 PMID:28826544

Santos, C. B. R. D., Lobato, C. C., de Sousa, M. A. C., Macêdo, W. J. D. C., & Carvalho, J. C. T. (2014). Molecular modeling: Origin, fundamental concepts and applications using structure-activity relationship and quantitative structure-activity relationship. *Reviews in Theoretical Science*, *2*(2), 91–115. doi:10.1166/rits.2014.1016

Saxena, A., Wong, D., Diraviyam, K., & Sept, D. (2009). The basic concepts of molecular modeling. *Methods in Enzymology*, *467*, 307–334. doi:10.1016/S0076-6879(09)67012-9 PMID:19897098

Schluttenhofer, C., & Yuan, L. (2017). Challenges towards revitalizing hemp: A multifaceted crop. *Trends in Plant Science*, *22*(11), 917–929. doi:10.1016/j.tplants.2017.08.004 PMID:28886910

Shen, P., Gao, Z., Fang, B., Rao, J., & Chen, B. (2021). Ferreting out the secrets of industrial hemp protein as emerging functional food ingredients. *Trends in Food Science & Technology*, *112*, 1–15. doi:10.1016/j.tifs.2021.03.022

Silva, T. B., Pereira, M. A., Malta, V. S., Bento, E. S., San-Miguel, M. A., Ziolli, R. L., & Taft, C. A. (2008). Study of the structure-activity relationship for theoretical molecular descriptors using density functional theory and chemometric methods in cannabinoid metabolites. *International Journal of Quantum Chemistry*, *108*(13), 2530–2539. doi:10.1002/qua.21696

Small, E., & Cronquist, A. (1976). A practical and natural taxonomy for Cannabis. *Taxon*, *25*(4), 405–435. doi:10.2307/1220524

Tang, C.-H., Ten, Z., Wang, X.-S., & Yang, X.-Q. (2006). Physicochemical and functional properties of hemp (Cannabis sativa L.) protein isolate. *Journal of Agricultural and Food Chemistry*, *54*(23), 8945–8950. doi:10.1021/jf0619176 PMID:17090145

Tuzun, B. (2020). Investigation of the molecules obtained from marijuana: Computational study of spectral, structural and docking. [IAU Iran]. *Journal of Physical & Theoretical Chemistry*, *16*, 59–74.

Vonapartis, E., Aubin, M.-P., Seguin, P., Mustafa, A. F., & Charron, J.-B. (2015). Seed composition of ten industrial hemp cultivars approved for production in Canada. *Journal of Food Composition and Analysis*, *39*, 8–12. doi:10.1016/j.jfca.2014.11.004

Wang, Q., Jiang, J., & Xiong, Y. L. (2018). High pressure homogenization combined with pH shift treatment: A process to produce physically and oxidatively stable hemp milk. *Food Research International*, *106*, 487–494. doi:10.1016/j.foodres.2018.01.021 PMID:29579952

Wang, Q., & Xiong, Y. L. (2019). Processing, nutrition, and functionality of hempseed protein: A review. *Comprehensive Reviews in Food Science and Food Safety*, *18*(4), 936–952. doi:10.1111/1541-4337.12450 PMID:33336999

Wang, X.-S., Tang, C.-H., Yang, X.-Q., & Gao, W.-R. (2008). Characterization, amino acid composition and in vitro digestibility of hemp (Cannabis sativa L.) proteins. *Food Chemistry*, *107*(1), 11–18. doi:10.1016/j.foodchem.2007.06.064

Xian-Sheng, W. (2007). Characterization. *Amino Acid Composition and in Vitro Digestibility of Hemp (Cannabis Sativa L.) Proteins. Food Chemistry*, *107*(1), 11–18.

Xu, J., Zhang, Y., Wang, W., & Li, Y. (2020). Advanced properties of gluten-free cookies, cakes, and crackers: A review. *Trends in Food Science & Technology*, *103*, 200–213. doi:10.1016/j.tifs.2020.07.017

Xu, X., Qiao, Y., Shi, B., & Dia, V. P. (2021). Alcalase and bromelain hydrolysis affected physicochemical and functional properties and biological activities of legume proteins. *Food Structure*, *27*, 100178. doi:10.1016/j.foostr.2021.100178

Zhang, H., Zhong, Z., & Feng, L. (2016). Advances in the performance and application of hemp fiber. *Int J Simul Syst Sci Technol, 17*(9), 18.11-18.15.

Chapter 8
Cannabis sativa: A Miracle Plant for Remediation of Soil Pollutants

Khursheed Ahmad Wani
https://orcid.org/0000-0001-5577-3455
Government Degree College Thindim Kreeri, Baramulla, India

Shivom Singh
ITM University, India

Siraj Yousuf
Government Degree College, Bijbehara, India

ABSTRACT

Phytoremediation is a plant-based technology that is both cost-effective and environmentally beneficial, and it is classified as an in-situ modification method. Using phytoremediation, on the other hand, results in the restoration of the preservation site's biological activity, physical structure, and chemical properties. Heavy metals can be found in a variety of places in the environment. Because most of these compounds are water soluble, they circulate quickly across the environment. Heavy metals and other pollutants in high concentrations can impair the body's physiology and biochemistry, resulting in health problems. This chapter will review the literature available in different data bases on Cannabis sativa for possible remediation of pollutants from different ecosystems.

INTRODUCTION

Cannabis sativa is a dioecious flowering plant with male and female reproductive organs on distinct plants (Desanlis, and Cerruti, 2013). Monoecious plants are ones that have both reproductive organs on the same plant. *Cannabis sativa* flourishes at temperatures ranging from 16 to 27 degrees Celsius (Adesina et al., 2020). This plant is a short-day plant that blossoms in 12 to 14 hours of daylight (Hall et al., 2012). The plants are tall (up to 6 metres) with deep roots (45–90 cm) (Desanlis & Cerruti, 2013).

DOI: 10.4018/978-1-6684-5718-4.ch008

The blooms take 10 to 16 weeks to develop, and during full blossoming, fibre production is at its highest (Amaducci & Gusovius, 2010). Fiber maturation at greater internodes is more advanced at full flowering, and fibre is more homogenous.

The release of various harmful pollutants into the environment, ozone depletion and global warming are some of the most pressing challenges (Mishra et al., 2019). The various heavy metals like Mg, Mo, Fe, Mn, Zn, Cu, and Ni which are indispensable for the plant growth but harmful to the environment at larger amounts in the soil are examples of inorganic pollutants. Rainwater runoff can leach these metals into nearby areas, causing serious environmental and health risk (Saxena et al., 2019). Metals having uncertain biological functions, such as Cadmium, Chromium, lead, Cobalt, silver, Selenium, and mercury, can accumulate and be hazardous in high doses (Hajar et al., 2018).

Phytoremediation is a low-cost, natural process that employs vegetation to eradicate dangerous pollutants from the soil (Cunningham et al., 1995; Bauddh et al., 2017). Many plants have been investigated and proven to be beneficial in the detoxification of contaminants from the top layer of the soil. On the other hand, most of the plants have been identified as phytoremediators. Withdrawal and throwing away procedures for these plants are not well characterized (Tangahu et al., 2011). *Cannabis sativa* has been discovered as a hyper accumulator (Linger et al., 2002; Linger et al., 2005; Shi et al., 2009). Metal deposition has been verified in both Cannabis roots and stem tissues in an earlier investigation, with no evident modifications in development of the plants. The technique of accumulation, on the other hand, has remained a mystery. *Cannabis sativa* is an ideal candidate for phytoremediation experiments because of its short growth cycle, minimal pesticide usage, and low plant care.

Cannabis proponents have long claimed that the plant was employed to assist decrease the harm caused by the tragic Chernobyl nuclear tragedy. The stories turned out to be correct. *Cannabis sativa* was cultivated in contaminated areas near the Chernobyl site by a team of Russian scientists headed by Ilya Raskin in the 1990s. The researchers sought to explore whether *Cannabis sativa* could extract heavy metals from the earth in a process known as "phytoremediation," according to Raskin. According to accounts, the team was successful, and the *Cannabis sativa* plants were able to cleanse the poisonous soil.

Traditional soil rehabilitation techniques involve expensive and ecologically dangerous physical and chemical treatments. However, scientists have mainly been unable to create biological answers to the issue that can scale to the requisite degree. In 2001, German scientists duplicated the experiment by cultivating *Cannabis sativa* on a sewage-contaminated patch of land. The team claims to have been able to extract lead, cadmium, and nickel from the earth. Phytoremediation is a practical, cost-effective, and long-term approach for cleansing contaminated soil. The technique of phytoremediation is the involvement of plants to remove harmful pollutants from different ecosystems (Cunningham, Berti,1993: Raskin et al 1997; Băbău et al., 2020; Băbău, 2021). Many plants have been discovered to collect metal pollutants, and their susceptibility to do so varies substantially across species and cultivars within a species. Small shrubs with shallow roots, which need special growth conditions (Kanwar et al., 2020; Küpper et al., 1999; Sumiahadi et al., 2018; Vázquez et al., 1992; Vögeli-Lange et al., 1990), make up the bulk of metal-accumulating plants. More than merely the top layer of soil must be cleaned of contaminants to be successful at soil remediation. Cannabis sativa' has deep roots capable to remove metals from soil, together with its economic potential, making it a great alternative for phytoremediation as a profit-generating crop.

Cannabis sativa has a lot of promise as a phytoremediator as it can be cultivated on polluted soil and creates important commodities such bioenergy, wood fiber, pulp, and feed (Cherney and Small, 2016; Chundawat et al., 2011; Hu and Lim, 2016; Zhao et al., *2020*). *Cannabis sativa* may be used to clean up metals, pesticides, solvents, explosives, crude oil, polyaromatic hydrocarbons, and toxins, among other things. Chendawat and colleagues (2011) found that *Cannabis sativa* harvested from remediation sites could be converted into ethanol and utilized as a biofuel without encountering any difficulties (Hu and Lim, 2016; Zhao et al. 2020). Various plants have been used as fuel over the decades that have decreased the stress on fossil fuels. However, lignocellulosic biomass has piqued interest as a promising, renewable source of bioethanol due to its widespread availability and low cost of feedstock (Chundawat et al., 2011). According to the results of a cost comparison, *Cannabis sativa* is a lucrative commodity.

It is not possible to utilize *Cannabis sativa* as a raw material in clothing or in the food supply chain due to the fact that it accumulates potentially toxic metals in all plant parts. It is possible to remove metals from leaves and stems that contain significant quantities of cadmium, lead, or nickel utilizing a number of techniques. Among the techniques used for the bioconversion of *Cannabis sativa* biomass into succinic acid is a process that comprises thermochemical pretreatment followed by enzymatic hydrolysis (Gunnarsson et al., 2015). Succinic acid is a biodegradable polymer that may be used to make food, fine chemicals, green solvents, and medications (Song and Lee, 2006). It is also a precursor to pharmaceuticals. Combined Cannabis sativa-hurd biomass and Ralstoniaeutropha are used in the production of poly-3-hydroxybutyrate (Khattab and Dahman, 2019). Metal contamination has no influence on the excellent quality of *Cannabis sativa* fibers and hurds, which allows them to be utilized in goods such as composite materials because of their great strength.

Salt et al., 1995 described how pollutant-rich plants are harvested and how the collected material is composted, disposed of as hazardous waste, or (more cheaply) employed for metal recovery after being harvested. Furthermore, since *Cannabis sativa* fibers are renewable, they may be used in the production of sustainable polymer matrix composites (Ku and Wang, 2011; Musio et al., 2018; Yan et al., 2013; Yan et al., 2013). *Cannabis sativa* fibers were used in resin matrix composites for the mechanical work on Henry Ford's vehicle and were "ten times stronger than steel. *Cannabis sativa* is a fast-growing plant with deep, broad roots that can be harvested quickly. It can grow in a wide range of climates and adapts to a wide range of soil conditions (Citterio et al., 2003), and it is quite adaptable. Numerous studies have shown that *Cannabis sativa* has a high level of tolerance to heavy metals. Industrial *Cannabis sativa* is capable of absorbing and storing a wide range of metals.

Plants employed for phytoremediation may acquire toxins in their roots, leaves, and stalks, according to research published in 2004 (Angelova et al., 2004). It is as a result of this that the leaves are no longer harvested for food or personal care, but the stalks can be used to produce building materials, paper, textiles, and biofuel (Ahmad and colleagues, 2016). Because of the 1986 Chernobyl nuclear accident (Charkowski, 2022), *Cannabis sativa* has been utilised to remediate soil toxins from agricultural areas that were severely harmed (Charkowski, 2022). In 2008, *Cannabis sativa* was grown to drain toxins such as dioxin from the soil in an Italian agricultural area damaged by a nearby steel factory (Roberts, 2022). The goal was to reduce soil contamination. In addition to causing cancer, dioxins have been shown to interfere with hormone synthesis and impair reproductive and developmental processes. (Morin-Crini and colleagues, 2019).

Heavy metal deposition in soil as a result of human activity is a significant cause of pollution. In addition to being nonbiodegradable, these potentially toxic components offer a long-term health risk to both people and the environment. Traditional cleanup approaches are both costly and possibly detrimental to the environment. They should be avoided if possible. The use of plants to gather metals from the environment, known as phytoremediation, is an alternative method of environmental remediation. In terms of phytoremediation, *Cannabis sativa* (industrial Cannabis sativa) is a promising contender. Its roots are robust, and it can survive the accumulation of a variety of metals over time. Furthermore, the crop biomass may be used for a number of economic purposes once it has been harvested. Aside from that, the newly published annotated genome sequence of *Cannabis sativa* offers an excellent platform for genetically modifying the plant for enhanced phytoremediation.

Because *Cannabis sativa* accumulates potentially hazardous metals in all of its plant components, it cannot be used as a raw material in clothing or as a component of the food chain. There are many procedures that may be used to remove metals from leaves and stems that contain significant amounts of cadmium, lead, or nickel, for example. One approach for the bioconversion of *Cannabis sativa* biomass into succinic acid, developed by Gunnarsson et al. (2015), involves the use of thermochemical pretreatment prior to enzymatic hydrolysis. Succinic acid is utilized as a precursor in the production of biodegradable polymers, food, fine chemicals, environmentally friendly solvents, and medicinal products. (Khattab & Dahman, 2019) report on the use of Cannabis sativa-hurd biomass in conjunction with Ralstoniaeutropha for the synthesis of poly-3-hydroxybutyrate. Metal contamination has no effect on the excellent quality of *Cannabis sativa* fibers and hurds, enabling them to be utilized in goods such as composite materials because of their high quality. This chapter analyzed the material on *Cannabis sativa* that was accessible in various data sources in order to determine if it might be used to remediate contaminants from various ecosystems.

PHYTOREMEDIATION

Phytoremediation Process

Metals that have the potential to be harmful to plants initially interact with them at the roots, where they are absorbed by mass flow and diffusion to the rest of the plant. These heavy metals are made available to plants through root secretion of metal-chelating compounds into the surrounding rhizosphere, metal reductase in the plasma membrane, and proton extrusion from roots, all of which occur as a result of root secretion of metal-chelating compounds into the surrounding rhizosphere. There are a variety of phytoremediation techniques available. In phytoextraction, soil contaminants are taken up by the roots and accumulate in the shoots as a result of the process. Plant tissue accumulation is often related with higher metal concentrations in the growing environment. A variety of disposal processes, including heat and extraction, are used to handle the contaminated shoot tissues after that point in the process. It is possible, for example, to harvest the tissues and burn them as hazardous waste (Cunningham and Berti, 1993; Raskin et al., 1997; Băbău et al., 2020; Băbău, 2021).

The biomass collected may be utilized as a bioenergy fuel or pyrolyzed to make biochar, depending on the application (Keller et al., 2005; McGrath et al., 2002; Sheora et al., 2013). Metallic contaminants are immobilized by root adsorption and metal precipitation and stabilized through the creation of complexes or a reduction in the amount of phytostabilization present in the environment. Immobilization and stabilization of metals occur inside the plant, resulting in the formation of a harmless state that does not interfere with cellular metabolism. By phytovolatilization, potentially dangerous metals are converted into more volatile forms, which are subsequently removed from the environment through transpiration and decomposition. (Andersson-Sköldet al., 2014; Huang et al., 2018; Schreurset al., 2011; Schröderet al., 2018; Baker et al., 1981; Ghosh et al., 2005).

Cannabis sativa as a Phytoremediator

Industrial *Cannabis sativa* is one of the most often investigated species for phytoremediation (*Cannabis sativa* L.). Due to the porous and hydrophilic surface structure, in-situ pollution treatment is possible. Using *Cannabis sativa* fibers as an example, lead (II), zinc (II), and cadmium ion remediation has been successful. Efficacy ranged from 17.5 to 39 percent in single/ternary ion metal(s) solutions with *Cannabis sativa* (Pejic et al., 2011). When it came to benzo(a)pyrene, Campbell et al. (2002) observed considerable drops (33,5 percent) in contaminated soil, but inconsistent findings on chrysene (-50 percent to 64 percent). It was also considered that contaminant accumulation was especially averse to *Cannabis sativa* components in general.

Cannabis sativa leaves, for example, have quantities of nickel, lead, and cadmium 4–12 times greater than those found in fibers, seeds, and plants (Linger et al., 2002). In accordance with the circular economy, it enables for the reuse and remanufacturing of *Cannabis sativa* components that are less polluted for the rest of the year, industrial *Cannabis sativa* might be utilized for non-food uses because of its quick maturity time and high biomass output (Kumar et al., 2017).

Chromium Phytoremediation

Cannabis sativa contains chromium (Cr) and other important elements, which are absorbed by the plant. For both seed and fiber varieties of Cannabis sativa, the root system (for both seed and fiber) collects the most chromium. Other plants have shown that Cr may be immobilized in root cells, which may explain why *Cannabis sativa's* roots accumulate so much of it (61, 62). Proline buildup and phenolic content increase significantly in the roots of *Cannabis sativa* growing in polluted environments. Protective effects of proline and phenolics may be seen in plants that have high levels of these compounds. Chlorophyll, carotenoids, and dry biomass levels are all dropping at the same time as Cr accumulates in root systems (Raimondi et al., *2010*)

Zinc Phytoremediation

As a result of its ability to handle high zinc (Zn) concentrations, *Cannabis sativa* is able to retain the bulk of the Zn it consumes in its roots. All photosynthetic and plant growth is unaffected by the Zn shoot limitation. Additionally, seeds are considered safe for human consumption since they contain low amounts of Zn (Ahmad et al., *2016*). Zn accumulates more in shoots than roots according to Malik et al.,2010. Zn concentrations in the order of Angelova et al. 2004 were as follows: It all starts with seeds and ends with fiber. Roots > Leaves > Fibers > Flowers.

Copper Phytoremediation

Only the *Cannabis sativa* leaves contain copper (Cu), not its fibers. Responsive oxygen species (ROS) formed under metal-stress circumstances protect plant cells from oxidative damage by inhibiting GSR and PLD, two antioxidant enzymes. It has been shown that GSR and PLD expression is raised in *Cannabis sativa* that has been enriched with copper. Researchers have shown that the NAD(P)H-dependent aldo-keto reductase enzyme was increased in *Cannabis sativa* cultivated under Cu stress (Arru et al., 2004; Bona et al., 2007; Elisa et al., 2007). To help in detoxification, the cell's capacity to remove toxins is increased by this reductase. Phytochelatins and other proteins interact with this protein to decrease ions, which then transports them to the vacuole, according to the scientists (Bona et al., 2007). Despite the fact that photosynthesis was unaffected, Cu treatment significantly reduced plant aerial sections and root system architecture in this research. Cu concentrations were found in the following order by Angelovaet et al.: flower > seeds > roots > stems > leaves > fiber.

Selenium Phytoremediation

Soil enriched with selenium may provide selenomethionine and methionine in *Cannabis sativa* seed embryos. Because of this, the seeds may be used as a source of selenium for both people and cattle. Besides the brain and spinal cord, various parts of the body that aren't underground contain Se. CBD and terpenes are not adversely affected by the presence of se in the flower and stems, where these metabolites are formed and removed. Crops that grow in soil with low levels of selenium may benefit from the Se in the leaves as a fertilizer (Stonehouseet al; 2020; Placido, 2022).

Cadmium, Nickel, and Lead Phytoremediation

Abandoned mine soils may have significant quantities of cadmium and nickel and lead that *Cannabis sativa* can absorb. Metal concentrations were greater in the leaves for all three of these elements. Another study found that the same metal contamination had no effect on the quality of the fibers and hurds, thus they could be utilized in goods like composite materials. Even while high Cd concentrations in the soil don't hinder Cannabis sativa's germination, Cd accumulates in the aerial parts, lowering photosynthesis and decreasing plant development. Roots acquired the highest Cd, although root development was unaffected by the contamination (Husain et al., 2019; Linger et al., 2002; Vandenhove & Van Hees, 2005)

CECs Degradation

Industrial Cannabis sativa's fiber production and medicinal value have been widely recognized thus far. However, because industrial *Cannabis sativa* has been prohibited in North America for a long time, its phytoremediation capacity has been largely unknown. The efficiency of Cannabis sativa's ability to remove heavy metals has been repeatedly proved in the limited industrial *Cannabis sativa* phytoremediation experiments available (Stonehouse et al., 2020; Praspaliauskas et al., 2020). *Cannabis sativa* outperformed other commonly used phytoremediation species like mustard and sunflower when it came to heavy metal removal (Meers et al., 2010).

For heavy metal removal, industrial *Cannabis sativa* is ideal because of its broad and porous surface structure, low nutritional needs, and high toxicity. As waste leachate and mining regions have shown, only a few agricultural plants can survive, *Cannabis sativa* can thrive in even the most hazardous of settings (Mihoc et al., 2012). As a nutritional form of heavy metal, accumulated heavy metal may be consumed, metabolized, and even excreted (Stonehouse et al. 2020). Industrial *Cannabis sativa* did an excellent job of removing CECs as well. For CECs with varying molecular weights and solubilities, *Cannabis sativa* was employed.

Cannabis sativa cultivation has been shown to improve soil remediation and microbiological activity, according to a number of studies. Cannabis sativa's roots emit potent allelopathic compounds that aid in the repair of the soil (Linger et al., 2002). Similarly, a research on Zea mays demonstrated that hydrocarbons in soil originate from biogenetic, rather than anthropogenic, origins (Grifoni et al., 2020). Isolated bacteria from Cannabis sativa, such as Achromobacter species, Pseudomonas species, and Alcaligenes species completely degraded the toxic chemicals phenol and benzene, showing the plant's high potential for phytoremediation (Iqbal et al., 2018). It is significantly more difficult to deal with heavy metal and CECs. Since heavy metals have a variety of roles and interact with organic pollutants, the outcomes of phytoremediation are controversial.

Studies have demonstrated that *Cannabis sativa* cultivation may promote soil remediation and microbiological activity, as well. During *Cannabis sativa* development, the root secretes powerful allelopathic chemicals that hasten soil restoration (Linger et al., 2002). The biogenetic rather than the anthropogenic causes of soil hydrocarbon concentrations were also discovered in research on Zea mays (Grifoni et al., 2020). A number of *Cannabis sativa*-derived bacteria, including Achromobacter sp., Pseudomonas sp., and Alcaligenes sp., completely eliminated the phenol and benzene, proving that *Cannabis sativa* has a high phytoremediation capability (Iqbal et al., 2018). Even more problematic are CECs and heavy metal. The phytoremediation results are contentious because of the varied roles played by heavy metals and the interactions between heavy metals and organic contaminants.

Figure 1. Removal of heavy metals by Cannabis sativa

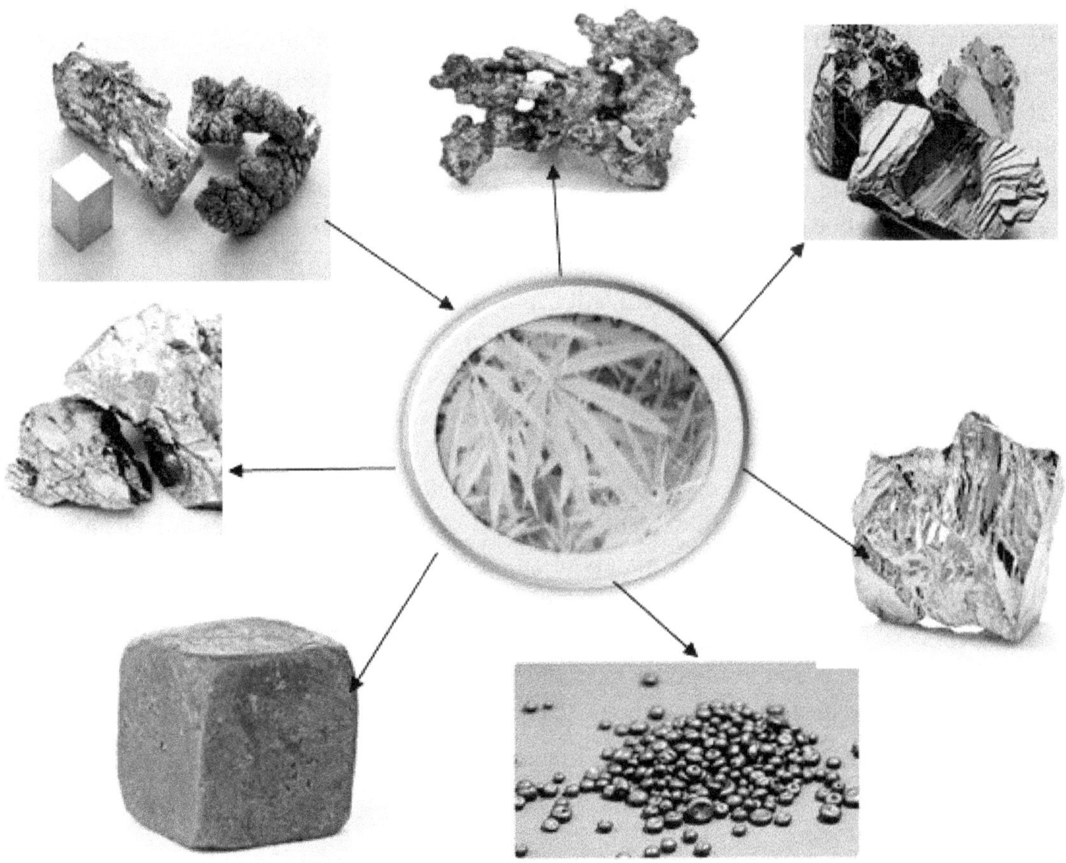

CONCLUSION

Industrial *Cannabis sativa* is a good choice for metal-contaminated soil phytoremediation. *Cannabis sativa* has been shown to absorb metals in a variety of conditions in multiple investigations. Metal absorption in various *Cannabis sativa* cultivars may be difficult to determine due to the wide range of variables (growth settings, tissue sampling, metal analysis, and phenotyping) utilized in these investigations. Research comparing metal concentrations and tissue localization in various cultivars under identical experimental settings is badly required. More comprehensive investigations. This endeavor is greatly aided by *Cannabis sativa* cultivation collections. However, as *Cannabis sativa* technology progresses, better cultivars will become available.

FUTURE SCOPE

Cannabis sativa crops that have undergone phytoremediation may be disposed of in a variety of ways, as stated in the previous research. However, there are still many unsolved questions about the use of industrial Cannabis sativa. It is difficult to conduct economic and environmental research on industrial *Cannabis sativa* disposal techniques since there is no commercial manufacturing line. LCA estimations, for example, are less reliable because they rely on published literature rather than experimental evidence, acceptable assumptions, and results from similar crops. Crop cultivation with industrial *Cannabis sativa* might have an adverse effect on the environment. Bioenergy production dramatically increases emissions of greenhouse gases, acidification, and eutrophication as a result of feedstock cultivation. For further information see Martnez et al.

Using a combination of 85 percent ethanol and fossil fuels contributed more than twice as much GHG to global warming as using conventional fuels, according to González-Garca et al. (2012). *Cannabis sativa* and fax for non-wood pulp mills were examined for their environmental consequences, and it was shown that 80 percent of greenhouse gas emissions were caused by fertilizer usage during *Cannabis sativa* growing (Gonzalez-Garcia et al. 2010). All *Cannabis sativa* pieces cannot be recycled. Since ash can only replace a tiny portion of fertilizer and consumes a comparable amount of energy, there is presently some controversy about whether *Cannabis sativa* ashes can be used as mineral fertilizer. A vital approach for ending the nutrition cycle, however, is ash recycling due to the depletion of phosphorus stores (Prade et al. 2012).

We don't know for sure whether mineral fertilizer ashes are safe to use. In fact, several studies have shown that biomass polluted with heavy metals is not only lighter, but also concentrates heavy metals in the ash/char part. There are no heavy metals in either its bio-oil/tar or gas pyrolysis products (Liu et al. 2012). Although metal valorization may be conceivable, the utilization of ashes is improbable. Finally, there are certain tactics that are uncompetitive in the market. The lack of widespread adoption of biofuels, for example, is due to ongoing technological developments. Biomass, which is abundant and cheap to get, is not everything that can be utilized for biofuel production because of the difficulties of cost-effective hydrolysis.

REFERENCES

Adesina, I., Bhowmik, A., Sharma, H., & Shahbazi, A. (2020). A review on the current state of knowledge of growing conditions, agronomic soil health practices and utilities of *Cannabis sativa* in the United States. *Agriculture, 10*(4), 129. doi:10.3390/agriculture10040129

Ahmad, R., Tehsin, Z., Malik, S. T., Asad, S. A., Shahzad, M., Bilal, M., Shah, M. M., & Khan, S. A. (2016). Phytoremediation potential of *Cannabis sativa* (*Cannabis sativa* L.): Identification and characterization of heavy metals responsive genes: Biotechnology. *CLEAN Soil Air Water*, *44*, 195–201. doi:10.1002/clen.201500117

Amaducci, S., & Gusovius, H. J. (2010). Cannabis sativa-cultivation, extraction and processing. In *Industrial Applications of Natural Fibers: Structure, Properties and Technical Applications* (pp. 109–134). John Wiley & Sons. doi:10.1002/9780470660324.ch5

Andersson-Sköld, Y., Hagelqvist, A., Crutu, G., & Blom, S. (2014). Bioenergy grown on contaminated land—A sustainable bioenergy contributor? *Biofuels*, *5*(5), 487–498. doi:10.1080/17597269.2014.996728

Angelova, V., Ivanova, R., Delibaltova, V., & Ivanov, K. (2004). Bioaccumulation and distribution of heavy metals in fibre crops (flax, cotton, and Cannabis sativa). *Industrial Crops and Products*, *19*(3), 197–205. doi:10.1016/j.indcrop.2003.10.001

Arru, L.; Rognoni, S.; Baroncini, M.; Bonatti, P.M.; Perata, P., (2004). Copper localization in *Cannabis sativa* L. grown in a copper-rich solution. *Euphytica140*, 33–38.

Băbău, A. M. C., Micle, V., Damian, G. E., & Sur, I. M. (2020). Preliminary investigations regarding the potential of *Robiniapseudoacacia* L. (leguminosae) in the phytoremediation of sterile dumps. *Journal of Environmental Protection and Ecology*, *21*, 46–55.

Băbău, A. M. C., Micle, V., Damian, G. E., & Sur, I. M. (2021). Sustainable ecological restoration of sterile dumps using *Robiniapseudoacacia. Sustainability*, *13*(24), 14021. doi:10.3390u132414021

Baker, A. J. M. (1981). Accumulators and excluders-strategies in the response of plants to heavy metals. *Journal of Plant Nutrition*, *3*(1-4), 643–654. doi:10.1080/01904168109362867

Bañuelos, G. S., & Ajwa, H. A. (1999). Trace elements in soils and plants: An overview. *Journal of Environmental Science and Health. Part A, Toxic/Hazardous Substances & Environmental Engineering*, *34*(4), 951–974. doi:10.1080/10934529909376875

Bauddh, K., Singh, B., & Korstad, J. (2017). *Phytoremediation potential of bioenergy plants*. Springer. doi:10.1007/978-981-10-3084-0

Bona, E., Marsano, F., Cavaletto, M., & Berta, G. (2007). Proteomic characterization of copper stress response in *Cannabis sativa* roots. *Proteomics*, *7*(7), 1121–1130. doi:10.1002/pmic.200600712 PMID:17352425

Chalot, M., Blaudez, D., Rogaume, Y., Provent, A.-S., & Pascual, C. (2012). Fate of trace elements during the combustion of phytoremediation wood. *Environmental Science & Technology*, *46*(24), 13361–13369. doi:10.1021/es3017478 PMID:23153074

Chandra, S., Lata, H., & ElSohly, M. A. (2017). *Cannabis sativa L.—Botany and Biotechnology*. Springer. doi:10.1007/978-3-319-54564-6

Charkowski, E. (1998). *Cannabis sativa* "eats" Chernobyl waste offers hope for Hanford. *Rediscover Cannabis sativa.* sativa.com/inspire/Cannabis sativa-eats-chernobyl-waste-offers-hope-for-hanford/

Cherney, J.; Small, E., (2016). Industrial *Cannabis sativa* in North America: Production, politics, and potential. *Agronomy, 6*, 58.

Chundawat, S. P. S., Beckham, G. T., Himmel, M. E., & Dale, B. E. (2011). Deconstruction of lignocellulosic biomass to fuels and chemicals. *Annual Review of Chemical and Biomolecular Engineering*, *2*(1), 121–145. doi:10.1146/annurev-chembioeng-061010-114205 PMID:22432613

Citterio, S., Santagostino, A., Fumagalli, P., Prato, N., Ranalli, P., & Sgorbati, S. (2003). Heavy metal tolerance and accumulation of Cd, Cr and Ni by *Cannabis sativa* L. *Plant and Soil, 256*(2), 243–252. doi:10.1023/A:1026113905129

Cunningham, S. D., & Berti, W. R. (1993). Remediation of contaminated soils with green plants: An overview. *Vitr. Cell. Dev. Biol. Plant*, *29*(4), 207–212. doi:10.1007/BF02632036

Cunningham, S. D., Berti, W. R., & Huang, J. W. (1995). Phytoremediation of contaminated soils. *Trends in Biotechnology*, *13*(9), 393–397. doi:10.1016/S0167-7799(00)88987-8

Desanlis, F., Cerruti, N., & Warner, P. (2013). *Cannabis sativa* agronomics and cultivation. In P. Bouloc, S. Allegret, & L. Arnaud (Eds.), *Cannabis sativa: Industrial Production and Uses* (pp. 98–124). CABI. doi:10.1079/9781845937935.0098

Elisa, B., Marsano, F., Cavaletto, M., & Berta, G. (2007). Copper stress in *Cannabis sativa* roots: Morphological and pro-teomic analysis. *Caryologia*, *60*(1-2), 96–101. doi:10.1080/00087114.2007.10589553

Feeney, M., & Punja, Z. K. (2003). Tissue culture and *Agrobacterium*-mediated transformation of *Cannabis sativa* (*Cannabis sativa* L.). *Vitr. Cell. Dev. Biol. Plant*, *39*(6), 578–585. doi:10.1079/IVP2003454

Garbisu, C., & Alkorta, I. (2001). Phytoextraction: A cost-effective plant-based technology for the removal of metals from the environment. *Bioresource Technology*, *77*(3), 229–236. doi:10.1016/S0960-8524(00)00108-5 PMID:11272009

Ghosh, M., & Singh, S. P. (2005). A review on phytoremediation of heavy metals and utilization of its byproducts. *Applied Ecology and Environmental Research*, *3*(1), 1–18. doi:10.15666/aeer/0301_001018

González-García, S., Hospido, A., Feijoo, G., & Moreira, M. T. (2010). Life cycle assessment of raw materials for non-wood pulp mills: *Cannabis sativa* and flax. *Resources, Conservation and Recycling*, *54*(11), 923–930. doi:10.1016/j.resconrec.2010.01.011

González-García, S., Luo, L., Moreira, M. T., Feijoo, G., & Huppes, G. (2012). Life cycle assessment of *Cannabis sativa* hurds use in second generation ethanol production. *Biomass and Bioenergy*, *36*, 268–279. doi:10.1016/j.biombioe.2011.10.041

Grifoni, M., Rosellini, I., Angelini, P., Petruzzelli, G., & Pezzarossa, B. (2020). The efect of residual hydrocarbons in soil following oil spillages on the growth of Zea mays plants. *Environmental Pollution, 265*, 114950. doi:10.1016/j.envpol.2020.114950 PMID:32554092

Gunnarsson, I. B., Kuglarz, M., Karakashev, D., & Angelidaki, I. (2015). Thermochemical pretreatments for enhancing succinic acid production from industrial *Cannabis sativa* (*Cannabis sativa* L.). *Bioresource Technology, 182*, 58–66. doi:10.1016/j.biortech.2015.01.126 PMID:25682224

Hajar EW, Sulaiman AZ, Sakinah AM., (2014). Assessment of heavy metals tolerance in leaves, stems and flowers of *Stevia rebaudiana* plant. *Procedia Environmental Sciences, 20*, 386–93.

Hall, J., Bhattarai, S. P., & Midmore, D. J. (2012). Review of flowering control in industrial Cannabis sativa. *Journal of Natural Fibers, 9*(1), 23–36. doi:10.1080/15440478.2012.651848

Hou, D., O'Connor, D., Igalavithana, A. D., Alessi, D. S., Luo, J., Tsang, D. C. W., Sparks, D. L., Yamauchi, Y., Rinklebe, J., & Ok, Y. S. (2020). Metal contamination and bioremediation of agricultural soils for food safety and sustainability. *Nat. Rev. Earth Environ., 1*(7), 366–381. doi:10.103843017-020-0061-y

Hu, R., & Lim, J.-K. (2016). Fabrication and mechanical properties of completely biodegradable *Cannabis sativa* fiber reinforced polylactic acid composites. *Journal of Composite Materials, 41*(13), 1655–1669. doi:10.1177/0021998306069878

Huang, H., Yao, W., Li, R., Ali, A., Du, J., Guo, D., Xiao, R., Guo, Z., Zhang, Z., & Awasthi, M. K. (2018). Effect of pyrolysis temperature on chemical form, behavior, and environmental risk of Zn, Pb and Cd in biochar produced from phytoremediation residue. *Bioresource Technology, 249*, 487–493. doi:10.1016/j.biortech.2017.10.020 PMID:29073559

Husain, R., Weeden, H., Bogush, D., Deguchi, M., Soliman, M., Potlakayala, S., Katam, R., Goldman, S., & Rudrabhatla, S. (2019). Enhanced tolerance of industrial *Cannabis sativa* (*Cannabis sativa* L.) plants on abandoned mine land soil leads to overexpression of cannabinoids. *PLoS One, 14*(8), e0221570. doi:10.1371/journal.pone.0221570 PMID:31465423

Iqbal, A., Arshad, M., Hashmi, I., Karthikeyan, R., Gentry, T. J., & Schwab, A. P. (2018). Biodegradation of phenol and benzene by endophytic bacterial strains isolated from refnery wastewater-fed Cannabis sativa. *Environmental Technology, 39*(13), 1705–1714. doi:10.1080/09593330.2017.1337232 PMID:28562230

Järup, L. (2003). Hazards of heavy metal contamination. *British Medical Bulletin, 68*(1), 167–182. doi:10.1093/bmb/ldg032 PMID:14757716

Kanwar, V. S., Sharma, A., Srivastav, A. L., & Rani, L. (2020). Phytoremediation of toxic metals present in soil and water environment: A critical review. *Environmental Science and Pollution Research International, 27*(36), 44835–44860. doi:10.100711356-020-10713-3 PMID:32981020

Keller, C., Ludwig, C., Davoli, F., & Wochele, J. (2005). Thermal treatment of metal-enriched biomass produced from heavy metal phytoextraction. *Environmental Science & Technology, 39*(9), 3359–3367. doi:10.1021/es0484101 PMID:15926590

Khattab, M. M., & Dahman, Y. (2019). Production and recovery of poly-3-hydroxybutyrate bioplastics using agro-industrial residues of *Cannabis sativa* hurd biomass. *Bioprocess and Biosystems Engineering, 42*(7), 1115–1127. doi:10.100700449-019-02109-6 PMID:30993443

Ku, H., Wang, H., Pattarachaiyakoop, N., & Trada, M. (2011). A review on the tensile properties of natural fiber reinforced polymer composites. *Composites. Part B, Engineering, 42*(4), 856–873. doi:10.1016/j.compositesb.2011.01.010

Küpper, H., & Zhao, J. (1999). Cellular compartmentation of zinc in leaves of the hyperaccumulator *Thlaspicaerulescens. Plant Physiology, 119*(1), 305–312. doi:10.1104/pp.119.1.305 PMID:9880373

Linger, P., Müssig, J., Fischer, H., & Kobert, J. (2002). Industrial *Cannabis sativa* (*Cannabis sativa* L.) growing on heavy metal contaminated soil: Fiber quality and phytoremediation potential. *Industrial Crops and Products, 16*, 33–42. doi:10.1016/S0926-6690(02)00005-5

Liu, C. F., Li, Y. H., & Shi, G. R. (2012). Utilize heavy metal-contaminated farmland to develop bioenergy. *Advanced Materials Research, 414*, 254–261. doi:10.4028/www.scientific.net/AMR.414.254

Malik, R. N., Husain, S. Z., & Nazir, I. (2010). Heavy metal contamination and accumulation in soil and wild plant species from industrial area of Islamabad, Pakistan. *Pakistan Journal of Botany, 42*, 291–301.

Martin, M., Svensson, N., Fonseca, J., & Eklund, M. (2014). Quantifying the environmental performance of integrated bioethanol and biogas production. *Renewable Energy, 61*, 109–116. doi:10.1016/j.renene.2012.09.058

McGrath, S. P., Zhao, J., & Lombi, E. (2002). Phytoremediation of metals, metalloids, and radionuclides. *Advances in Agronomy, 75*, 1–56. doi:10.1016/S0065-2113(02)75002-5

Meers, E., Van Slycken, S., Adriaensen, K., Ruttens, A., Vangronsveld, J., Du Laing, G., Witters, N., Thewys, T., & Tack, F. M. G. (2010). The use of bio-energy crops (Zea mays) for 'phytoattenuation' of heavy metalson moderately contaminated soils: A fieldexperiment. *Chemosphere, 78*(1), 35–41. doi:10.1016/j.chemosphere.2009.08.015 PMID:19837447

Mihoc, M., Pop, G., Alexa, E., & Radulov, I. (2012). Nutritive quality of romanian *Cannabis sativa* varieties (*Cannabis sativa* L.) with special focus on oil and metal contents of seeds. *Chemistry Central Journal, 6*(1), 122. doi:10.1186/1752-153X-6-122 PMID:23088580

Mishra, S., Bharagava, R. N., More, N., Yadav, A., Zainith, S., & Mani, S. (2019). *Heavy Metal Contamination: An Alarming Threat to Environment and Human Health Environmental Biotechnology: For Sustainable Future*. Springer.

Morin-Crini, N., Staelens, J. N., Loiacono, S., Martel, B., Chanet, G., & Crini, G. (2019). Simultaneous removal of Cd, Co, Cu, Mn, Ni, and Zn from synthetic solutions on a Cannabis sativa-based felt. III. Real discharge waters. *Journal of Applied Polymer Science, 137*(24), 48823. doi:10.1002/app.48823

Musio, S., Müssig, J., & Amaducci, S. (2018). Optimizing *Cannabis sativa* fiber production for high performance composite applications. *Front. Plant Sci., 9*, 1702. doi:10.3389/fpls.2018.01702 PMID:30532760

Placido, D. F., & Lee, C. C. (2022). Potential of Industrial *Cannabis sativa* for Phytoremediation of Heavy Metals. *Plants, 11*(5), 595. doi:10.3390/plants11050595 PMID:35270065

Prade, T., Svensson, S.-E., & Mattsson, J. E. (2012). Energy balances for biogas and solid biofuel production from industrial Cannabis sativa. *Biomass and Bioenergy, 40*, 36–52. doi:10.1016/j.biombioe.2012.01.045

Praspaliauskas, M., Žaltauskaitė, J., Pedišius, N., & Striūgas, N. (2020). Comprehensive evaluation of sewage sludge and sewage sludge char soil amendment impact on the industrial *Cannabis sativa* growth performance and heavy metal accumulation. *Industrial Crops and Products, 150*, 112396. doi:10.1016/j.indcrop.2020.112396

Raimondi, G., Rodrigues, J., Maucieri, C., Borin, M., & Bona, S. (2020). Phytomanagement of chromium-contaminated soils using *Cannabis sativa* (L.). *Agronomy (Basel), 10*(9), 1223. doi:10.3390/agronomy10091223

Raskin, I., Smith, R. D., & Salt, D. E. (1997). Phytoremediation of metals: Using plants to remove pollutants from the environment. *Current Opinion in Biotechnology, 8*(2), 221–226. doi:10.1016/S0958-1669(97)80106-1 PMID:9079727

Roberts, C. (2017). How Cannabis Cleans Up Nuclear Radiation and Toxic Soil. *High Times*. https://hightimes.com/news/how-cannabis-cleans-up-nuclear-radiation-and-toxic-soil/

Salt, D. E., Blaylock, M., Kumar, N. P. B. A., Dushenkov, V., Ensley, B. D., Chet, I., & Raskin, I. (1995). Phytoremediation: A novel strategy for the removal of toxic metals from the environment using plants. *Nature Biotechnology, 13*(5), 468–474. doi:10.1038/nbt0595-468 PMID:9634787

Saxena, G., Purchase, D., Mulla, S. I., Saratale, G. D., & Bharagava, R. N. (2019). *Phytoremediation of Heavy Metal-Contaminated Sites: Eco-environmental Concerns, Field Studies, Sustainability Issues, and Future Prospects*. Springer.

Schreurs, E., Voets, T., & Thewys, T. (2011). GIS-based assessment of the biomass potential from phytoremediation of contaminated agricultural land in the Campine region in Belgium. *Biomass and Bioenergy, 35*(10), 4469–4480. doi:10.1016/j.biombioe.2011.09.005

Schröder, P., Beckers, B., Daniels, S., Gnädinger, F., Maestri, E., Marmiroli, N., Mench, M., Millan, R., Obermeier, M. M., Oustriere, N., Persson, T., Poschenrieder, C., Rineau, F., Rutkowska, B., Schmid, T., Szulc, W., Witters, N., & Sæbø, A. (2018). Intensify production, transform biomass to energy and novel goods and protect soils in Europe—A vision how to mobilize marginal lands. *The Science of the Total Environment, 616–617*, 1101–1123. doi:10.1016/j.scitotenv.2017.10.209 PMID:29132720

Sheoran, V., Sheoran, A. S., & Poonia, P. (2013). Phytomining of gold: A review. *Journal of Geochemical Exploration, 128*, 42–50. doi:10.1016/j.gexplo.2013.01.008

Shi, G., & Cai, Q. (2009). Cadmium tolerance and accumulation in eight potential energy crops. *Biotechnology Advances, 27*(5), 555–561. doi:10.1016/j.biotechadv.2009.04.006 PMID:19393309

Ślusarkiewicz-Jarzina, A., Ponitka, A., & Kaczmarek, Z. (2005). Influence of cultivar, explant source and plant growth regulator on callus induction and plant regeneration of *Cannabis sativa* L. *Acta Biologica Cracoviensia. Series; Botanica, 47*, 145–151.

Song, H., & Lee, S. Y. (2006). Production of succinic acid by bacterial fermentation. *Enzyme and Microbial Technology, 39*(3), 352–361. doi:10.1016/j.enzmictec.2005.11.043

Stonehouse, G. C., McCarron, B. J., Guignardi, Z. S., El Mehdawi, A. F., Lima, L. W., Fakra, S. C., & Pilon-Smits, E. A. H. (2020). Selenium metabolism in *Cannabis sativa* (*Cannabis sativa* L.)—Potential for phytoremediation and biofortification. *Environmental Science & Technology*, *54*(7), 4221–4230. doi:10.1021/acs.est.9b07747 PMID:32182043

Sumiahadi, A., & Acar, R. (2018). A review of phytoremediation technology: Heavy metals uptake by plants. *IOP Conference Series. Earth and Environmental Science*, *142*, 012023. doi:10.1088/1755-1315/142/1/012023

Tangahu, B. V., Abdullah, S., Rozaimah, S., Basri, H., Idris, M., & Anuar, N. (2011). A review on heavy metals (As, Pb, and Hg) uptake by plants through phytoremediation. *International Journal of Chemical Engineering*, *2011*, 1–31. doi:10.1155/2011/939161

Vandenhove, H., & Van Hees, M. (2005). Fiber crops as alternative land use for radioactively contaminated arable land. *Journal of Environmental Radioactivity*, *81*(2-3), 131–141. doi:10.1016/j.jenvrad.2005.01.002 PMID:15795030

Vázquez, M. D., Barceló, J., Poschenrieder, C., Mádico, J., Hatton, P., Baker, A. J. M., & Cope, G. H. (1992). Localization of zinc and cadmium in *Thlaspicaerulescens* (Brassicaceae), a metallophyte that can hyperaccumulate both metals. *Journal of Plant Physiology*, *140*(3), 350–355. doi:10.1016/S0176-1617(11)81091-6

Vögeli-Lange, R., & Wagner, G. J. (1990). Subcellular localization of cadmium and cadmium-binding peptides in tobacco leaves: Implication of a transport function for cadmium-binding peptides. *Plant Physiology*, *92*(4), 1086–1093. doi:10.1104/pp.92.4.1086 PMID:16667375

Wahby, I., Caba, J. M., & Ligero, F. (2013). *Agrobacterium* infection of *Cannabis sativa* (*Cannabis sativa* L.): Establishment of hairy root cultures. *Journal of Plant Interactions*, *38*(4), 312–320. doi:10.1080/17429145.2012.746399

Yan, Z. L., Wang, H., Lau, K. T., Pather, S., Zhang, J. C., Lin, G., & Ding, Y. (2013). Reinforcement of polypropylene with *Cannabis sativa* fibres. *Composites. Part B, Engineering*, *46*, 221–226. doi:10.1016/j.compositesb.2012.09.027

Zhao, J., Xu, Y., Wang, W., Griffin, J., Roozeboom, K., & Wang, D. (2020). Bioconversion of industrial *Cannabis sativa* biomass for bioethanol production: A review. *Fuel*, *281*, 118725. doi:10.1016/j.fuel.2020.118725

Chapter 9
Heavy Metals and Pesticides on Contaminants of Concern in Cannabis

Asma Zafar
University of Kashmir, India

Sheema Zaffar
University of Kashmir, India

Ab Qayoom Mir
Government Degree College, Hajin, India

Irfan Jamila
Government Degree College for Women, Srinagar, India

Waseem Yaseen
Government Degree College, Kangan, India

ABSTRACT

Cannabis is cultivated in different parts of the world for different purposes. Potential dangers from microbiological contamination exist for cannabis users. Opportunistic infections in immunocompromised patients can be brought on by bacteria and fungi. Allergies and asthma can be brought on by even dead germs. Shigla toxin and aflatoxins are two examples of microbial overload-related toxins that might be problematic, though it's unlikely. There is currently work being done to identify the diverse microbiome that the cannabis plant supports. Because of how readily heavy metals bioaccumulate in the tissues of cannabis, hemp crops have been employed in bioremediation. Because heavy metals are linked to a wide range of human ailments, it is important to keep them to a minimum in crops grown for human consumption. The chapter discusses interlinkage of heavy metals and pesticides associated with cannabis.

DOI: 10.4018/978-1-6684-5718-4.ch009

INTRODUCTION

Evidence suggests that Neolithic people from the Near East arrived in Ireland during the fourth millennium BCE (Cassidy et al., 2016), but little is known about the food and fibre plants they used at this time. Carbonized seeds of hemp (Cannabis sativa L.) were discovered at a Celtic archaeological site in what is now Hungary, dating back to the 1st century BCE (Dalnoki & Jacomet 2002). Archaeological and pollen records suggest that cannabis first arrived in the British Isles no later than the Roman period, when it quickly gained importance as a staple crop, a source of fibre, and a medicine (Dark 2000). The Lacnunga, an Anglo-Saxon medico-religious document from the 10th century, had a "Rite for Salve, Partly Irish" that used hemp as one of several topical herbal elements (Grattan & Singer 1952). (p. 123). Despite this one mention, it is challenging to document any other uses of hemp in the folk medicine or ethnobotany of Ireland. Although its relative, *Humulus lupulus*, was widely used at an early date, (Allen & Hatfield, 2004), no information on hemp is included in this reference. Neither does a classic work on the ethnobotany of Ireland (Moloney 1919).

In the early 19th century, hemp was produced in Ireland for fibre; at the time, it was estimated that 14,000 tonnes were necessary to supply Great Britain in a year of peace (Besnard 1816), with the author recommending that Ireland contribute more to its provision as a superior crop than flax linen. A local hemp fabric sample was also praised with the following praise: "This hemp [grown in Bunratty, Ireland] has all the properties of the Italian, and was especially well fitted for exquisite Works." As a result of human activity, the annual herb cannabis (*Cannabis sativa* L.) can now be found and grown in almost every biome on Earth, from the tropics to the foothills of the Himalayas. Seed oil, intoxicating resin, medicine, and textile fibre all come from this ancient plant (Kriese et al. 2004; Zuardi 2006). According to archaeological evidence, Cannabis was first cultivated in China for its fibre, and then it was exported to the Middle East, Europe, and South America in the early 16th century (Nelson 1996; Schultes et al. 1974). For thousands of years, people have been dispersing and altering this species, making it impossible to trace back its original range. The Canadian settlement of Port Royal was responsible for introducing hemp growing to the New World in 1606 (Small & Marcus 2002).

Throughout history, people have turned to the healing properties of cannabis. A history of medicinal cannabis usage dates back to at least the sixth century BCE, and it was first used to treat epilepsy, tetanus, rheumatism, migraine, asthma, trigeminal neuralgia, tiredness, insomnia, and other conditions after being brought to Western Europe in the early nineteenth century (Figure 1). Currently, federal law in the United States classifies cannabis as a schedule 1 substance, making the growing of the plant illegal and subject to strict regulations.

Both classification (the process of identifying and grouping various species) and nomenclature are part of taxonomy (the naming and describing of organisms). There are two recognised subspecies of Cannabis, both of which are included in the official botanical taxonomy established by Small and Cronquist (1976). Some botanists classify *Cannabis sativa* and *Cannabis indica* as two separate species (Hillig & Mahlberg 2004; Clarke & Merlin 2013).

These days, the terms "Sativa" and "Indica" often lead to misunderstandings (Small 2007; Erkelens & Hazekamp 2014; McPartland 2014; Russo 2016). An alternate method, "from cultivar to chemovar," is advocated by Hazekamp and Fischedick (2012), in which plants are classified according to their chemical fingerprint rather than a fanciful name.

Over 100,000 acres were devoted to industrial hemp cultivation in Italy every year a century ago (Ranalli & Casarini 1988). Farmers bred their own seed to use in planting. Through a process of "mass

Figure 1. Medicinal properties of cannabis

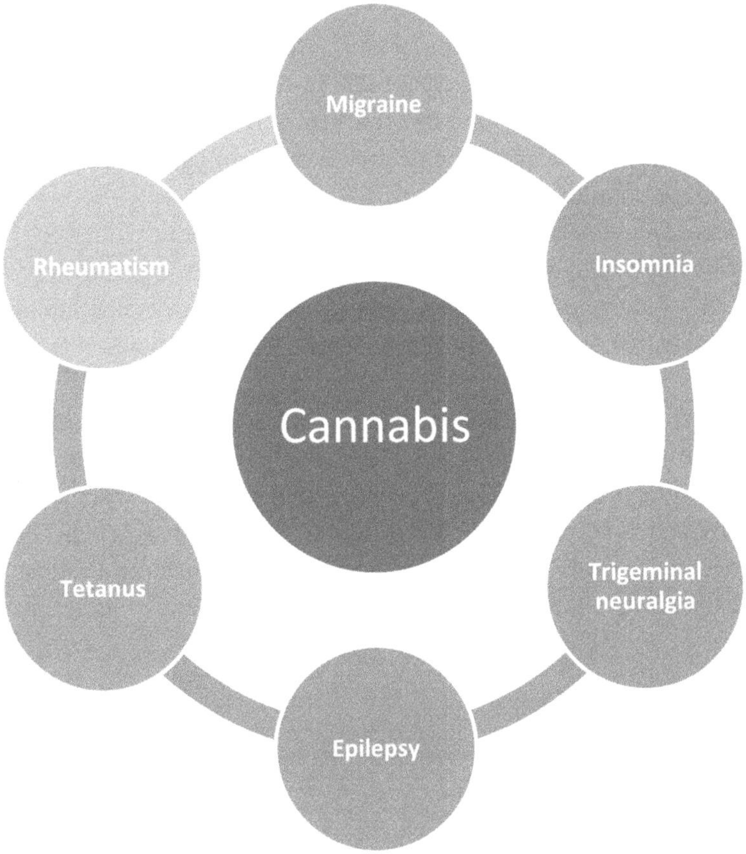

selection," in which several individuals displaying favourable phenotypes were chosen and their seeds collected, desirable traits were systematically increased. Because of the manual nature of harvesting, taller and heavier females were left in the field after fertilisation was complete. Many provinces contributed to the development of landraces, and these varieties are now known by their provincial names: Ferrara, Bologna, Modena, Rovigo, and Carmagnola, to mention a few. The first hybrid Cannabis cultivars were established when professional breeders started crossing different landraces and then subjecting the offspring to repeated selection. To create 'Ferramington,' Dewey (1928) mated Ferrara to an inbred group of Chinese landraces. Fleischmann (1931) created "F-hemp" by inbreeding landraces from Bologna and Ferrara in Hungary. For the purpose of studying morphological differences in Carmagnola and non-Italian types, Crescini (1934) proposed crossing and selfing, using both sexes.

Cannabis is a very diverse plant species that is pollinated by the wind and exhibits strong allogamy. Cannabis is dioecious, meaning that if grown from seed, it will produce male and female flowers on different plants. On rare occasions, it reveals its true hermaphrodite (monoecious) nature. Cannabis taxonomy remains a point of contention. Disagreement exists in the field of taxonomy, or the study of plant classification, over the proper naming of the many kinds of cannabis, each of which has its own unique physical and chemical characteristics. Chemical research into C. sativa has resulted in the isolation and identification of a large number of naturally occurring compounds across a wide variety of chemical classes, as reported in recent literature. In 1980, Turner et al. reported the isolation and identification of 423 different chemicals (1980).

In 1995, this number was raised to 483 compounds (Ross & ElSohly 1995). Between the years of 1995 and 2005, the list grew by 7. (ElSohly & Slade 2005). As of 2016, 565 unique chemicals have been extracted and characterised from *C. sativa*, a fact that was summarised by ElSohly et al. It is possible to divide these substances into two classes: cannabinoids and non-cannabinoids (alkaloids, flavonoids, terpenoids, amino acids and others).

In this plant, the cannabinoids are the most distinct class of chemicals due to their composition as C21 terpenophenolics, which are connected to the terpenes due to their geranyl pyrophosphate-derived ring structure. Due to the widespread production and usage of synthetic cannabinoids, the name "Phyto-cannabinoids" has emerged to describe the naturally separated cannabinoids (Pate 1999). Cannabinoids have 11 distinct chemical classes.

Heavy metals and pesticides are dangerous to human health, thus any cannabis grown for human use must have as little of these pollutants as possible. Effectively removing metals from the soil is one of cannabis' many benefits. Plants used for bioremediation remove harmful substance like heavy metals and pesticides from the soil and store them in their tissues until they are harvested. There is no "other side of the coin" when it comes to pesticide residues; they are always harmful. Pesticide use has increased dramatically as the cannabis business has expanded from outdoor hippy gardens to inside commercial warehouses.

HEAVY METALS AND CANNABIS

Heavy metals pose a risk to human health because they accumulate in the body, making contamination by them a matter for worry. They are poisonous, may cause cancer, and contribute to the development of a wide range of disorders. Cadmium, mercury, lead, arsenic, and nickel are some examples of elements that are particularly hazardous. The presence of radionucleotides in the environment may also result in the contamination of plants and increase the chance of developing lung cancer. In Hawaii, where the volcanic soil naturally contains naturally high quantities of mercury, Siegel et al. (1988) detected 440 ng of mercury per gramme of cannabis in that state. Siegel argues that the lungs are capable of absorbing mercury at a rate that is ten times more effective than the stomach. Volcanic soil also includes substantial quantities of cadmium. According to Grant et al. (2004), this is due to the increased amounts of cadmium found in tobacco and cannabis that was cultivated in Jamaica. On the other hand, the majority of cadmium comes from human activity, namely the burning of fossil fuels and various mining and smelting processes.

According to findings published by Singani and Ahmadi (2012), *C. sativa* quickly absorbs lead and cadmium from soils that have been treated with polluted cow and poultry manures. Even fertiliser that is said to be "clean" seems to enhance the amount of cadmium that *Cannabis sativa* may take in (Ahmad et al. 2015). The most common kind of heavy metal contamination is carried by phosphate ions, and hydroponic fertilisers are especially susceptible to contamination (Karadjov 2014).

There are specific issues with arsenic in phosphate fertilisers marketed at cannabis cultivators (also known as "bud blooms"), which may be anywhere from 10–50 ppm (N. Palmer, pers. common. 2016). There is also the potential for contamination in rockwool, also known as mineral wool fibre, which is utilised as a growth medium in hydroponic systems.According to the findings of Mihoc et al. (2012) research on hemp seeds, there is a concern with cadmium contamination. The researchers detected amounts ranging from 1.3–4.0 mg/kg. In their study, Eboh and Thomas (2005) found that the quantities of arsenic, cadmium, chromium, iron, nickel, lead, and mercury in the leaf material were higher than those found in the seeds. Heavy metals such as mercury, cadmium, lead, chromium, nickel, arsenic, and selenium were found in marijuana smoke according to research conducted by Moir et al. (2008) [Figure 2]. Heavy metals were breathed in at a deeper level, which is characteristic of marijuana users. This resulted in an increased risk of adverse health effects.

Figure 2. Heavy metals reported in C Sativa

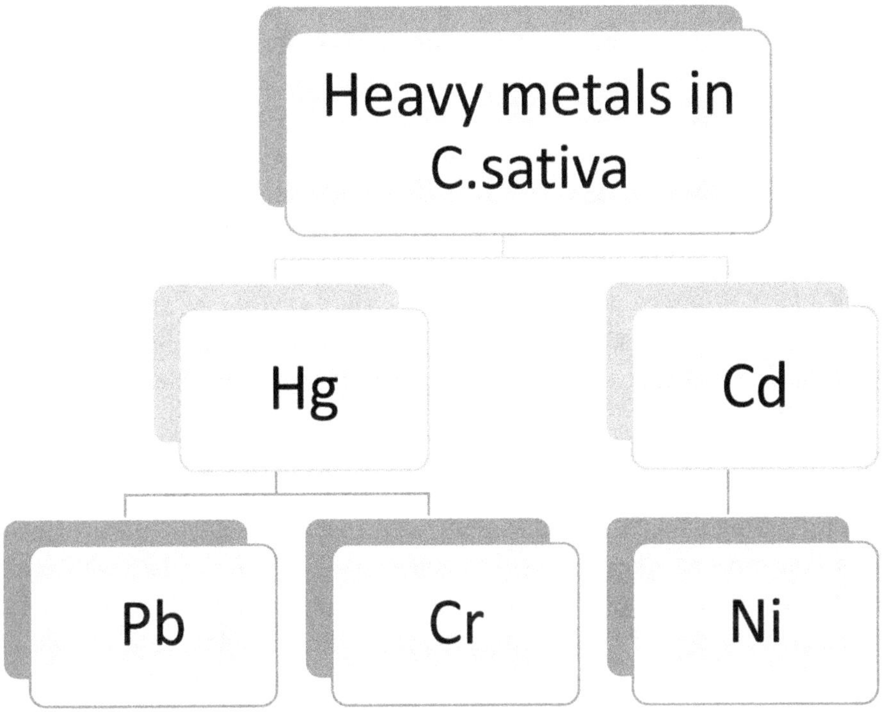

BIOREMEDIATION AND ACCUMULATION OF TOXIC COMPOUNDS

Plants may be used in a phytoremediation process to either eliminate or reduce the bioavailability of elemental contaminants in soil (Berti & Cunningham, 2000). To survive, plants need to take in nutrients from the soil, and their root systems can take in ionic substances even at low quantities. Plants recover damaged soil by sending their roots deep into the soil to build a rhizosphere ecosystem, which accumulates heavy metals and reduces their bioavailability (Ali et al., 2013; Jacob et al., 2018; DalCorso et al., 2019). Phytoremediation has benefits such as I its cheap cost and ease of management due to the fact that it is a solar-powered autotrophic system; (ii) its potential to improve air quality and reduce water pollution; and (iii) its potential to reduce greenhouse gas emissions. Among its many benefits are (ii) its low impact on the ecosystem and environment; (iii) its wide range of application; (iv) its ability to stabilise heavy metals and prevent erosion and leaching, thereby lowering the likelihood of contamination spreading;

and (v) its ability to boost soil fertility through the release of a variety of organic matter (Aken et al., 2009; Wuana & Okieimen, 2011; Jacob et al., 2018). Research into the molecular processes of heavy metal tolerance and methods to increase the efficacy of phytoremediation have been actively pursued for decades. In this overview, we explain the detoxifying methods (avoidance and tolerance) employed by plants in response to heavy metals, and we detail the processes by which heavy metals are taken up and translocated inside plants. The major goal is to provide an overview of the most current developments in phytoremediation methods, with a special focus on tactics to enhance heavy metal bioavailability, tolerance, and accumulation. Enhanced plant performance during phytoremediation is also highlighted, as is the use of genetic engineering.

Cannabis has been dubbed a "bioremediation crop" due to its remarkable ability to absorb and store toxic metals. Bioremediation is a process where plants or microorganisms are used to clean up polluted areas. For example, *Thlaspicaerulescens* (= *T. alpestre*) plants are able to draw poisons from the ground and store them in their tissues. Toxins are extracted from the plants before harvest. Although the quantity of metal taken up by Cannabis is negligible compared to *T. caerulescens* (Giovanardi et al. 2002; Löser et al. 2002; Citterio et al. 2003; Meers et al. 2005), it is an attractive option for bioremediation (Shi & Cai 2009).

Lithium levels in hemp (1.04 mg/kg) were found to be much greater than those found in any of the other crop plants studied by Jurkowska et al. (1990), which included barley, maize, mustard, oats, radish, rape, sorrel, spinach, sunflower, and wheat. Growing cannabis on cadmium and copper-contaminated waste dumps in Silesia. Seeds are collected and then leached with hydrochloric acid to extract the metals (Kozlowski 1995).

Heavy metals are stored in hemp both in its roots (Giovanardi et al. 2002; Citterio et al. 2003; Shi and Cai 2009) and in its leaves (Giovanardi et al (Giovanardi et al. 2002; Arru et al. 2004). Mycorrhizal plants, in which fungus colonise the roots, are more likely to absorb heavy metals via their foliage (Citterio et al. 2005). Plants that have been infected with mycorrhizal fungi may be healthier overall, making them more resistant to the toxic effects of metal stress. Fiber plants of the 'Fibranova' kind were shown to have bioremediation potential by Ciurli et al. (2002), since they could thrive in soil polluted with zinc. They also demonstrated the necessity to do such tests on soil as opposed to a hydroponic screening test. Plants grown in soil were far more resistant to zinc salts than those grown in hydroponics.

Although chloride is a necessary nutrient and sodium is good in tiny levels, cannabis bioaccumulates sodium chloride, which kills it. Hemp is easily stunted by the salty air near the ocean. The ability of several Italian cultivars to thrive in a saline water environment with a concentration of 2.5% NaCl is now being investigated (Grassi, 2016). Toxic polycyclic aromatic hydrocarbons found in soil, such as benzo[a] pyrene and chrysene, may be extracted by cannabis (Campbell et al. 2002). In addition to caesium-137 and strontium-90, cannabis is capable of removing these radioactive elements from contaminated soil (Vandenhove & Van Hees 2005; Hoseini et al., 2012). Near the Chernobyl site, hemp crops were cultivated to harvest radionucleotides (Anonymous 2000).

PESTICIDES AND CANNABIS

It is estimated that around 9,000 species of insects and mites, 50,000 species of plant diseases, and 8,000 species of weeds cause harm to crops throughout the world. It is estimated that insect pests alone are responsible for 14% of losses and weeds for another 13%. When it comes to food production, pesticides are essential. A third or more of all food grown uses pesticides. With no use of pesticides, fruit, vegetable, and cereal yields would drop by 78%, 54%, and 32%, respectively, due to insect damage. When pesticides are employed, crop loss may be reduced by 35%-42%.

In contrast to other agricultural goods, cannabis is often smoked and inhaled, putting users at an uncertain danger from pesticide residues. Pesticides may be detected in smoked cannabis at up to 69.5% levels (Sullivan et al. 2013). Illegal pesticide usage is a growing problem and a sign of moral collapse. According to research by Voelker and Holmes (2015), about half of the cannabis sold in Oregon dispensaries has pesticide residues.

Irresponsible and careless Pesticides sold at hardware shops and garden centres are used in the cannabis cultivation process. Some of them can only be used on ornamental plants and cannot be consumed. Hydroponic stores resell bifenazate and abamectin, two insecticides used for decorative plants, to Cannabis farmers (McLean 2010). Guardian, a "100% natural" miticide, was promoted by a questionable company while containing undeclared abamectin, which led to the recall of cannabis in a number of states (Associated Press, 2016).

Based on interviews with farmers and research in the field, McPartland et al. (2000) compiled a list of pesticides used in agriculture. This concoction of synthetic pyrethroids and other pesticides includes such ingredients as abamectin, acephate, benomyl, carbaryl, carboxin, chlorpyrifos, chlorothalonil, diazinon, dichlorvos, dicofol, dimethoate, fenbutatin oxide, iprodione, malathion, maneb, parathion, vinclozolin Researchers at British Columbia's Centre for Disease Control looked at the history of marijuana cultivation in private residences. They detected chlorpyrifos, diazinon, and 11 synthetic pyrethroids among the pesticide residues in previous crops (NCCEH, 2009). Synthetic pyrethroids, paclobutrazol, and diazinon were found in medical cannabis grown in southern California (Sullivan et al., 2013) [Figure 3].

Up to 49.3 percent of cannabis samples tested positive for the presence of 12 pesticides and growth regulators in a study conducted in central California (Wurzer 2016). Myclobutanil was the most popular (40%) followed by bifenazate (20%), spiromesifen (15%), imidacloprid (4.6%), spinodad (1.3%), abamectin (3%), acequinocyl (2%), bifenazate (2%), daminozide (1%), fenoxycarb (1%), pyrethrum (1%), and spirotetramat (1%). Cannabis may potentially be tainted by fertilisers. N-nitrosamines are very carcinogenic and may be produced when liquid fertilisers are sprayed on plants (Farnsworth and Cordell 1976). Four police officers had pulmonary histoplasmosis while removing marijuana plants, as reported by Ramrez (1990). The plants were probably fertilised by Histoplasma capsulatum-infected bird guano. Outbreaks of hepatitis virus infections have been linked to the usage of human faeces (Cates & Warren 1975; Alexander 1987).

The Environmental Protection Agency (EPA) says it hasn't reviewed the safety of any pesticide on marijuana since it "has yet to receive any applications for pesticide usage on marijuana" (EPA 2016). Due to the lack of federal oversight, states and interested parties have developed their own set of rules.

Mostly botanicals (including rosemary oil, thyme oil, garlic oil, corn gluten meal, and eugenol) and other compounds like 2-phenylethyl propionate and potassium sorbate are included in this category of minimal-risk pesticides exempted by the EPA (EPA 2015). Expanded lists of legal pesticides have been provided by the agriculture departments of Colorado and Washington (CDA 2016, WSDA 2016). The majority of these pesticides are uthorized for use on The National List of materials approved by the Organic Foods Production Act of 1990. Botanical poisons (such neem oil, garlic oil, azadirachtin, pyrethrins), minerals (like potassium salts, copper, sulphur), and biological control organisms are all examples (e.g., *Bacillus thuringiensis, Streptomyces griseoviridis*). Piperonyl butoxide was legal in both of the states. All of these topics have been extensively covered elsewhere (McPartland et al. 2000).

Figure 3. Pesticides reported in C Sativa

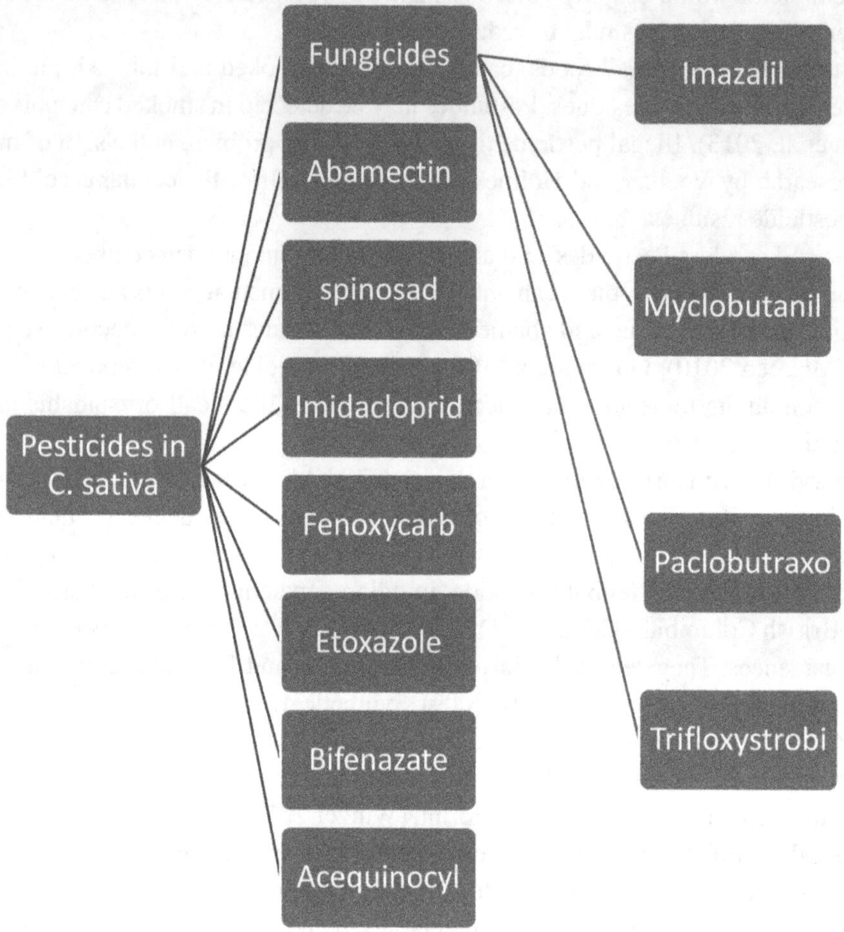

CONCLUSION

C sativa is now grown in almost every part of the world although it has several legal considerations. This plant absorbs different types of toxic substances that add additional risk to its consumers. The prominent toxic substances that have been reported are heavy metals and pesticides that may cause serious health concerns to the consumers, be whatever form they may take it. Hence there is a need to address these issues before it can be used for any beneficial purposes.

REFERENCES

Ahmad, A., Hadi, F., & Ali, N. (2015). Effective phytoextraction of cadmium (Cd) with increasingconcentration of total phenolics and free proline in Cannabis sativa (L.) plant under varioustreatments of fertilizers, plant growth regulators and sodium salt. *International Journal of Phytoremediation*, *17*(1–6), 56–65. doi:10.1080/15226514.2013.828018 PMID:25174425

Alexander, T. (1987) Hepatitis outbreak linked to imported pot. *Sinsemilla Tips.*

Anonymous. (2000) *Phytoremediation: using plants to clean soil.* McGraw Hill Botany. www.mhhe.com/biosci/pae/botany/botany_map/articles/article_10.html

Arru, L., Rognoni, S., Baroncini, M., Bonatti, P. M., & Perata, P. (2004). Copper localization in Cannabissativa L. grown in a copper-rich solution. *Euphytica, 140*(1-2), 33–38. doi:10.100710681-004-4752-0

Associated Press. (2016) Oregon, other states stop sales of pot pesticide due to labeling problem. *USA Today.*

Baca, R., & Migoya, D. (2015) Denver issues ninth pot product recall in 10 weeks. *The Denver Post.*

Bell J (1857) On the haschisch or cannabis indica. *Boston Med Surg J 56*(209–216), 229–236.

Doctor, B. (1993). Stash alert: How to preserve pot potency. *High Times, 213*, 75–79.

Busse, F. P., Fiedler, G. P., Leichtle, A., Hentschel, H., & Stumvoll, M. (2008). Lead poisoning due toadulterated marijuana in Leipzig. *Deutsches Ärzteblatt International, 105*, 757–762. PMID:19623274

Caligiani, A., Palla, G., & Bernardelli, B. (2006). GC-MS analysis of hashish samples: A case ofadulteration with colophony. *Journal of Forensic Sciences, 51*(5), 1096–1100. doi:10.1111/j.1556-4029.2006.00202.x PMID:17018088

Cao, H. X., Schmutzer, T., Scholz, U., Pecinka, A., Schubert, I., & Vu, G. T. (2015). Metatranscriptomeanalysis reveals host-microbiome interactions in traps of carnivorous Genlisea species. *Frontiers in Microbiology, 6*, 526. doi:10.3389/fmicb.2015.00526 PMID:26236284

Cates, W. C., & Warren, J. W. (1975). Hepatitis B in Nuremberg, Germany. Epidemiology of adrug-associated epidemic among US Army soldiers. *Journal of the American Medical Association, 234*(9), 930–934. doi:10.1001/jama.1975.03260220034014 PMID:1242490

Cescon, D. W., Page, A. V., Richardson, S., Moore, M. J., Boerner, S., & Gold, W. L. (2008). Invasive pulmonaryaspergillosis associated with marijuana use in a man with colorectal cancer. *Journal of Clinical Oncology, 26*(13), 2214–2215. doi:10.1200/JCO.2007.15.2777 PMID:18445848

Campbell, S., Paquin, D., Awaya, J. D., & Li, Q. X. (2002). Remediation of benzo[a]pyrene andchrysene-contaminated soil with industrial hemp (Cannabis sativa). *International Journal of Phytoremediation, 4*(2), 157–158. doi:10.1080/15226510208500080 PMID:12655808

CDA. (2016) *Pesticide use in Cannabis production information.* Colorado Department of Agriculture. https://www.colorado.gov/pacific/agplants/pesticide-use-cannabisproduction-information

Citterio, S., Santagostino, A., Fumagalli, P., Prato, N., Ranalli, P., & Sgorbati, G. (2003). Heavy metaltolerance and accumulation of Cd, Cr and Ni by Cannabis sativa L. *Plant and Soil, 256*(2), 243–252. doi:10.1023/A:1026113905129

Citterio, S., Prato, N., Fumagalli, P., Aina, R., Massa, N., Santagostino, A., Sgorbati, G., & Berta, G. (2005). The arbuscular mycorrhizal fungus Glomus mosseae induces growth and metal accumulation-changes in Cannabis sativa L. *Chemosphere, 59*(1), 21–29. doi:10.1016/j.chemosphere.2004.10.009 PMID:15698640

Ciurli, A., Alpi, A., & Perata, P. (2002). Impiegodellacanapanellafitodepurazione da metallipesanti [Use of hemp in phytodepuration from heavy metals]. *Agroindustria*, *1*(1), 64–60.

Chusid, M. J., Gelfand, J. A., Nutter, C., & Fauci, A. S. (1975). Pulmonary aspergillosis, inhalation ofcontaminated marijuana smoke, chronic granulomatous disease. *Annals of Internal Medicine*, *82*(5), 682–683. doi:10.7326/0003-4819-82-5-682 PMID:1094876

Eboh, L. O., & Thomas, B. E. (2005). Analysis of heavy metal content in Cannabis leaf and seedcultivated in southern part of Nigeria. *Pakistan Journal of Nutrition*, *4*(5), 349–351. doi:10.3923/pjn.2005.349.351

EPA. (2015) *Active ingredients eligible for minimum risk pesticide products*. United States Environmental Protection Agency. https://www.epa.gov/sites/production/files/ 2015-12/documents/minrisk-active-ingredients-tolerances-2015-12-15.pdf

EPA. (2016) *Pesticide use on marijuana*. United States Environmental Protection Agency. https://www.epa.gov/pesticide-registration/pesticide-use-marijuana

Farnsworth, N. R., & Cordell, G. A. (1976). New potential hazard regarding use of marijuana treatmentof plants with liquid fertilizers. *Journal of Psychedelic Drugs*, *8*(2), 151–155. doi:10.1080/02791072.1976.10471844

Farrer, D. G. (2015). *Technical report: Oregon health authority's process to determine which types ofcontaminants to test for in cannabis products*. Oregon Health Authority.

Feldman, J. (2015). Pesticide use in marijuana production: Safety issues and sustainable options. *Pesticides You*, *34*(4), 14–23.

Gautam, A. K., Kant, M., & Thakur, Y. (2013). Isolation of endophytic fungi from Cannabis sativa andstudy their antifungal potential. *Archiv für Phytopathologie und Pflanzenschutz*, *46*(6), 627–635. doi:10.1080/03235408.2012.749696

Giovanardi, R., Marchiol, L., Mazzocco, G. T., & Zuliani, F. (2002). Possibilità di impiegodellacanapanellafitoestrazione di metallipesanti in terrenicontaminati: Primirisultati [Possibility of using hemp in the phytoextraction of heavy metals in contaminated soils: First results.]. *Agroindustria*, *1*(1), 69–73.

Grant, C. N., Lalor, G. C., & Vutchkov, M. K. (2004). Trace elements in Jamaican tobacco. *The West Indian Medical Journal*, *53*(2), 66–70. PMID:15199713

Gzebenyuk, N. V. (1984). The occurrence of fungi on hemp stems. *Mikologiâ i Fitopatologiâ*, *18*(4), 322–326.

Hazekamp, A. (2006). An evaluation of the quality of medicinal grade cannabis in the Netherlands. *Cannabinoids*, *1*(1), 1–9.

Hazekamp, A. (2016). Evaluating the effects of gamma-irradiation for decontamination of medicinalcannabis. *Frontiers in Pharmacology*, *7*, 108. doi:10.3389/fphar.2016.00108 PMID:27199751

Health Canada. (2008) *Product information sheet on dried marihuana (cannabis)*. Health Canada. www.hc-sc.gc.ca/dhp-mps/marihuana/about-apropos/dried-information-sechee-eng.php

Holmes M, Vyas JM, Steinbach W, McPartland J (2015) *Microbiological safety testing of cannabis.*

Hoseini, P. S., Poursafa, P., Moattar, F., Amin, M. M., & Rezaei, A. H. (2012). Ability of phytoremediation forabsorption of strontium and cesium from soils using Cannabis sativa. *International Journal of Environmental Health Engineering*, *1*(1), 17. doi:10.4103/2277-9183.96004

Government Central Printing Office, Simla-Jurgensen C.W., & Madsen, A. (2009). Exposure to the airborne mould Botrytis and its health effects. *Annals of Agricultural and Environmental Medicine*, *16*, 183–186. PMID:20047250

Jurkowska, H., Rogóz, A., & Wojciechowicz, T. (1990). The content of lithium in some species of plantsfollowing differentiated doses of nitrogen. *Polish Journal of Soil Science*, *23*, 195–199.

Kagen, S. L., Kurup, V. P., Sohnle, P. G., & Fink, J. N. (1983). Marijuana smoking and fungal sensitization. *The Journal of Allergy and Clinical Immunology*, *71*(4), 389–3893. doi:10.1016/0091-6749(83)90067-2 PMID:6833678

Karadjov, J. (2014) Eliminating heavy-metal toxicity in medical marijuana. *Advanced Nutrients*. www.advancednutrients.com/heavymetal//Eliminating-Heavy-Metal-Toxicity-in-Medical-Marijuana.pdf

Kozlowski, R. (1995). Interview with Professor R. Kozlowski, director of the Institute of NaturalFibres. *J Int Hemp Assoc*, *2*(2), 86–87.

Kurup, V. P., Resnick, A., Kagen, S. L., Cohen, S. H., & Fink, J. N. (1983). Allergenic fungi and actinomycetesin smoking materials and their health implications. *Mycopathologia*, *82*(1), 61–64. doi:10.1007/BF00436948 PMID:6348548

Kusari, P., Kusari, S., Spiteller, M., & Kayser, O. (2013). Endophytic fungi harbored in Cannabis sativaL.: Diversity and potential as biocontrol agents against host plant-specific phytopathogens. *Fungal Biodiversity*, *60*(1), 137–151. doi:10.100713225-012-0216-3

Levitz, S. M., & Diamond, R. D. (1991). Aspergillosis and marijuana. *Annals of Internal Medicine*, *115*(7), 578–579. doi:10.7326/0003-4819-115-7-578_2 PMID:1652910

Llamas, R., Hart, D. R., & Schneider, N. S. (1978). Allergic bronchopulmonary aspergillosis associatedwith smoking moldy marihuana. *Chest*, *73*(6), 871–872. doi:10.1378/chest.73.6.871 PMID:657864

Llewellyn, G. C., & O'Rear, C. O. (1977). Examination of fungal growth and aflatoxin production onmarijuana. *Mycopathologia*, *62*(2), 109–112. doi:10.1007/BF01259400 PMID:414138

Löser, C., Zehnsdorf, A., Fussy, M., & Stärk, H. J. (2002). Conditioning of heavy metal-polluted riversediment by Cannabis sativa L. *International Journal of Phytoremediation*, *4*(1), 27–45. doi:10.1080/15226510208500071

Lucas, P. G. (2008). Regulating compassion: An overview of Canada's federal medical cannabispolicy and practice. *Harm Reduction Journal*, *5*(1), 5. doi:10.1186/1477-7517-5-5 PMID:18226254

Martyny, J. W., Serrano, K. A., Schaeffer, J. W., & Van Dyke, M. V. (2013). Potential exposures associatedwith indoor marijuana growing operations. *Journal of Occupational and Environmental Hygiene*, *10*(11), 622–639. doi:10.1080/15459624.2013.831986 PMID:24116667

McKernan, K., Spangler, J., Zhang, L., Tadogotla, V., Helbert, Y., Foss, T., & Smith, D. (2015). Cannabismicrobiome sequencing reveals several mycotoxic fungi native to dispensary grade cannabisflowers. *bioRxiv*.

Mclean, K. (2010). Pot and pesticides: A bustling illegal trade. The Bay Citizen.

McPartland, J. M. (1984). Pathogenicity of Phomopsis ganjae on Cannabis sativa and the fungistaticeffect of cannabinoids produced by the host. *Mycopathologia*, *87*, 149–153.

McPartland, J. M. (1989). Storage molds associated with post-harvest Cannabis decay. CoverIllustration. *Mycol Soc Am Newsl*, *40*(1), 1.

McPartland, J. M. (1992). The Cannabis pathogen project: Report of the second five-year plan. *MycolSoc Am Newsl*, *43*(1), 43.

McPartland, J. M. (1994a). Microbiological contaminants of marijuana. *J Int Hemp Assoc*, *1*, 41–44.

McPartland, J. M. (1994b). Cannabis pathogens X: Phoma, Ascochyta and Didymella species. *Mycologia*, *86*(6), 870–878. doi:10.1080/00275514.1994.12026492

McPartland, J. M. (2002). Contaminants and adulterants in herbal Cannabis. In F. Grotenhermen & E. Russo (Eds.), *Cannabis and Cannabinoids pharmacology, toxicology and therapeuticpotential* (pp. 337–343).

McPartland, J. M. (2003). Byssinosis in hemp mill workers. *J Int Hemp Assoc*, *8*(1), 33–44. doi:10.1300/J237v08n01_04

McPartland, J. M., & Cubeta, M. A. (1997). New species, combinations, host associations and locationrecords of fungi associated with hemp (Cannabis sativa). *Mycological Research*, *101*(7), 853–857. doi:10.1017/S0953756297003584

McPartland, J. M., & Pruitt, P. (1997). Medical marijuana and its use by the immunocompromised. *Alternative Therapies in Health and Medicine*, *3*(3), 39–45. PMID:9141290

McPartland JM, West D (1999) Killing Cannabis with mycoherbicides. *J Int Hemp Assoc* *6*(1), 1,4–8

McPartland, J. M., Clarke, R. C., & Watson, D. P. (2000). *Hemp diseases and pests management and biological control*. CABI Publishing.

McPartland, J. M., Blanchon, D., & Musty, R. E. (2008). Cannabimimetic effects modulated by cholinergic compounds. *Addiction Biology*, *13*(3-4), 411–415. doi:10.1111/j.1369-1600.2008.00126.x PMID:18782385

Meers, E., Ruttens, A., Hopgood, M., Lesage, E., & Tack, F. M. (2005). Potential of Brassicrapa, Cannabissativa, Helianthus annuus and Zea mays for phytoextraction of heavy metals from calcareous-dredged sediment derived soils. *Chemosphere*, *61*(4), 561–572. doi:10.1016/j.chemosphere.2005.02.026 PMID:16202810

Mihoc, M., Pop, G., Alexa, E., & Radulov, I. (2012). Nutritive quality of Romanian hemp varieties(Cannabis sativa L.) with special focus on oil and metal content of seeds. *Chemistry Central Journal*, *6*(1), 122. doi:10.1186/1752-153X-6-122 PMID:23088580

Mikuriya, T. H., North, W., Lucido, F., Jaffee, R., & Weirick, J. (2005) Cerebrospinal delayed allergicreaction to pesticide residue. In: *Conference proceedings, international association forCannabis as medicine*, (p 14). Springer.

Moir, D., Rickert, W. S., Levasseur, G., Larose, Y., Maertens, R., White, P., & Desjardins, S. (2008). Acomparison of nainstream and sidestream marijuana and tobacco cigarette smoke producedunder two machine smoking conditions. *Chemical Research in Toxicology*, *21*(2), 494–502. doi:10.1021/tx700275p PMID:18062674

Moody, M., Wharton, R. C., Schnaper, N., & Schimpff, S. C. (1982). Do water pipes prevent transmission offungi from contaminated marijuana? *The New England Journal of Medicine*, *306*(24), 1492–1493. doi:10.1056/NEJM198206173062424 PMID:7078603

NCCEH. (2009). *Recommendations for safe re-occupancy of marijuana grow operations*. NationalCollaborating Centre for Environmental Health.

NJMMP. (2011) *Medicinal marijuana program rules*. New Jersey Medicinal Marijuana Program.: www.nj.gov/health/medicalmarijuana/documents/final_rules.pdf

Ondrej, M. (1991). Vyskyt hub nastonínchkonopi [Occurrence of hemp fungus]. *Len a Konopí*, *21*, 51–57.

Perry, D. C. (1977). Street drug analysis and drug use trends 1969-1975. Part II. *PharmChem Newsletter*, *6*(4), 1–3.

Ramírez J (1990) Acute pulmonary histoplasmosis: new recognized hazard of marijuana planthunters. *Am J Med 88*(5, Suppl.), 60 N.

Ross, S. A., & ElSohly, M. A. (1996). The volatile oil composition of fresh and air-dried buds of Cannabissativa. *Journal of Natural Products*, *59*(1), 49–51. doi:10.1021/np960004a PMID:8984153

Ruchlemer, R., Amit-Kohn, M., Raveh, D., & Hanuš, L. (2015). Inhaled medicinal cannabis and theimmunocompromised patient. *Supportive Care in Cancer*, *23*(3), 819–822. doi:10.100700520-014-2429-3 PMID:25216851

Russo, E. (2016) Pesticide contamination of cannabis in the legal market. In: *Proceedings of the26th Annual Symposium on the Cannabinoids*. International Cannabinoid Research Society.

Safari Singani, A. A., & Ahmadi, P. (2012). Manure application and Cannabis cultivation influence onspeciation of lead and cadmium by selective sequential extraction. *Soil & Sediment Contamination*, *21*(3), 305–321. doi:10.1080/15320383.2012.664186

Samson, R. A., Hoekstra, E. S., & Frisvad, J. C. (Eds.). (2004). Introduction to food- and airborne fungi.CentraalbureauvoorSchimmelcultures, UtrechtScheel AH, Kraus D, Haars H, Schmitz I, Junker K (2012) Talcum induced pneumoconiosisfollowing inhalation of adulterated marijuana. *Diagnostic Pathology*, *7*, 26.

Taylor, D. N., Wachsmuth, I. K., Shangkuan, Y. H., Schmidt, E. V., Barrett, T. J., Schrader, J. S., Scherach, C. S., McGee, H. B., Feldman, R. A., & Brenner, D. J. (1982). Salmonellosis associated with marijuana: Amultistate outbreak traced by plasmid fingerprinting. *The New England Journal of Medicine*, *306*(21), 1249–1253. doi:10.1056/NEJM198205273062101 PMID:7070444

Turner, T. R., James, E. K., & Poole, P. S. (2013). The plant microbiome. *Genome Biology*, *14*(6), 209. doi:10.1186/gb-2013-14-6-209 PMID:23805896

Ungerleider, J. T., Andrysiak, T., Tashkin, D. P., & Gale, R. P. (1982). Contamination of marijuana cigaretteswith pathogenic bacteria. *Cancer Treatment Reports*, *66*(3), 589–590. PMID:7060050

Upton, R., Craker, L., ElSohly, M., Romm, A., Russo, E., & Sexton, M. (Eds.). (2013). *Cannabis inflorescence,Cannabis spp. Standards of identity, analysis, and quality control*. American HerbalPharmacopoeia.

Vandenhove, H., & Van Hees, M. (2005). Fibre crops as alternative land use for radioactivelycontaminated arable land. *Journal of Environmental Radioactivity*, *81*(2-3), 131–141. doi:10.1016/j.jenvrad.2005.01.002 PMID:15795030

Venhuis, B. J., & de Kaste, D. (2008). Sildenafil analogs used for adulterating marihuana. *Forensic Science International*, *182*(1-3), e23–e24. doi:10.1016/j.forsciint.2008.09.002 PMID:18945564

Verweij, P. E., Kerremans, J. J., Voss, A., & Meis, J. F. (2000). Fungal contamination of tobacco andmarijuana. *Journal of the American Medical Association*, *284*(22), 2875. doi:10.1001/jama.284.22.2869 PMID:11147983

Wilson, D., Steinegger, P., & Parkin, D. P. (1989). Effects of cannabis smoked together with a substancesold as Mandrax. *South African Medical Journal*, *76*(11), 636. PMID:2595497

Winston, M. E., Hampton-Marcell, J., Zarraonaindia, I., Owens, S. M., Moreau, C. S., Gilbert, J. A., Hartsel, J. A., Kennedy, S. J., & Gibbons, S. M. (2014). Understanding cultivar-specificity and soildeterminants of the cannabis microbiome. *PLoS One*, *9*(6), e99641. doi:10.1371/journal.pone.0099641 PMID:24932479

Wurzer, J. (2016) *Safety testing of medicinal cannabis*. In: Proceedings of the 2006 CannmedConference. Medical Genomics, Woburn, MA.

Wyatt, K. (2015). Marijuana subject to product liability claim in Colorado. *U.S. News & World Report*.

Chapter 10
Cannabis sativa and Its Ability to Combat Climate Change:
Unravelling Sustainable Benefits of Cannabis and Its Derivatives

Zahid Nabi
Central University of Jammu, India

Shivali Kundan
Central University of Jammu, India

Neha Verma
Central University of Jammu, India

Dinesh Kumar
Central University of Jammu, India

ABSTRACT

Cannabis sativa plant is a multifunctional crop having multiple uses, including for food, fibre, fuel, and construction materials. This makes it a valuable resource for farmers, as it provides multiple income streams and reduces the need for mono-cropping. In addition, hemp has the potential to play a significant role in promoting carbon sequestration and sustainable land use practices. By using hemp for carbon sequestration, for harvesting bioenergy and making of bioplastics, we can help to mitigate the effects of climate change, improve soil health, and promote sustainable agriculture practices. With continued research and investment, this chapter assess different possibilities that could be explored to harvest environmental benefits of Cannabis sativa.

DOI: 10.4018/978-1-6684-5718-4.ch010

INTRODUCTION

Cannabis sativa L. (C. sativa), popularly called Indian hemp, is an herbaceous annual plant that has been growing since ancient times in Central Asia (India and China) (Russo et al., 2008). Cannabis sativa (often known as "Cannabis") is an angiosperm in the Cannabaceae family. Cannabis sativa has been farmed for more than 5000 years for fibres and seed oil (Lash, 2010, Leizer et al., 2000), as well as medical (Zuardi, 2006 and Clarke and Merlin, 2013;) and recreational usage (Small, 2017). (Burstein, 1997 and Cota et. al., 2003). The plant is known for its medicinal and recreational uses and is often referred to as marijuana or hemp. Cannabis sativa contains a variety of chemical compounds, including cannabidiol (CBD) and tetrahydrocannabinol (THC), which are responsible for its medicinal and psychoactive effects. The plant is also used for its fibres, which are used to make textiles, paper, and other products. Cannabis sativa plant has a wide range of uses including medicinal, recreational, industrial, and horticultural uses. Cannabis sativa is a species of the Cannabis genus of plants. It is a tall, slender, and fibrous plant that is typically grown for its seeds, leaves, and flowers, which contain compounds known as cannabinoids. Cannabis sativa is a plant species that has a wide range of uses. The most well-known use of the plant is for the production of marijuana, which is used for its psychoactive effects. However, there are many other uses for the plant as well, including:

MEDICINAL USE

Cannabis sativa has been used for medicinal purposes for centuries. The plant contains compounds called cannabinoids, which have been found to have therapeutic properties. Tetrahydrocannabinol (THC) and cannabidiol are the two principal cannabinoids present in the plant (CBD). The psychoactive qualities of marijuana are caused by the chemical THC, whereas CBD is non-psychoactive and has been shown to have anti-inflammatory, analgesic, and anti-anxiety properties. Medicinally, it can be used to help with conditions such as pain, anxiety, and insomnia. Recreationally, it can be consumed in various forms, such as smoking, vaporizing, and edibles.

Industrial Use

The fibres from the stem of the cannabis sativa plant can be used to make paper, textiles, and rope. The plant's seeds are also rich in oil and can be used for food and cosmetics. Industrially, it can be used to make a variety of products such as textiles, paper, and bioplastics. And horticulturally, it can be used as a cash crop or as a source of food.

Recreational Use

As mentioned before, the most well-known use of Cannabis sativa is for the production of marijuana, which is used for its psychoactive effects. These effects are caused by THC, a compound found in the plant. The plant is consumed in different forms such as dried flowers, resin, oil, or edibles.

Environmental Use

Cannabis sativa is known to be a hyper accumulator of heavy metals and other toxins. This means that the plant can be grown in contaminated soils to remove pollutants and clean the soil. Like all plants, hemp absorbs carbon dioxide from the atmosphere through the process of photosynthesis. When hemp is grown for industrial use, it can absorb large amounts of carbon, which can be stored in the plant's biomass. This process, known as carbon sequestration, can help to reduce the amount of greenhouse gases in the atmosphere, which can contribute to climate change. Hemp can be used to create a variety of products, including bioplastics. These are plastics made from plant materials, rather than fossil fuels. Bioplastics are more environmentally friendly than traditional plastics because they are biodegradable and can be composted. This reduces the amount of plastic waste in the environment, which can contribute to climate change. Hemp can also be used as a construction material. Hempcrete, a mixture of hemp and lime, is a lightweight, insulating material that can be used to build homes and other structures. It is also fire-resistant, durable, and sustainable. Using hempcrete instead of traditional building materials can reduce the amount of carbon emissions associated with the construction process. Biofuel: Hemp oil can also be used to create biofuel. Biofuels are fuels made from plant materials, and they can be used to power cars, trucks, and other vehicles. They are more environmentally friendly than traditional fossil fuels because they produce fewer greenhouse gas emissions. Growing hemp can also help to regenerate soil. Hemp plants have deep roots and can help to aerate the soil, which can improve its structure and fertility. This can lead to better crop yields and can help to reduce the need for synthetic fertilizers, which can contribute to climate change. The water quality of nearby waterways is improved by cannabis production. Unlike to other speciality crops, cannabis typically requires only a small amount of pesticide and fertiliser use to grow the crop successfully. Less usage of synthetic fertilisers and pesticides means less chemical seepage or runoff into adjacent rivers from the farm's irrigation system. As a result, less pesticide and fertiliser chemical pollution of vulnerable streams is possible. An outline of Environmental uses of Cannabis has been shown in Figure 1.1; these environmental have been described in detail in the upcoming sections.

Figure 1. An outline of environmental uses of cannabis

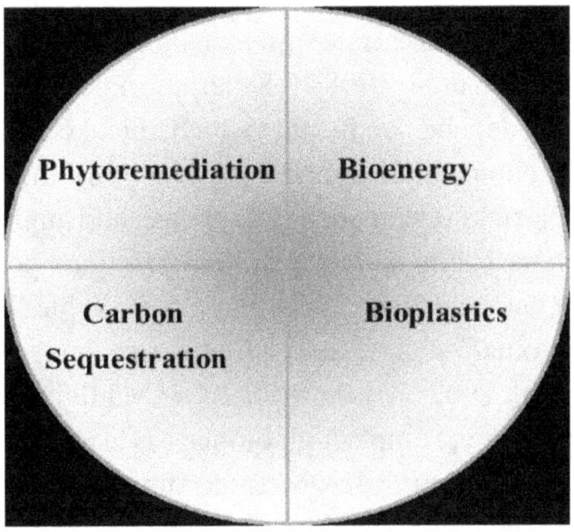

BIOREMEDIATION BY *CANNABIS SATIVA*

The plant's capacity to accumulate heavy metal in its body is the fundamental requirement for phytoremediation, but choosing plants that can store significant amounts of metal and are highly beneficial for the environment and the economy, highly resistant to contaminated soil and other environmental pollution (Angelova et al. 2004). Since hemp has a high tolerance to metals and produces a lot of biomasses, it is regarded as a promising candidate for soil phytoremediation. Hemp is a desirable plant for phytoremediation because of its high biomass output, great adaptability under a wide range of agro-ecological circumstances, and potential use of its biomass in non-food sectors (Linger et al. 2002; Citterio et al. 2003; Arru et al. 2004). Application of the changes had a big impact on the build-up of heavy metals. While EDDS caused larger amounts of Cu and Ni in the shoot, EDTA treatment showed increased lead and cadmium build up. In the case of Zn, no discernible difference was found. The authors backed the idea that applying amendments before harvest improves extraction results. Vandenhove and Hees (2005) explored the feasibility of the production of C. sativa on radionuclide-contaminated areas for the purpose of examining the transfer of radiocaesium from contaminated soil to the hemp, tests were conducted over a well-known radionuclide called radiocaesium in sandy soil under greenhouse and lysimeter settings. Additionally studied was the spread of radiocaesium during crop conversion. In the stem, straw, and fibres of the hemp plant, the translocation factor (TF) was determined to be 0.6 103 m2 / kg, 0.5 103 m2 / kg, and 1.0 103 m2 / kg, respectively. For the effective remediation of two polycyclic aromatic hydrocarbons, namely benzo[a]pyrene and chrysene, industrial hemp (Cannabis sativa) has been employed (Campbell et al. 2006).

BIOENERGY PRODUCTION ABILITY OF *CANNABIS SATIVA*

Industrial hemp, commonly known as Cannabis sativa, is currently a very promising source for the generation of bioenergy. It is a practical choice with little negative effects on the environment (Li et al. 2010). Hemp's cellulose concentration is quite high (around 44%) compared to agricultural lignocellulosic materials like corn stover and wheat straw, which comprise about 37% (dry mass or cellulose) (Öhgren et al., 2005; Linde et al. 2008). Hemp is a crop that has a significant potential for use in the production of bioethanol due to its high cellulose content and high biomass output. The two primary components of the hemp stem are a woody core with a much greater lignin concentration and bast fibres with a high cellulose content (Garcia-Jaldon et al. 1998). The appropriateness and usability of fuel produced from energy crops as solid biofuel depends on its physico-chemical characteristics. Physical treatments including milling, grinding, and compaction can be used to modify the physical characteristics of the fuel, including its bulk density, particle size, tendency to bridge, and angle of repose (Mattsson & Briere 1984). When burning hemp fuel, the chemical fuel qualities of sodium, potassium, magnesium, calcium, silicon, chlorine, aluminium, sulphur, and phosphorus play a crucial role (Baxter et al. 1998). Hemp seeds have an oil content that ranges from 26 to 38%, and a higher percentage of polyunsaturated fatty acids are present in this oil (Oomah et al. 2002; Kriese et al. 2004; Matthäus & Brühl 2008; Latif & Anwar, 2009). As a different form of bioenergy, hemp's high biomass is also used to produce biogas. In order to produce energy commercially, hemp biomass has been the subject of several studies (Castleman 2006; Burczyk et al. 2008; Rice 2008). The biomass output and, consequently, the amount of energy produced are influenced by the stage of plant growth. The amount of lignin and structural carbohydrates rises as the plant ages, while the degradation of the carbohydrates (cellulose and hemicellulose) begins (Jones 1970). Biodiesel is a sustainable power choice to hydrocarbon based energizes. Biodiesel can be used for transportation fuel and power creation with next to no alteration. Business creation of biodiesel has previously been begun utilizing different feedstock oils like soybean oil, rapeseed oil and palm oil in US, Europe and Southeast Asia. It comprises of monoalkyl esters of long chain unsaturated fats which are removed from different inexhaustible lipid feedstocks. These lipids are trans-esterified utilizing compound (corrosive/base)

BIOPLASTICS FORM *CANNABIS SATIVA*

Hemp-based plastic is biodegradable, making it a sustainable alternative to traditional petroleum-based plastics. This biodegradable plastic can decompose within 6 months, reducing the need for landfills and the release of harmful chemicals. biodegradable plastic made from hemp is a promising solution for reducing the impact of plastic waste on the environment. Its durability, renewability, and low carbon footprint make it an attractive alternative to traditional petroleum-based plastics. Unlike traditional petroleum-based plastics, hemp-based biodegradable plastic will break down and decompose over time when exposed to the environment. This makes it an environmentally friendly alternative to traditional plastics, as it does not contribute to plastic waste in landfills or the ocean. Hemp-based biodegradable plastic has comparable durability to traditional petroleum-based plastic, making it a suitable alternative for everyday use. It is also resistant to heat and moisture, making it a suitable option for food packaging and other applications where the plastic may be exposed to these elements (Rajak et al., 2022).

Renewability: Unlike petroleum, which is a finite resource, hemp is a fast-growing and renewable resource, making it an environmentally sustainable option for producing biodegradable plastic.

Carbon Footprint: Hemp has a low carbon footprint compared to other materials, as it requires less energy and fewer resources to produce, making it a more environmentally friendly option. Additionally, the process of making biodegradable plastic from hemp releases fewer greenhouse gases compared to traditional petroleum-based plastic production (Prade et al., 2012)

CARBON SEQUESTRATION USING *CANNABIS SATIVA*

Cannabis sativa has the potential to play a role in carbon sequestration, which is the process of removing carbon dioxide from the atmosphere and storing it in a long-term sink. One way to utilize Cannabis sativa in carbon sequestration is through the use of industrial hemp. Industrial hemp is a variety of Cannabis sativa that is grown specifically for its fiber, which can be used to make a wide range of products, including textiles, building materials, and biofuels. Because it is a fast-growing and high-yielding crop, industrial hemp is able to sequester large amounts of CO2 from the atmosphere over the course of its growth cycle (Ingrao et al.,2015). Another way to utilize Cannabis sativa for carbon sequestration is through the use of agroforestry systems, which combine the cultivation of cannabis plants with the cultivation of other crops, such as fruit and nut trees, and perennial grasses. The combination of different plant species in these systems can help to increase the overall carbon sequestration potential of the land (Ingrao et al.,2015).

It is important to note that these are theoretical ways and not yet implemented on a large scale, and more research needs to be done to determine the potential of cannabis plants for carbon sequestration, as well as the legal and practical issues surrounding their cultivation.

The use of hemp for carbon sequestration is a promising solution for reducing the impact of carbon dioxide on the environment. Its fast growth rate, carbon dioxide absorption, and long-term carbon storage make it a valuable tool for mitigating the effects of climate change (Glé et al., 2011). With continued research and investment, hemp has the potential to play a significant role in creating a more sustainable future by following measures:

Soil Carbon Sequestration

When hemp plants are harvested, the organic matter that was formed during photosynthesis remains in the soil. This organic matter helps to improve the soil's fertility and structure, and acts as a carbon sink, storing carbon in the soil for an extended period of time.

Long-Term Carbon Storage

The carbon that is stored in the soil through the use of hemp can remain in the soil for many years, providing a long-term carbon sink. Additionally, the use of hemp-based products, such as building materials and textiles, can also help to reduce the amount of carbon in the atmosphere by replacing traditional products that have a higher carbon footprint.

Carbon Footprint

The production of hemp has a low carbon footprint compared to other materials, as it requires less energy and fewer resources to produce, making it an environmentally friendly option.

Sustainable Land Use

The cultivation of hemp can also help to promote sustainable land use practices. Hemp is a hardy and versatile crop that can be grown in a variety of climates and soil types, and requires less water and pesticides compared to other crops. This makes it an ideal crop for farmers looking to implement sustainable land use practices.

Soil Health

Hemp has a deep root system that helps to improve soil health by preventing soil erosion, promoting soil aeration, and increasing the soil's organic matter content. This leads to a healthier and more resilient soil, which is better able to absorb and store carbon.

Rotational Cropping

Hemp can also be used as a rotational crop, which means that it can be grown in rotation with other crops, such as wheat, corn, or soybeans. Rotational cropping helps to maintain soil health and fertility, as well as to reduce the build-up of pests and diseases. This makes it an ideal crop for farmers looking to implement sustainable agriculture practices.

Reforestation

In addition to promoting sustainable land use practices, the use of hemp for carbon sequestration can also help to support reforestation efforts. By reducing the demand for traditional products that contribute to deforestation, such as paper and lumber, hemp has the potential to play a role in preserving forests and their role as carbon sinks.

Multifunctional Crops

Hemp is a multifunctional crop, meaning that it has multiple uses, including for food, fibre, fuel, and construction materials. This makes it a valuable resource for farmers, as it provides multiple income streams and reduces the need for mono-cropping. Apart from the above-mentioned applications, some more sustainable uses of Cannabis have been tabulated below in Table 1.

Table 1. Environmentally benefical uses of cannabis

Use of Cannabis	Detailed Informantion
Paper	In terms of making paper, hemp has the potential to take the place of trees, containing the consequences of deforestation. When compared to traditional wood paper, hemp paper is stronger, longer, and finer. Also, compared to trees, which take years to grow, the plant produces more paper in a shorter amount of time because to its rapid pace of growth.
Textiles	Hemp fibre is an environmentally beneficial product because it is cultivated and processed without the use of pesticides or chemicals. Hemp fibre has several important qualities, some of which are: eco-friendly and sustainable; strong and resilient fibre; ability to stop bacteria from growing by absorbing moisture; recyclable; and ability to block UV radiation.
Cosmetics	Hemp seed-derived essential oils are highly valued on the market. With its all-natural components, hemp oil has the potential to replace petroleum-based cosmetics and other skincare products. Hand soap, shower cream, lip balm, face cream, foot cream, and many other cosmetic products are made from hemp. Customers who care about the environment and who have sensitive well-being are drawn to these oil-based goods by their therapeutic effects and other advantages.
Phytoremediation	Hemp effectively enhances the soil's health and quality. Phytoremediation, or the capacity of a plant to remove undesirable and harmful toxins from air, soil, and water, is one of the key characteristics of hemp. Heavy metals like cadmium, lead, and nickel are absorbed by plants, minimising the impact of harmful metals on human health and the environment.

Source: Nath, M. K. (2022).

CONCLUSION

Cannabis, apart from being a plant that has multiple uses, has the potential to play a significant role in promoting carbon sequestration and sustainable land use practices. By using it for carbon sequestration, we can help to mitigate the effects of climate change, improve soil health, and promote sustainable agriculture practices. Cannabis can be used for making bioplastics which would degrade easily leaving no toxic components in the soil. Biofuel can also be extracted from cannabis products which can be used to meet increasing energy demands. With continued research and investment, hemp has the potential to become a valuable tool for creating a more sustainable and resilient future.

REFERENCES

Öhgren K, Galbe M, Zacchi G (2005) Optimization of steam pretreatment of SO2 impregnated corn stover for fuel ethanol production. *Appl Biochem Biotechnol*

Angelova, V., Ivanova, R., Delibaltova, V., & Ivanov, K. (2004). Bioaccumulation and distribution of heavy metals in fibre crops (flax, cotton, and hemp). *Industrial Crops and Products*, *19*(3), 197–205. doi:10.1016/j.indcrop.2003.10.001

Arnaud, L., & Gourlay, E. (2012). Experimental study of parameters influencing mechanical properties of hemp concretes. *Construction & Building Materials*, *28*(1), 50–56. doi:10.1016/j.conbuildmat.2011.07.052

Arru, L., Rognoni, S., Baroncini, M., Bonatti, P. M., & Perata, P. (2004). Copper localization in Cannabis sativa L. grown in a copper-rich solution. *Euphytica*, *140*(1-2), 33–38. doi:10.100710681-004-4752-0

Baxter, L. L., Miles, T. R., Miles, T. R. Jr, Jenkins, B. M., Milne, T., Dayton, D., Bryers, R. W., & Oden, L. L. (1998). The behavior of inorganic material in biomass-fired power boilers: Field and laboratory experiences. *Fuel Processing Technology*, *54*(1–3), 47–78. doi:10.1016/S0378-3820(97)00060-X

Burczyk, H., Grabowska, L., Kolodziej, J., & Strybe, M. (2008). Industrial hemp as a raw material for energy production. *Journal of Industrial Hemp*, *13*(1), 37–48. doi:10.1080/15377880801898717

Campbell, S., Paquin, D., Awaya, J. D., & Li, Q. X. (2006). Remediation of Benzo[a]pyrene and chrysenecontaminated soil with industrial hemp (Cannabis sativa). *International Journal of Theoretical Physics*, *4*(2), 157–168. PMID:12655808

Castleman, T. (2006). *Hemp biomass for energy*. Fuel and Fiber Company.

Citterio, S., Santagostino, A., Fumagalli, P., Prato, N., Ranalli, P., & Sgorbati, S. (2003). Heavy metal tolerance and accumulation of Cd, Cr and Ni by Cannabis sativa L. *Plant and Soil*, *256*(2), 243–252. doi:10.1023/A:1026113905129

Clarke, R., & Merlin, M. (2013). 1. Introduction to the Multipurpose Plant Cannabis. In *Cannabis* (pp. 1–12). University of California Press.

Cota, D., Marsicano, G., Lutz, B., Vicennati, V., Stalla, G. K., Pasquali, R., & Pagotto, U. (2003). Endogenous cannabinoid system as a modulator of food intake. *International Journal of Obesity*, *27*(3), 289–301. doi:10.1038j.ijo.0802250 PMID:12629555

Garcia-Jaldon, C., Dupeyre, D., & Vignon, M. R. (1998). Fibers from semiretted hemp bundles by steam explosion treatment. *Biotechnology and Bioengineering*, *14*, 251–260.

Glé, P., Gourdon, E., & Arnaud, L. (2011). Acoustical properties of materials made of vegetable particles with several scales of porosity. *Applied Acoustics*, *72*(5), 249–259. doi:10.1016/j.apacoust.2010.11.003

Ingrao, C., Giudice, A. L., Bacenetti, J., Tricase, C., Dotelli, G., Fiala, M., & Mbohwa, C. (2015). Energy and environmental assessment of industrial hemp for building applications: A review. *Renewable & Sustainable Energy Reviews*, *51*, 29–42. doi:10.1016/j.rser.2015.06.002

Jones, D. I. H. (1970). Cell-wall constituents of some grass species and varieties. *Journal of the Science of Food and Agriculture*, *21*(11), 559–562. doi:10.1002/jsfa.2740211104

Kriese, U., Schumann, E., Weber, W. E., Beyer, M., Bruhl, L., & Matthäus, B. (2004). Oil content, tocopherol composition and fatty acid patterns of the seeds of 51 Cannabis sativa L. genotypes. *Euphytica*, *137*(3), 339–351. doi:10.1023/B:EUPH.0000040473.23941.76

Latif, S., & Anwar, F. (2009). Physicochemical studies of hemp (Cannabis sativa) seed oil using enzymeassisted cold pressing. *European Journal of Lipid Science and Technology*, *111*(10), 1042–1048. doi:10.1002/ejlt.200900008

Linde, M., Jakobsson, E. L., Galbe, M., & Zacchi, G. (2008). Steam pretreatment of dilute H2SO4 – impregnated wheat straw and SSF with low yeast and enzyme loadings for bioethanol production. *Biotechnology and Bioengineering*, *32*, 326–332.

Linger, P., Mussig, J., Fischer, H., & Kobert, J. (2002). Industrial hemp (Cannabis sativa L.) growing on heavy metal contaminated soil: Fibre quality and phytoremediation potential. *Industrial Crops and Products*, *16*(1), 33–42. doi:10.1016/S0926-6690(02)00005-5

Matthäus, B., & Brühl, L. (2008). Why it is so difficult to produce high quality virgin rapeseed oil for human consumption? *European Journal of Lipid Science and Technology*, *110*(7), 611–617. doi:10.1002/ejlt.200700275

Mattsson, J. E., & Briere, D. M. (1984) External biomass characteristics for efficient energy conversion-some considerations. Biomass characteristics for efficient energy conversion. In: R.L. Gambles (ed) *Proceedings of joint workshop of IEA/FE programme Groups B, C and D, Uppsala, Sweden.* Canadian Forestry Service, Ottawa, Canada

Meers, E., Ruttens, A., Hopgood, M., Lesage, E., & Tack, F. M. G. (2005). Potential of Brassica rapa, Cannabis sativa, Helianthus annuus and Zea mays for phytoextraction of heavy metals from calcareous dredged sediment derived soils. *Chemosphere*, *61*(4), 561–572. doi:10.1016/j.chemosphere.2005.02.026 PMID:16202810

Nath, M. K. (2022). Benefits of Cultivating Industrial Hemp (Cannabis sativa ssp. sativa)—A Versatile Plant for a Sustainable Future. *Chemistry Proceedings*, *10*(1), 14.

Oomah, B. D., Busson, M., Godfrey, D. V., & Drover, J. C. G. (2002). Characteristics of hemp (Cannabis sativa L.) seed oil. *Food Chemistry*, *76*(1), 33–43. doi:10.1016/S0308-8146(01)00245-X

Pittau, F., Krause, F., Lumia, G., & Habert, G. (2018). Fast-growing bio-based materials as an opportunity for storing carbon in exterior walls. *Building and Environment*, *129*, 117–129. doi:10.1016/j.buildenv.2017.12.006

Prade, T., Svensson, S. E., & Mattsson, J. E. (2012). Energy balances for biogas and solid biofuel production from industrial hemp. *Biomass and Bioenergy*, *40*, 36–52. doi:10.1016/j.biombioe.2012.01.045

Rajak, N. (2022). Hemp Usage as a Green Building Material, Plastic, and Fuel. In *Revolutionizing the Potential of Hemp and Its Products in Changing the Global Economy* (pp. 157–167). Springer International Publishing. doi:10.1007/978-3-031-05144-9_8

Rice, B. (2008). Hemp as a feedstock for biomass-to-energy conversion. *Journal of Industrial Hemp, 13*(2), 145–156. doi:10.1080/15377880802391274

Small, E. (2017). Classification of Cannabis sativa L. in relation to agricultural, biotechnological, medical, and recreational utilization. In *Cannabis sativa L.-Botany and biotechnology* (pp. 1–62). Springer. doi:10.1007/978-3-319-54564-6_1

Vandenhove, H., & Hees, M. V. (2005). Fibre crops as alternative land use for radioactively contaminated arable land. *Journal of Environmental Radioactivity, 81*(2-3), 131–141. doi:10.1016/j.jenvrad.2005.01.002 PMID:15795030

Zuardi, A. W. (2006). History of cannabis as a medicine: A review. Brazilian. *Journal of Psychiatry, 28*, 153–157. PMID:16810401

Chapter 11
Marijuana, i.e., *Cannabis sativa*: The Quandary of Being an Amalgamate of a Useful and Abusive Medicinal Herb

Javid Manzoor
https://orcid.org/0000-0002-2821-206X
Shri JJT University, India

Sajood Ahmad Bhat
Government Degree College, Bhaderwah, India

Anuradha Sharma
Government Degree College, Bhaderwah, India

ABSTRACT

Cannabis sativa, popularly known as "marijuana," poses a problem since it may have both beneficial and harmful effects. Cannabis has long been used for medicinal and recreational purposes, which demonstrates its value as a plant. Instead of this, enough evidence suggests that abusing this wonder herb can have negative effects on a number of organs and organ systems, such as the pulmonary system, the body's defense system, the cardiovascular system, etc. Additionally, it may affect both male and female potency and may also have clastogenic effects. Yet, it cannot be ruled out that there are some benefits to using marijuana responsibly, since it has been shown to be a miraculous treatment for atrophy, acute pain, a loss of muscular tone, motion sickness, and insomnia. This chapter will attempt to provide a thorough understanding of the various health effects of the herb and its extracted active bioactive ingredients.

INTRODUCTION

'Marijuana' in Mexican dialect implies the therapeutic part of Cannabis, which often found its application for smoking purpose by armed forces of New-Spain (Johnson, N., 2017). Dioecian, infrequently synoicous, and dimorphous in behaviour (Rupasinghe et al. 2020). It is an annual anemophilic plant. This herb is implicitly believed to have originated from the great grass lands of Central Asia and more pioneeringly

DOI: 10.4018/978-1-6684-5718-4.ch011

in the areas specially lying in Mongolia and southern Siberia (McPartland et al. 2019). The scientific records evaluated about the annual herbaceous plant suggest that its cultivation dates back almost to 12 millennia which can be a good argument for claiming, that it is one of the oldest cultivated profitable herbs (Peltzer and Pengpid, 2017). On a historical basis the use of marijuana dates as far as back to six millennia of the common era, when the seeds of the plant were used for edible purpose in mainland China, even though the weaving material drawn from the plant in hemp dates back to four millennia of the pre-Christian era (Monotony, et al., 2021). The earliest recorded use of Cannabis on pharmaceutical grounds was in 2727 of the common eras in mainland China (Hand, et al., 2016). The records suggest that the plant was used in old (TCM) typically for intestinal disorders, jungle fever, joint aches as well as acute pains occurring during labour (Anand, et al., 2019). The literary perspectives suggest that cannabis was frequently sown as a viable source of food and yarn in and around 1500 BC (Deguchi et al., 2020). The plant has innumerable advantages of use like that as yarn, mash, pharmaceutical, concrete purpose, oil derivate, permeable fabrics, bedding use for domestic animals, toiletries, etc. (Stasilowicz, " et al", 2021). The traditional usage of cannabis is not only puffing in cigarettes, obtained after sun-drying the flora and leaflets of cannabis, but it has also got constructive uses (Small, 2015). The explorations carried have suggested with enough evidence that the wide variety of non-nutritive chemical substances of Cannabis acts as a deterrent against several ailments, indicating its broad-spectrum medicinal library of possible lead compounds. Hence, the present literary review will be substantial to comprehend the medicinal benefits of marijuana, but also at the same time of constant and recurrent changing face of therapeutical marijuana landscape, experts and the people who are directly or indirectly related to the marijuana should evolve themselves from time to time about the existing information about the positive use and abuse of marijuana. Though it is imperious to assess probable benefits achieved in an ailment, as there is not substantive study to reach a conclusion as most prospective studies that measure the effectiveness of a new intervention or treatment are lacking (Breijyeh, et al., 2021). So, an approach is needed where there can be a clear line of demarcation between possible health hazards and health benefits due to the short peer-quality evidence and dearth of directives. From several decades scholars have explored and carried trails to assess benefits of several bioactive compounds present in marijuana, but a comprehensive study regarding the possible potentially helpful compounds present in cannabis is lacking. Hence, the present endeavour attempts to accumulate, comprehend the different statics related to this herbaceous plant and chart out the guidelines to highlight the need for novel methods and policies to channelise the good use of cannabis. Also, the current endeavour aims to provide a general apprise on numerous wide varieties of non-nutritive chemical compounds found in this herb including their bio-screening for their probable medicinal benefits. This appraisal also abridges the cannabis withdrawal by deep learning about its conduct, observation in addition to blockages.

MEDICINAL USES OF BIOCHEMICAL CONSTITUENTS OF CANNABIS SP

The medicinal use of Marijuana is recorded in primeval texts from numerous diasporas and ethnic lore's (Brand and Zhao, 2017). The versatility of this herb has can be argued by the remedial properties of cannabinoids and its associated derivatives. Up till now 113 (the potentially helpful compounds) phytonutrients and some odd 120 volatile unsaturated hydrocarbons found in the essential oils of plants have identified after their high throughput screening, (Calvi, et al., 2018) but an in-depth extent the collaborative action of polyphenolics has not yet been studied in such a detail. The each and every part of marijuana is rich in a variety of compounds which have different pharmacologic properties substantiated by researchers who have worked out the complex biosynthetic pathways of these the potentially helpful compounds, their collaborative action of use, separation, in addition to identification and homoeopathic uses (Andre, et al., 2016). Polycyclic aromatic amides, prenylated flavonoids, and hydroxylated fractions of stilbene established the potential positive biological screening properties and have proved an imperative antagonist for various types of microbial attacks (Pollastro, et al., 2018). The natural occurring chemicals with variable phenolic structures, like kaempferol, apigenin, vitexin, isovitexin, luteolin were tested for their repressing potential against lipoxygenase and prostaglandin endoperoxide synthase and their role in abrogation or delay in the onset of cancer (Birt, et al., 2001). The great void which occurs for explorations of marijuana phytochemicals is their incomplete structural analysis of the library of active compounds which occur in different cultivated varieties of cannabis which can fit in the window of medicinal or 'official drug list'. Different cultivars of the herb vary to a considerable extent in both cannabis specific bioactive compounds and chemical constituents common to the most of the plants. Whether a particular cultivating variety of cannabis can be deemed to contain the medicinal, narcotic or sedative constituent, it stands necessary to evaluate profile of chemical ingredients using a sophisticated characterization technique on quantitative and qualitatively. Some sophisticated characterization techniques like assessing the change in the optical rotation of a chemical constituent of a plant (ORD) and analysing the extent of absorption of oppositely circular polarized lights through ECD, chromatographic techniques (LC, GC-HRMS), Proton-NMR, C-13 and Mass spectral (MS) based structural profiling are very important in profiling the content of bioactive molecule in different cultivable species (Calvi, et al., 2018). The qualitative analysis for the Marinol and Epidiolex in any cultivated species is equally imperative to be suggested for a 'legally safe' approval (Raderman, 2016). It is to be noted that the varieties which are cultivated on the commercial basis must be evaluated thoroughly, while a synergistic approach is adopted for the human and active constituents' interactions, present to evaluate the innocuous usage of marijuana as a beneficial remedial herbaceous plant (Jin, et al., 2017).

TOBACCO VS. MARIJUANA AND TETRAHYDROCANNABINOL (THC)

The analytical studies carried on the constituents of smoke of cannabis and Tobacco have concluded that both do contain that the similar constituents with chemical substances which are toxic to the pulmonary system of humans (Melamede, 2005). The main particulate constituent of the tobacco and cannabis abuse i.e., tar is common to both the substances while the presence of Marinol and other analogous structural compounds is present only in cannabis, when an analysis is carried on the comparative scale (Sharma, et al., 2012). The nicotine present in tar of tobacco is unique to it while at the same time cannabis lacks it, but, at the same time it cannot be argued that marijuana is not carcinogenic due to lack of nicotine, as the presence of chemical constituents like benzo[a]pyrene, which acts as a connecting link for the pulmonary oncogenesis (Do, et al., 2018). The difference in puffing of cigarettes laden with tobacco which contain a filter which reduces the tar content, while at the same time marijuana cigarettes does not contain any filter which increases the risk of tar content two-fold (Aldington, et al., 2008). Moreover, the process of moving air in and out, while puffing of marijuana laden cigarettes increases almost over sixty six percent and the amount of smoke after the breathing in is 40% larger. Cannabis, includes concoction of dry leaflets, stems, flowers, and seeds tattered from the herbaceous plant, do not pose any serious harm but its toxic effects cannot be negated (DeFilippis, et al., 2020). The herb is deemed to have deleterious effects because it contains mood-altering ingredients, named (6aR,10aR)-delta-9-Tetrahydrocannabinol;(−)-trans-Δ^9- trade named as Marinol (Roychoudhury, et al., 2021). More the concentration of Marinol present in a particular variety of cannabis more mood altering can be it classified. The important parts of the herb are quite often puffed by stuffing into a ciggy known as 'joint' and also smoked by means of cigars (Cooper and Haney, 2009). In research carried in the year 2001 in USA on 12th grade students enumerated that 19% were puffing cigarettes, 5.8% puffed cannabis, and 3.6% were addicted to liquor abuse on a day-to-day basis. The research further revealed that almost 49% senior secondary grade students has had an abuse of cannabis at least once in their life (Grucza and Bierut, 2006). The distress which arises due to use of cannabis by younger generation further exposes the buddies towards more dangerous drugs like cocaine and heroin (Volkow, et al., 2014). It was observed that almost more than sixty percent of adolescents belonging to the age group of 12-17 reported the marijuana abuse while the rest who reported the marijuana abuse belong to the young adult age group of 18-25 (Ellickson, et al., 2005).

BIOCHEMICAL INTERACTION OF MARINOL

Cannabis has an ephemeral history of consumption either for distress relieving or for achieving medicinal benefits. The contemporary research has given significant insights to comprehend the biochemical processes of Cannabis and the bioactive compounds present in it i.e., cannabinoids, which alter the typical functioning of the human body (Fin, et al., 2021). Cannabinoids is broad spectrum term in terms of psychoactive chemical constituents which comprises almost 21 carbon alkaloids that are unique to the marijuana plant. Cannabis smoke comprise almost five dozen different cannabinoids (Bridgeman and Abazia, 2017) and main among them is the Marinol which is chemically (6aR,10aR)-delta-9-Tetrahydrocannabinol;(−)-trans-Δ^9- (**Figure 1.**) is the key culprit behind the addiction and abuse associated with cannabis (Gaoni and Mechoulam, 1964), (Seely, et al., 2011). The alteration of mood and biological changes associated with canniboid abuse are linked with broad-based interactions and less likely linked to explicit membrane-bound targets present on lipid bi-layer of a cell. Out of these two main target receptors for psychoactive drugs present in cannabis are CB1 and CB2 (Glogauer and Blay, 2021), while at the same time the first target receptor i.e., CB1 is where the most of the interactions take place (Fig.2) and these targets are found in almost all primates (Silver, 2019). The chemical constituents present in cannabis cause many negative effects in the brain of humans i.e., they reduce the capacity to learn, analyse and also lessen the capacity of information storing in hippocampus, control of locomotion action and reduce hunger inducing ability in the hypothalamus (Reggio, 2010). The signals triggered by cannabinoids is quite antagonistic to the action induced by Bacopa monnieri bacosides, 'tonic for the human brain', which enhances the memory (Banerjee, et al., 2021), besides, the mode of action of psychoactive chemicals in enhancing memory and their application in immediate future for brain ailments (Halder, et al., 2021).

Figure 1. Chemical structure of (6aR,10aR)-delta-9-Tetrahydrocannabinol

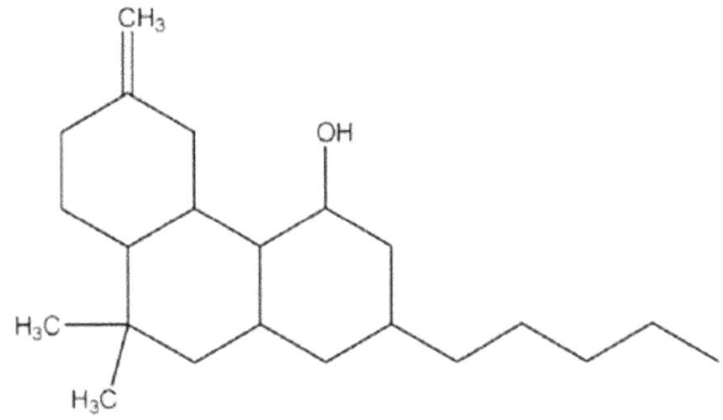

Marinol acts analogously like naturally occurring endocannabinoids, synthesized in the brain and has a sturdy influence. CB target receptors mostly occur in the frontal region of the outer most layer of brain and areas of brain like subcortical nuclei, little brain, anterior cingulate cortex (Zou and Kumar, 2018). Several signalling molecules namely ACh, Revivan, γ-Aminobutyric acid, 2-Aminopentanedioic acid and l-1-(3,4-Dihydroxyphenyl)-2-aminoethanol are repressed by the action of Marinol, whereas maximum of the time endogenous lipid-based retrograde neurotransmitters (ECS) are rendered into inaction owing to the enzyme (FAAH) (Atakan, 2012). While externally sourced psychoactive substances like Marinol remain in the body for a longer time resulting in alteration of normal functioning of body (Wyrofsky, et al., 2019). The resultant action flanked by Marinol and CB targets transpires in the presynaptic neurons which carries the signal to stimulate G-proteins, and thereupon they pass the information in, to either trigger or deactivate several information signals linked with genetic transfer pathways. The guanine nucleotide-binding proteins is responsible for the reticence of sodium (Na_V) and calcium (Ca_V) channels which, when repressed, result in stimulation of mitogen-activated protein kinase pathway. A total of emblematic four ailments i.e., analgesia, muscular rigidity, inhibition of behavioural or locomotor activity and incessant low body temperature, arises due to the formation of bioactive agonists (Manzanares, et al., 2006). Some additional disorders due to consumption of marijuana are nociception, trouble in achieving concentration, hyperactivity of senses, palpitations and unwanted appetite which jointly are responsible for cognitive impairment, impairment in information storage and locomotive and cognitive skills (Goncalves, et al., 2020). Severe mental breakdowns and anxiety are the deleterious effects which evolve usually observed in younger generation which metamorphoses into chronic psychiatric disorders in them in some cases (Radhakrishnan, "et, al", 2014).

GATEWAY HYPOTHESIS AND ITS LINKS WITH MARIJUANA

The model, which sheds on light on the substance is called escalation hypothesis. This principle is based on the fact that use of less effective drugs may lead to the substance abuse of dangerous nature and resultant anti-social acts (Nkansah, et al., 2016). It is a well-known fact that persons who were marijuana or liquor users once are addicted now to dangerous drugs however another study illustrates that uncommon vivacious medication users have used several drugs before consuming liquor or Marijuana (Budney, et al., 2007). Hence, the gateway drug effect decrees that the use of marijuana can ultimately result into use of dangerous drugs. Most of the experts are of the opinion that marijuana acts as a stepping-stone to various drugs because of its links with many social aspects (Secades, et al., 2015).

Figure 2. Deleterious ill effects of Herb (Cannabis sativa) and (6aR,10aR)-delta-9-Tetrahydrocannabinol on the humanoid brain

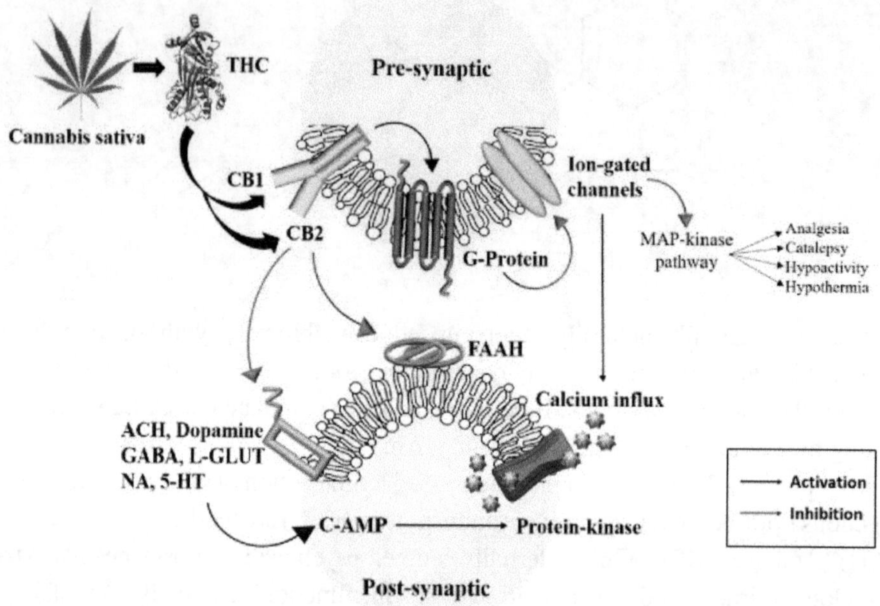

Figure 3. Multi-layered deleterious traits of cannabis

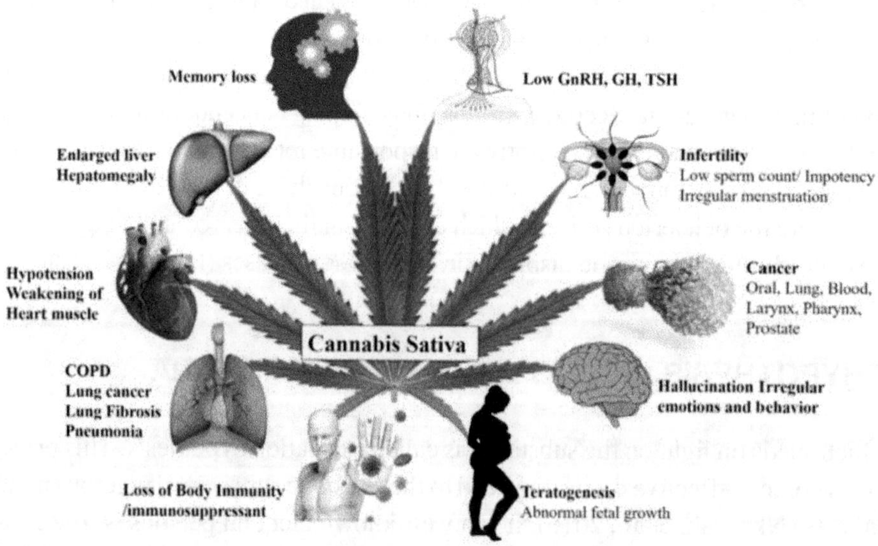

MARIJUANA AND HEALTH EFFECTS: CONTRADICTORY BUT STIMULATING CONSEQUENCES

Mammals other than humans are exposed to cannabis due to unintentional ingestion. The standard studies enumerate, that in the case of abuse by men the quantitative peak for concentration of Marinol is experienced in blood plasma for approximately 5 to 12 min, whereas the effect lasts for hrs. once consumed. The outcome is felt immediately within a span of 6–12 min after puffing and ranges between half hour and hour duration when ingested through the mouth (Huestis,2007). On assessment, the cases examined by APCC concluded that clinical traits were displayed inside two hours after ingesting. A case examined by APCC where a canine gulped 3g of cannabis displayed motor ataxia, head jogging, in addition to that vocalization. Correspondingly slower heart rate and dyssynergia were experienced in a canine whose weight ranged around 17 kg who had guzzled merely 1 tsp of cannabis. The assessment of the cases subjectively drew that the effects of marijuana ingestion commenced in a span of 30 to 90 minutes and lasted for three days. The psychoactive compounds present in cannabis are soluble in lipids in case of humans, although 97–99% are amino acids and distributed to several parts of body that include the brain, heart, kidneys, liver, and salivary glands. The moment Marinol is gulped, it has a considerable first-pass effect and is absorbed by microsomes by process of hydroxylation and is also processed by non-microsomal oxidation in the liver. The pathway adopted for excretory purpose passes through bile. As cannabis is ingested, within 3 days almost 35% is excreted as after taking of abusive substance within 72 h, around 35% of abusive substance consumed orally is expelled as non-conjugated metabolites, even though a fractional percentage is passed out through urine as acidic fractions and conjugates while still a large portion is passed out unchanged through urine. The resultant exposure to marijuana abuse 85% of it is passed out after five days (Fitzgerald, et al., 2013). It has been analyzed that when canines are exposed to 3,000-9,000 mg /kg of Marinol was not fatal. Moreover, majority of the canines behaved well after just one day. Rats reported minor to intensified lacerations with an effective dosage of 3600 mg /kg of Marinol and also thickening of adrenal gland with fat, blood loss, accumulation of mucus in the lungs, lung inflammation, splenic hypocellularity, thymus apoplexy (Taffe, 2012), (Thompson, et al., 1973).The research explorations on those who have experienced a continued exposure to the Marinol feel less appetite and less urge for sexual activity an advance in behavioral acceptance, a waning in stimulated hostile conduct (Colizzi, et al. 2018a), (Zamberletti, et al., 2012). The continued exposure to marijuana results in brain damage and metal disturbances as associated with continued abuse of liquor (Mandelbaum and Suzanne, 2017). Those who have a continued exposure of the marijuana are highly vulnerable and extremely susceptible to the risk of respiratory failure as a basis of fatality (**Figure 3**). Cannabis abuse is not associated with diseases alone but also disturbs the social life of an individual and in addition to the above negatives, it lessens the activity of an individual if he is a student, or a worker and makes an individual sluggish. The cannabis addiction leads to a monetary crisis and provokes a man to take the extreme step.

MODULATION OF THE IMMUNE SYSTEM AND LINK WITH CANNABIS: HAZARD VERSUS ADVANTAGE

The puffing of cannabis is related to inflammatory reactions. Dust cells have been separated from the pulmonary system of persons who are accused of cannabis and nicotine abuse, two out of three in contrast to individuals who do not smoke. Also, the deleterious effects induced both by nicotine abuse and cannabis abuse were almost similar (Cabral and Staab, 2005). The studies have suggested that recurrent cannabis smokers trigger the tissue damage, resulting in the build-up of dust cells in higher concentration in pulmonary regions. White blood cells separated from the pulmonary tract of marijuana or tobacco smokers showed an extensive surge in size because of particulate matter due to smoking displaying intricacy amongst the inclusion lying within gelatinous fluid of cell. While on the other hand the dust cells of both cannabis and nicotine users were found to be entirely embedded by inclusion bodies (Tanasescu and Constantinescu, 2010). The newer studies stresses on recognizing the Marinol receptors in the WBC as Marinol has swaying effects on the defence system. The examination carried on variety of defence cells like WBC's, large granular lymphocytes, and T lymphocyte of mammals, specified that Marinol has an immune regressing effect (Randall, 2007). In addition, WBCs of cannabis puffers are not able to secrete cytokines to bring a pro-inflammatory signal. Accordingly, these studies somewhat imply cannabis as an immune retainer hindering the defence mechanism of the man and intensifies the various risks in persons who suffer cancer, HIV-AIDS and those who have gone transplantation because they have a weak defence mechanism. Consequently, cannabis is not said to be good for health because of hazards allied with it, such as HIV-AIDS, (Tashkin & Roth, 2007) greater likelihood of unscrupulous contamination additionally Kaposi's sarcoma (Tashkin & Roth, 2019).

The decrease in the quantity of surface receptors of the neural inflammation process in animal models of cerebral palsy was checked by the usage of Epidiolex related to D9-THC, lessened pain of muscles and stiffness of muscles in persons affected by cerebral palsy. Besides, the behaviour affecting disadvantages of Marinol were diminished when taken along with Epidiolex (Goncalves et al., 2020). The homolog of Epidiolex (CBDV) displayed probable colon reducto-inflammatory influences in kids with active ulcers by supressing the cytokine signalling in intestinal cultures of infant patients (Pagano et al., 2019). The inoculation of endotoxin generated depressing activity was repressed by terpene alcohol by moderating the intropin target receptor site i.e., type 2 (D2R), the cannabinoid target site i.e., type 1 (CB1R), and also the target receptor site i.e., type 2 (CB2R) (Vieira et al., 2020).

CANNABIS AND REDUCED POTENCY: ALLEGORY AS AGAINST GENUINENESS

The feminine primates established the similar outcome of psychoactive compounds of cannabis on sexual organs akin to their nearest counterparts. Marinol was responsible for decline of lutropin almost ranging from 50–80% in apes. Insinuation of LNRH discharge was seen in direct and oblique ways. Reticence of gonadotropin release was experienced because of interference in the periods (John, et al., 2018). The research carried at reproductive psychology department at the University of Buffalo quantified about the persons who are addicted to cannabis experience lower concentration of seminal fluid and lower count of spermatozoa with unhealthy sperm affecting their impotency to a considerable extent (Hallak et al., 2019). The spermatozoa of cannabis puffers could swim in uterus displaying an anomalous trait. This unusual trait is also characterized by hyperactivity of spermatozoa of cannabis smokers in preliminary stage in cervix area, but in lateral stage its activity of swimming across the uteral fluid gets lowered and does not reach the ovum (Rajanahally et al., 2019). The persons who occasionally smoke cannabis also experience a reduction in impotency by delaying ejection. Rats and canines experienced reduction of gonadal size when they were fed with preparation of extracts of cannabis. The weakening of the seminiferous tubules of the gonads is the main reason for this problem and also the of the regular working of interstitial cells of gonadal region (Barak & Baker, 2016), (Kasman, et al., 2018b). The adverse outcome of cannabis results in lower spermatozoa due to lesser formation. The extreme users of cannabis experienced almost 60% decline in spermatozoa in seminal fluid with little intervention in lutropin and testosterone (Sharma, 2017). Females who puff cannabis lie at extreme end of risk of fertility because of unbalanced periods. The bioactive compound Marinol was assessed in the reproductive system along with the cervical fluid of females puffing cannabis (Lammert et al., 2018). The bioactive components of cannabis, tobacco and other psychoactive substances can be evaluated. Cannabis puffing enhances Marinol to reach female's fallopian tube. The effects of Marinol have even been experienced in those couples if the female is reported of cannabis abuse, the male gemmates are hindered by Marinol in cervix, uterine tube and reducing the motility of the sperm in cervical fluid (Kasman et al., 2018a), (Kasman et al., 2018b). There are evidences which suggest that excessive abuse of cannabis results in irregular release of ova from ovary (Dubovis & Muneyyirci, 2020).

A CRITICAL ANALYSIS OF THE STUDY: SUMMARY OF THE ANTAGONISTIC EFFECTS OF CANNABIS AND THE PROBABLE MEDICINAL USE

The main chemical constituents extracted from cannabis have been extensively researched in relation to their behaviour in humans i.e., epidiolex and dronabinol. Nevertheless, while dealing with cannabis, the ill effects of its active component i.e., Marinol are large. Marinol is one of the extremely effective bioactive chemical constituent that signals the release of molecules from brain; consequently, it somewhat intercedes in neural signalling activity, endorses a high ecstasy and a exposure on larger basis or 'drug relapse syndrome' is coupled with many behavioural problems, which involves change in brain structure ultimately reducing the mental capability (Moore et al., 2007), (Bhattacharyya, et al., 2010), (Meier, et al., 2012), (Leweke, et al., 2012). But controlled case studies have demonstrated positive effects of Marinol where it relieved pain in persons with neuropathic ailments and good results were seen which involved decrease of queasiness, lack of sleep, reduction in shallow breathing during sleep and recovery of good balance of hunger. The researches have demonstrated that of its probable positive effect in reducing cerebral palsy, pigmentary dispersion syndrome, PTSD and many others. The active components of cannabis have demonstrated effective role in inflammatory bowel syndrome by fluctuating the immune response that is, affecting ~5–25 kDa, immune gamma globulin release (Martinez et al., 2020). In a thorough study conducted the researcher's hand-delivered surveys to one hundred consecutive patients who were returning for yearly re-certification for therapeutic cannabis use in Hawai'i in order to assess benefits and antagonistic effects perceived by therapeutic Marijuana patients. The general response rate was 94%. The mean age was 49.3 years, and the average age was 51. The researchers did not assess the respondents on the basis of sex or race/origin. Virtually almost all respondents (97%) used therapeutic cannabis mainly for respite for lingering pain. The average reported pain respite from therapeutic cannabis was significant and average pre-treatment pain on a zero to ten scale was 7.8, while average post-treatment pain was 2.8, giving a reported average improvement of 5 points which roughly translates to a 64% average comparative reduction in pain. The additional testified benefits comprised respite from stress/anxiety (50% of respondents), relief of insomnia (45%), improved appetite (12%), diminished nausea (10%), increased focus/concentration (9%) and reprieve from depression (7%). Some of the respondents wrote notes relating that cannabis helped them to decrease or discontinue medications for pain, anxiety, and insomnia. Comments included the following: "Therapeutic Marijuana substituted my need for oxycodone. A majority (71%) testified no adverse effects, while 6% reported a cough and/or throat irritation and 5% reported a fear of arrest. Altogether other antagonistic effects were less than 5%. On no account serious antagonistic effects were reported (Charles and Sandra, 2014). Though, there are differences in approach towards the medicinal benefits of cannabis herb as whole (behavioral or therapeutic studies) and its main component i.e. of the and its main active compound Marinol (Wilkinson, et al., 2016). This dilemma has given rise to a conundrum where the active compounds from cannabis should be rather used as investigational medicines rather as legalized medicines. There is a disturbing survey report that after legalization there was an increase of almost 65% abuse of cannabis use in teenagers (Rocky Mountain HIDTA,2015). But, beneficial use of active components which include CBN, Epidiolex, (+)-CBT, (S, S)-9,10-Dihydroxy-$\Delta^{6a(10a)}$-THC, CBL, 2-Methyl-2-(4-methylpent-3-enyl)-7-pentyl-5-chromenol, CBE and additional assorted active compounds may perhaps be authenticated by carrying 'arbitrative, DUH-bul-blind STUH-dee, dummy and active-controlled medical tests' after recognition, separation and systematic quantification (Elsohly & Slade, 2005), (Wilkinson et al., 2016). **(Table 2.)**

Remarkably, within-subject research concluded that the administration of THC, lowers the dependency in humans when studied with a mood changer, divalproex, which intuitively aggravated perceptive performance and produced undesirable reactions, naming a few i.e., exasperation, nervousness, despair, and exhaustion so on (Haney et al., 2004). Moreover, combinatorial medicinal therapeutic action comprising lofexidine and Marinol assured towards an auspicious outcome of marijuana withdrawal (Haney, et al., 2008) The deleterious effects of the herb are a matter of research from several decades and ratification of the herb, has forced the health and health related people to adopt a conventional approach. Even though there exist some studies which suggest that using the herb in a constructive way produces positive results, but the differences of opinion still exist. The herb is commonly used for smoking purpose and as a food additive whose foundations lie on brew-tea oil or in the form of hashish, which has its derivation in the term 'assassin', and it is palpable to conclude that what part can it play in those persons who are reported of constant abuse of the herb. The addictiveness induced by the abuse of the herb is the foremost deleterious effect of cannabis where rehabilitation towards a normal social life takes a long time (Volkow, et al., 2014a) **(Table 1.)**

CONCLUSION

The methodical assessment of the bulk literary studies in context of the deleterious effects of Marijuana on humans and its association to various noxious substances, which have an antagonistic effect on men and other organisms alike, the extensive research have suggested to drop the word used for the herb as 'medical marijuana'. Puffing of cannabis is allied to enhanced deleterious results and it is quite reasonable that the cannabis cannot be used a therapeutic agent against ailments when talking of outnumbered patients. The positive effect of the active fraction of the herb i.e., Marinol would be unwise to ignore especially in persons who report acute pain, predominantly in persons who have Encephalomyelitis dis-

Table 1. Adverse effects of short-term use and long-term or heavy use of marijuana

Table 1. **Adverse Effects of Short-Term Use and Long-Term or Heavy Use of Marijuana.**
Effects of short-term use
Impaired short-term memory, making it difficult to learn and to retain information
Impaired motor coordination, interfering with driving skills and increasing the risk of injuries
Altered judgment, increasing the risk of sexual behaviors that facilitate the transmission of sexually transmitted diseases
In high doses, paranoia and psychosis
Effects of long-term or heavy use
Addiction (in about 9% of users overall, 17% of those who begin use in adolescence, and 25 to 50% of those who are daily users)*
Altered brain development*
Poor educational outcome, with increased likelihood of dropping out of school*
Cognitive impairment, with lower IQ among those who were frequent users during adolescence*
Diminished life satisfaction and achievement (determined on the basis of subjective and objective measures as compared with such ratings in the general population)*
Symptoms of chronic bronchitis
Increased risk of chronic psychosis disorders (including schizophrenia) in persons with a predisposition to such disorders

* The effect is strongly associated with initial marijuana use early in adolescence.

seminata. Cannabis is an extremely safe and effective medication for many patients with chronic pain. In stark contrast to opioids and other available pain medications, cannabis is relatively non-addicting and has the best safety record of any known pain medication (no deaths attributed to overdose or direct effects of medication). Adverse reactions are mild and can be avoided by titration of dosage using

Table 2. The positive effects of cannabinoids

Health Effects of Marijuana	THC	THC-A	THC-V	CBN	CBD	CBD-A	CBC	CBC-A	CBG	CBG-A	Benefits
Pain relief	■			■	■		■		■		Analgesis
Reduces inflammation		■			■	■	■		■	■	Anti-inflamatory
Supresses appetite			■								Anoretic
Stimulates appetite	■				■						Appetite stimulant
Reduces vomiting and nausea	■				■						Antimetic
Reduces contractions of small intestine					■						Intestinal antiprokinetic
Relieves anxiety					■						Anxiolytic
Tranquilizing / psychosis management					■						Antipsychotic
Reduces seizures and convulsions		■	■		■						Antiepileptic
Suppresses muscle spasms	■			■	■						Antispasmodic
Aides sleep				■							Anti-insomnia
Reduces efficacy of immune system					■						Immunosuppresive
Reduces blood sugar levels			■		■						Anti-diabetic
Prevents nervous system degeneration					■						Neuroprotective
Treats psoriasis					■						Antipsioratic
Reduces risk of artery blockage					■						Anti-ischemic
Kills or slows bacteria growth					■		■	■	■		Anti-bacterial
Treats fungal infection								■	■		Anti-fungal
Inhibits cell growth in tumours / cancer		■			■	■	■		■		Anti-proliferative
Promotes bone growth			■		■		■		■		Bone-stimulant

Note: Tetrahydrocannabinol, or THC, 2. THC-A is the acidic form of THC known as tetrahydrocannabinolic acid. THC-A is the biosynthetic precursor for THC,3. Tetrahydrocannabivarin, or THC-V, is a homologue of THC found naturally in the Cannabis plant. THC-V has a propyl side chain group on the molecule which can affect your body much differently than THC., 4. Cannabinol, abbreviated as CBN, stems from cannabigerolic acid.,5. Cannabidiol cannabinoid, known as CBD. 6. Other common Cannabidiol cannabinoids include CBD-A, CBC, CBC-A, CBG and CBG-A.

smokeless vaporizers. More research needs to be pursued to discover degrees of efficacy in other areas of promise such as in treating anxiety, depression, bipolar disorder, autism, nausea, vomiting, muscle spasms, seizures, and many neurologic disorders. Patients deserve to have cannabis released from its current federal prohibition so that scientific research can proceed and so that physicians can prescribe cannabis with the same freedom accorded any other safe and effective medications. Though, we cannot deny that constant use of herb (especially Marinol) has numerous ill effects on nervous system. The shortcomings ascribed to cannabis usage are short- and long-term memory damage combine with different mental disorders. Besides its ill effects of mental breakdown, it too intensifies the probabilities of lung carcinoma or still it can cause result in dangerous effects in some users. Also, the key anxiety is the lateral effects cause on heart, endocrine glands, defensive mechanism of body and cerebral functions. The research has concluded that pregnant ladies, who are reported of cannabis abuse results in leads to a decrease of rational aptitude of the new-borns experienced at a certain stage also increasing the risks of severe mental breakdowns. When a balanced approach is adopted, it suggests that cannabis is not good option for treatment of certain diseases even if a registered medical practitioner suggests it. The younger folks find a thrill in consuming cannabis and consume it recreationally under pressure of their buddies. This disturbs their general wellbeing and sets their future at stake.

REFERENCES

Aldington, S., Harwood, M., Cox, B., Weatherall, M., Beckert, L., Hansell, A., Pritchard, A., Robinson, G., & Beasley, R. (2008). Cannabis use and risk of lung cancer: A case- control study. *The European Respiratory Journal*, *31*(2), 280–286. doi:10.1183/09031936.00065707 PMID:18238947

Anand, U., Jacobo-Herrera, N., Altemimi, A., & Lakhssassi, N. (2019). A Comprehensive Review on Medicinal Plants as Antimicrobial Therapeutics: Potential Avenues of Biocompatible Drug Discovery. *Metabolites*, *9*(11), 258. doi:10.3390/metabo9110258 PMID:31683833

Andre, C. M., Hausman, J. F., & Guerriero, G. (2016). Cannabis sativa: The plant of the thousand and one molecules. *Front. Plant Sci*, *7*, 19. doi:10.3389/fpls.2016.00019 PMID:26870049

Atakan, Z. (2012). Cannabis, a complex plant: Different compounds and different effects on individuals. *Therapeutic Advances in Psychopharmacology*, *2*(6), 241–254. doi:10.1177/2045125312457586 PMID:23983983

Banerjee, S., Anand, U., Ghosh, S., Ray, D., Ray, P., Nandy, S., Dewaji Deshmukh, G., Tripathi, V., & Dey, A. (2019). Bacosides from Bacopa monnieri extract: An overview of the effects on neurological disorders. *Phytotherapy Research*, 1–12. doi:10.1002/ptr.7203 PMID:34254371

Barak, S., & Baker, H. (2016). *Clinical Management of Male Infertility*. Endotext.

Bhattacharyya, S., Morrison, P. D., Fusar-Poli, P., Martin-Santos, R., Borgwardt, S., Winton-Brown, T., Nosarti, C., O' Carroll, C. M., Seal, M., Allen, P., Mehta, M. A., Stone, J. M., Tunstall, N., Giampietro, V., Kapur, S., Murray, R. M., Zuardi, A. W., Crippa, J. A., Atakan, Z., & McGuire, P. K. (2010). Opposite effects of D-9- tetrahydrocannabinol and cannabidiol on human brain function and psychopathology. *Neuropsychopharmacology*, *35*(3), 764–774.

Birt, D. F., Hendrich, S., & Wang, W. (2001). Dietary agents in cancer prevention: Flavonoids and isoflavonoids. *Pharmacology & Therapeutics*, *90*(2-3), 157–177. doi:10.1016/S0163-7258(01)00137-1 PMID:11578656

Brand, E.J. & Zhao, Z., (2017). Cannabis in Chinese medicine: Are some traditional indications referenced in ancient literature related to cannabinoids. *Front. Pharmacol*, *8*, 108.. doi:10.3389/fphar.2017.00108

Breijyeh, Z., Jubeh, B., Bufo, S. A., Karaman, R., & Scrano, L. (2021). Cannabis: A Toxin- Producing Plant with Potential Therapeutic Uses. *Toxins*, *13*(2), 117. doi:10.3390/toxins13020117 PMID:33562446

Bridgeman, M. B., & Abazia, D. T. (2017). Medicinal cannabis: History, pharmacology, and implications for the acute care setting. *Pharm. Therap.*, *42*(3), 180. PMID:28250701

Budney, A., Roffman, R., Stephens, R., & Walker, D. (2007). Marijuana dependence and its treatment. *Addiction Science & Clinical Practice*, *4*(1), 4–16. doi:10.1151/ASCP07414 PMID:18292704

Cabral, G.A., Staab, A., (2005). Effects on the immune system. *Cannabinoids,* 385–423. . doi:10.1007/3-540-26573-2_13

Calvi, L., Pentimalli, D., Panseri, S., Giupponi, L., Gelmini, F., Beretta, G., Vitali, D., Bruno, M., Zilio, E., Pavlovic, R., Giorgi, A., (2018). Comprehensive quality evaluation of medical Cannabis sativa L. inflorescence and macerated oils based on HS-SPME coupled to GC–MS and LC-HRMS (q-exactive orbitrap®) approach. *J. Pharm. Biomed. Anal., 150*, 208–219. doi:. jpba.2017.11.073. doi:10.1016/j

Calvi, L., Pentimalli, D., Panseri, S., Giupponi, L., Gelmini, F., Beretta, G., Vitali, D., Bruno, M., Zilio, E., Pavlovic, R., & Giorgi, A. (2018). Comprehensive quality evaluation of medical Cannabis sativa L. inflorescence and macerated oils based on HS-SPME coupled to GC–MS and LC-HRMS (q-exactive orbitrap) approach. *J.Pharm.Biomed.Anal*, *150*, 208–219.. doi:10.1016/j.jpba.2017.11.073

Charles W. Webb and Sandra M. Webb RN, (2014), Therapeutic Benefits of Cannabis: A Patient Survey, *Hawai'i Jour. Of Med. & Pub. Health,73*(4).

Colizzi, M., McGuire, P., Giampietro, V., Williams, S., Brammer, M., & Bhattacharyya, S. (2018). Modulation of acute effects of delta-9-tetrahydrocannabinol on psychotomimetic effects, cognition and brain function by previous cannabis exposure. *European Neuropsychopharmacology*, *28*(7), 850–862. doi:10.1016/j.euroneuro.2018.04.003 PMID:29935939

Cooper, Z. D., & Haney, M. (2009). Comparison of subjective, pharmacokinetic, and physiological effects of marijuana smoked as joints and blunts. *Drug and Alcohol Dependence*, *103*(3), 107–113. doi:10.1016/j.drugalcdep.2009.01.023 PMID:19443132

DeFilippis, E. M., Bajaj, N. S., Singh, A., Malloy, R., Givertz, M. M., Blankstein, R., Bhatt, D. L., & Vaduganathan, M. (2020). Marijuana use in patients with cardiovascular disease: JACC review topic of the week. *Journal of the American College of Cardiology*, *75*(3), 320–332. doi:10.1016/j.jacc.2019.11.025 PMID:31976871

Deguchi, M., Kane, S., Potlakayala, S., George, H., Proano, R., Sheri, V., Curtis, W. R., & Rudrabhatla, S. (2020). Metabolic Engineering Strategies of Industrial Hemp (Cannabis sativa L.): A Brief Review of the Advances and Challenges. *Front. Plant Sci.*, *11*, 580621. Advance online publication. doi:10.3389/fpls.2020.580621 PMID:33363552

Do, E. P. B. (2018). Medicinal Properties of Cannabinoids, Terpenes, and Flavonoids in Cannabis, and Benefits in Migraine, Headache, and Pain: An Update on Current Evidence and Cannabis Science. *Wiley Online Library*, *58*(7), 1139–1186. doi:10.1111/head.13345

Dubovis, M., & Muneyyirci-Delale, O. (2020). Effects of marijuana on human reproduction. *Reprod. Toxicol. 94*, 22–30. . reprotox.2020.04.071. doi:10.1016/j

Ellickson, P. L., D'Amico, E. J., Collins, R. L., & Klein, D. J. (2005). Marijuana use and later problems: When frequency of recent use explains age of initiation effects (and when it does not). *Substance Use & Misuse*, *40*(3), 343–359. doi:10.1081/JA-200049356 PMID:15776981

Elsohly, M. A., & Slade, D. (2005). Chemical constituents of marijuana: The complex mixture of natural cannabinoids. Elsevier. https://doi.org/ 10.1016/j.lfs.2005.09.011.

Finn, D. P., Haroutounian, S., Hohmann, A. G., Krane, E., Soliman, N., & Rice, A. S. (2021). Cannabinoids, the endocannabinoid system, and pain: A review of preclinical studies. *Pain*, *162*, S5–S25. doi:10.1097/j.pain.0000000000002268 PMID:33729211

Fitzgerald, K. T., Bronstein, A. C., & Newquist, K. L. (2013). Marijuana Poisoning. *Topical Review Marijuana Poisoning. Elsevier*, *28*(1), 8–12. doi:10.1053/j.tcam.2013.03.004 PMID:23796481

Gaoni, Y., & Mechoulam, R. (1964). Isolation, Structure, and Partial Synthesis of an Active Constituent of Hashish. *Journal of the American Chemical Society*, *86*(8), 1646–1647. doi:10.1021/ja01062a046

Glogauer, J. & Blay, J. (2021). Cannabinoids, their cellular receptors, and effects on the invasive phenotype of carcinoma and metastasis. *Cancer Reports,* e1475.

Gonçalves, E. C., Baldasso, G. M., Bicca, M. A., Paes, R. S., Capasso, R., & Dutra, R. C. (2020). Terpenoids, cannabimimetic ligands, beyond the cannabis plant. *Molecules (Basel, Switzerland)*, *25*(7), 1567. doi:10.3390/molecules25071567 PMID:32235333

Gonçalves, E. C., Baldasso, G. M., Bicca, M. A., Paes, R. S., Capasso, R., & Dutra, R. C. (2020). Terpenoids, cannabimimetic ligands, beyond the cannabis plant. *Molecules (Basel, Switzerland)*, *25*(7), 1567. doi:10.3390/molecules25071567 PMID:32235333

Grucza, R. A., & Bierut, L. J. (2006). Cigarette smoking and the risk for alcohol use disorders among adolescent drinkers. *Alcoholism, Clinical and Experimental Research*, *30*(12), 2046–2054. doi:10.1111/j.1530-0277.2006.00255.x PMID:17117970

Halder, S., Anand, U., Nandy, S., Oleksak, P., Qusti, S., Alshammari, E.M., El-Saber Batiha, G., Koshy, E.P. & Dey, A. (2021). Herbal drugs and natural bioactive products as potential therapeutics: A review on pro-cognitives and brain boosters' perspectives. *Saudi Pharm. J. 29* (8), 879–907. doi:. jsps.2021.07.003. doi:10.1016/j

Hallak, J., Teixeira, T. A., Pariz, J. R., Iori, I., Costa, E., & Saldiva, P. H. (2019). MP75-09 Marijuana consumption has a direct deleterious effect on spermatozoa by increasing intracellular reactive oxygen species levels 20 times more than tobacco smoking: Reasons for concern on widespread use. *The Journal of Urology*, *201*(4).

Hand, A., Blake, A., Kerrigan, P., Samuel, P., & Friedberg, J. (2016). History of medical cannabis. *Journal of Pain Management*, *9*(4), 387–394.

Haney, M., Hart, C. L., Vosburg, S. K., Comer, S. D., Reed, S. C., & Foltin, R. W. (2008). Effects of THC and lofexidine in a human laboratory model of marijuana withdrawal and relapse. *Psychopharmacology 197* (1), 157–168. s00213-007-1020-8. doi:10.1007/

Haney, M., Hart, C. L., Vosburg, S. K., Nasser, J., Bennett, A., Zubaran, C., & Foltin, R. W. (2004). Marijuana withdrawal in humans: effects of oral THC or divalproex. *Neuropsychopharmacology 29* (1), 158–170. . npp.1300310. doi:10.1038/sj

Huestis, M. (2007). Human cannabinoid pharmacokinetics. *Chemistry & Biodiversity*, *4*(8), 1770–1804. doi:10.1002/cbdv.200790152 PMID:17712819

Jin, D., Jin, S., Yu, Y., Lee, C., & Chen, J. (2017). Classification of Cannabis Cultivars Marketed in Canada for Medical Purposes by Quantification of Cannabinoids and Terpenes Using HPLC-DAD and GC-MS Analytical & Bioanalytical Techniques. *Journal of Analytical & Bioanalytical Techniques*, *8*(01), 1. doi:10.4172/2155-9872.1000349

John, W. S., Martin, T. J., Solingapuram Sai, K. K., Nader, S. H., Donald Gage, H., Mintz, A., & Nader, M. A. (2018). Chronic d9-THC in rhesus monkeys: Effects on cognitive performance and dopamine D2/D3 receptor availability. *The Journal of Pharmacology and Experimental Therapeutics*, *364*(2), 300–310. doi:10.1124/jpet.117.244194 PMID:29203575

Johnson, N. (2017). Workers' weed: Cannabis, sugar beets, and landscapes of labour in the American West, 1900–1946. *Agricultural History*, *91*(3), 320–341. doi:10.3098/ah.2017.091.3.320

Kasman, A., Thoma, M., McLain, A., & Eisenberg, M. (2018a). PD09-09 Association between use of marijuana and infertility in men and women: findings from the national survey of family growth. *J. Urol. 199* (4). . juro.2018.02.606. doi:10.1016/j

Kasman, A. M., Thoma, M. E., McLain, A. C., & Eisenberg, M. L. (2018b). Association between use of marijuana and time to pregnancy in men and women: Findings from the National Survey of Family Growth. *Fertility and Sterility*, *109*(5), 866–871.

Kasman, A. M., Thoma, M. E., McLain, A. C., & Eisenberg, M. L. (2018b). Association between use of marijuana and time to pregnancy in men and women: Findings from the National Survey of Family Growth. *Fertility and Sterility*, *109*(5), 866–871.

Lammert, S., Harrison, K., Tosun, N., & Allen, S. (2018). Menstrual Cycle in Women Who Co-use Marijuana and Tobacco. *Journal of Addiction Medicine*, *12*(3), 207–211.

Leweke, F. M., Piomelli, D., Pahlisch, F., Muhl, D., Gerth, C. W., Hoyer, C., Klosterkötter, J., Hellmich, M., & Koethe, D. (2012). Cannabidiol enhances anandamide signaling and alleviates psychotic symptoms of schizophrenia. *Translational Psychiatry*, *2*(3), e94.

Mandelbaum, D. E., & Suzanne, M. (2017). Adverse structural and functional effects of marijuana on the brain: Evidence reviewed. *Pediatric Neurology*, *66*, 12–20. doi:10.1016/j.pediatrneurol.2016.09.004 PMID:27789118

Manzanares, J., Julian, M., & Carrascosa, A. (2006). Role of the Cannabinoid System in Pain Control and Therapeutic Implications for the Management of Acute and Chronic Pain Episodes. *Current Neuropharmacology*, *4*(3), 239–257. doi:10.2174/157015906778019527 PMID:18615144

Martínez, V., Iriondo De-Hond, A., Borrelli, F., Capasso, R., Del Castillo, M. D., & Abalo, R. (2020). Cannabidiol and Other Non-Psychoactive Cannabinoids for Prevention and Treatment of Gastrointestinal Disorders: Useful Nutraceuticals. *International Journal of Molecular Sciences*, *21*(9), 3067.

McPartland, J. M., Hegman, W., & Long, T. (2019). Cannabis in Asia: Its center of origin and early cultivation, based on a synthesis of subfossil pollen and archaeobotanical studies. *Vegetation History and Archaeobotany*, *28*(6), 691–702. doi:10.100700334-019-00731-8

Meier, M. H., Caspi, A., Ambler, A., Harrington, H., Houts, R., Keefe, R. S. E., Mcdonald, K., Ward, A., Poulton, R., & Moffitt, T. E. (2012). Persistent cannabis users show neuropsychological decline from childhood to midlife. *Nat. Acad Sci.*, *109*, 15980. doi:10.1073/pnas.1206820109

Melamede, R. J. (2005). Cannabis and tobacco smoke are not equally carcinogenic. *Harm Reduction Journal*, *2*(1), 21. doi:10.1186/1477-7517-2-21 PMID:16232311

Monthony, A. S., Page, S. R., Hesami, M., & Jones, A. M. P. (2021). The past, present and future of Cannabis sativa tissue culture. *Plants, 10*(1), 185. doi:10.3390/plants10010185 PMID:33478171

Moore, T. H., Zammit, S., Lingford-Hughes, A., Barnes, T. R., Jones, P. B., Burke, M., & Lewis, G. (2007). Cannabis use and risk of psychotic or affective mental health outcomes: A systematic review. *Lancet, 370*(9584), 319–328. https://doi.org/ 10.1016/S0140-6736(07)61162-3

Nkansah-Amankra, S. & Minelli, M. (2016). ''Gateway hypothesis'' and early drug use: Additional findings from tracking a population-based sample of adolescents to adulthood. *Prevent. Med. Reports, 4*, 134–141. doi:. pmedr.2016.05.003. doi:10.1016/j

Pagano, E., Romano, B., Iannotti, F. A., Parisi, O. A., D'Armiento, M., Pignatiello, S., Coretti, L., Lucafò, M., Venneri, T., Stocco, G., Lembo, F., Orlando, P., Capasso, R., Di Marzo, V., Izzo, A. A., & Borrelli, F. (2019). The non-euphoric phytocannabinoid cannabidivarin counteracts intestinal inflammation in mice and cytokine expression in biopsies from UC pediatric patients. *Pharmacological Research, 149*, 104464. doi:10.1016/j.phrs.2019.104464 PMID:31553934

Peltzer, K., & Pengpid, S. (2017). Cannabis and Amphetamine Use Among Adolescents in Five Asian Countries. *Central Asian Journal of Global Health, 6*(1). doi:10.5195/cajgh.2017.288 PMID:30881756

Pollastro, F., Minassi, A., & Fresu, L. G. (2018). Cannabis Phenolics and their Bioactivities. *Current Medicinal Chemistry, 25*(10), 1160–1185. doi:10.2174/0929867324666170810164636 PMID:28799497

Raderman, J.M., (2016). *Method for modifying THC content in a lipid-based extract of Cannabis.*

Radhakrishnan, R., Wilkinson, S. T., & D'Souza, D. C. (2014). Gone to pot-a review of the association between cannabis and psychosis. *Frontiers in Psychiatry*, 5. doi:10.3389/fpsyt.2014.00054 PMID:24904437

Rajanahally, S., Raheem, O., Rogers, M., Brisbane, W., Ostrowski, K., Lendvay, T., & Walsh, T. (2019). The relationship between cannabis and male infertility, sexual health, and neoplasm: A systematic review. *Andrology, 7*(2), 139–147. https:// doi.org/10.1111/andr.2019.7.issue-210.1111/andr.12585

Randall, M. D. (2007). Endocannabinoids and the haematological system. *British Journal of Pharmacology, 152*(5), 671–675. doi:10.1038j.bjp.0707420 PMID:17704826

Reggio, P. (2010). Endocannabinoid Binding to the Cannabinoid Receptors: What Is Known and What Remains Unknown. *Current Medicinal Chemistry, 17*(14), 1468–1486. doi:10.2174/092986710790980005 PMID:20166921

Rocky Mountain High Intensity Drug Trafficking Area. (2015). The legalization of marijuana in Colorado: *The impact, 3.* http://www.rmhidta.org/html/2015%20 PREVIEW%20Legalization%20of%20MJ%20 in%20Colorado%20the% 20Impact.pdf (Retrieved 30 October 2020).

Roychoudhury, P., Wang, N. N., & Narouze, S. N. (2021). Phytocannabinoids: Tetrahydrocannabinol (THC). In S. N. Narouze (Ed.), *Cannabinoids and Pain* (pp. 71–77). Springer. doi:10.1007/978-3-030-69186-8_10

Rupasinghe, H. P., Davis, A., Kumar, S. K., Murray, B., & Zheljazkov, V. D. (2020). Industrial hemp (Cannabis sativa subsp. sativa) as an emerging source for value-added functional food ingredients and nutraceuticals. *Molecules (Basel, Switzerland)*, *25*(18), 4078. doi:10.3390/molecules25184078 PMID:32906622

Secades-Villa, R., Garcia-Rodríguez, O., Jin, C. J., Wang, S., & Blanco, C. (2015). Probability and predictors of the cannabis gateway effect: A national study. *The International Journal on Drug Policy*, *26*(2), 135–142. doi:10.1016/j.drugpo.2014.07.011 PMID:25168081

Seely, K. A., Prather, P. L., James, L. P., & Moran, J. H. (2011). Marijuana-based drugs: Innovative therapeutics or designer drugs of abuse. *Molecular Interventions*, *11*(1), 36–51. doi:10.1124/mi.11.1.6 PMID:21441120

Sharma, A. (2017). Male infertility; evidences, risk factors, causes, diagnosis and management in human. *Annals of Clinical and Laboratory Research*, *5*(3), 188.

Sharma, P., Murthy, P., & Bharath, M. S. (2012). Chemistry, metabolism, and toxicology of cannabis: Clinical implications. *Iranian Journal of Psychiatry*, *7*(4), 149. PMID:23408483

Silver, R. J. (2019). The endocannabinoid system of animals. *Animals (Basel)*, *9*(9), 686. doi:10.3390/ani9090686 PMID:31527410

Small, E. (2015). Evolution and Classification of Cannabis sativa (Marijuana, Hemp) in Relation to Human Utilization. *Botanical Review*, *81*(3), 189–294. doi:10.100712229-015-9157-3

Stasiłowicz, A., Tomala, A., Podolak, I., & Cielecka-Piontek, J. (2021). Cannabis sativa L. as a natural drug meeting the criteria of a multitarget approach to treatment. *International Journal of Molecular Sciences*, *22*(2), 778. doi:10.3390/ijms22020778 PMID:33466734

Taffe, M. A. (2012). d 9-Tetrahydrocannabinol attenuates MDMA-induced hyperthermia in rhesus monkeys. *Neuroscience*, *201*, 125–133. doi:10.1016/j.neuroscience.2011.11.040 PMID:22138434

Tanasescu, R., & Constantinescu, C.S. (2010). Cannabinoids and the immune system: An overview. *Elsevier,215*(8), 588–597.

Tashkin, D. P. & Roth, M.D. (2007). Effects of Marijuana on the Lung and Immune Defenses. *Marijuana and the Cannabinoids,* 253–275. . doi:10.1007/978-1-59259-947-9_11

Tashkin, D. P., & Roth, M. D. (2019). Pulmonary effects of inhaled cannabis smoke. *The American Journal of Drug and Alcohol Abuse*, *45*(6), 596–609. doi:10.1080/00952990.2019.1627366 PMID:31298945

Thompson, G. R., Rosenkrantz, H., Schaeppi, U. H., & Braude, M. C. (1973). Comparison of acute oral toxicity of cannabinoids in rats, dogs and monkeys. *Toxicology and Applied Pharmacology*, *25*(3), 363–372. doi:10.1016/0041-008X(73)90310-4 PMID:4199474

Vieira, G., Cavalli, J., Gonçalves, E. C., Braga, S. F., Ferreira, R. S., Santos, A. R., Cola, M., Raposo, N. R., Capasso, R., & Dutra, R. C. (2020). Antidepressant-like effect of terpineol in an inflammatory model of depression: Involvement of the cannabinoid system and D2 dopamine receptor. *Biomolecules*, *10*(5), 792. doi:10.3390/biom10050792 PMID:32443870

Volkow, N. D., Baler, R. D., Compton, W. M., & Weiss, S. R. B. (2014a). Adverse health effects of marijuana use. *The New England Journal of Medicine*, *370*(23), 2219–2227. doi:10.1056/NEJMra1402309 PMID:24897085

Volkow, N. D., Baler, R. D., Compton, W. M., & Weiss, S. R. B. (2014a). Adverse health effects of marijuana use. *The New England Journal of Medicine*, *370*(23), 2219–2227.

Wilkinson, S. T., Radhakrishnan, R., & D'Souza, D. C. (2016). A systematic review of the evidence for medical marijuana in psychiatric indications. *The Journal of Clinical Psychiatry*, *77*(08), 1050–1064. https://doi.org/10.4088/JCP.15r10036

Wilkinson, S. T., Radhakrishnan, R., & D'Souza, D. C. (2016). A systematic review of the evidence for medical marijuana in psychiatric indications. *The Journal of Clinical Psychiatry*, *77*(08), 1050–1064. https://doi.org/10.4088/JCP.15r10036

Wyrofsky, R.R., Reyes, B.A.S., Zhang, X.-Y., Bhatnagar, S., Kirby, L.G., & Van Bockstaele, E.J. (2019). Endocannabinoids, stress signaling, and the locus coeruleus-norepinephrine system. *Neurobiol. Stress*, *11*. doi:. ynstr.2019.100176. doi:10.1016/j

Zamberletti, E., Prini, P., Speziali, S., Gabaglio, M., Solinas, M., Parolaro, D., & Rubino, T. (2012). Gender-dependent behavioral and biochemical effects of adolescent delta-9-tetrahydrocannabinol in adult maternally deprived rats. *Neuroscience*, *204*, 245–257. doi:10.1016/j.neuroscience.2011.11.038 PMID:22178986

Zou, S., & Kumar, U. (2018). Cannabinoid receptors and the endocannabinoid system: Signalling and function in the central nervous system. *International Journal of Molecular Sciences*, *19*(3), 833. doi:10.3390/ijms19030833 PMID:29533978

Compilation of References

. Pedersen, W., Sandberg, S., (2013). The medicalisation of revolt: a sociological analysis of medical cannabis users. *Sociol. Health Illn.* 35, 17–32. doi:. 1467-9566.2012.01476.x. doi:10.1111/j

Abbasi, A. M., Khan, S. M., Ahmad, M., Khan, M. A., Quave, C. L., & Pieroni, A. (2013). Botanical ethnoveterinary therapies in three districts of the Lesser Himalayas of Pakistan. *Journal of Ethnobiology and Ethnomedicine*, *9*(1), 84. doi:10.1186/1746-4269-9-84 PMID:24359615

Abdulsalami, I. O., Adeoye, M. D., Alabi, K. A., Abdulsalami, B. A., & Abolurin, N. O. (2018). Comparative Analysis of Theoretical and Empirical Data of Synthetic Cannabinoids. *Fountain Journal of National Ad Applied Sciences*, *7*(1), 29–41. doi:10.53704/fujnas.v7i1.247

Abel, E. L. (1980). *Marijuana: The First Twelve Thousand Years*. Springer. doi:10.1007/978-1-4899-2189-5

Abi-Jaoude, E., Chen, L., Cheung, P., Bhikram, T., Sandor, P. (2017). Preliminary evidence on cannabis effectiveness and tolerability for adults with tourette syndrome. *J. Neuropsychiatry Clin. Neurosci.* 29, 391–400. doi:. neuropsych.16110310. doi:10.1176/appi

Abrams, D. I., Jay, C. A., Shade, S. B., Vizoso, H., Reda, H., Press, S., Kelly, M. E., Rowbotham, M. C., & Petersen, K. L. (2007). Cannabis in painful HIV-associated sensory neuropathy: A randomized placebo-controlled trial. *Neurology*, *68*(7), 515–521. doi:10.1212/01.wnl.0000253187.66183.9c PMID:17296917

Adams, T. K., & Masondo, N. A. (2021). Malatsi, P.; Makunga, N.P.Cannabissativa: FromTherapeutic Uses to Micro-propagation and Beyond. *Plants*, *10*, 2078. doi:10.3390/plants10102078 PMID:34685890

Adesina, I., Bhowmik, A., Sharma, H., & Shahbazi, A. (2020). A review on the current state of knowledge of growing conditions, agronomic soil health practices and utilities of *Cannabis sativa* in the United States. *Agriculture*, *10*(4), 129. doi:10.3390/agriculture10040129

Adhikary, D., Kulkarni, M., El Mezawy, A., Mobini, S., Elhiti, M., Gjuric, R., Ray, A., Polowick, P., Slaski, J. J., Jones, M. P., & Bhowmik, P. (2021). Medical Cannabis and Industrial Hemp Tissue Culture: Present Status and Future Potential. *Front. PlantSci.*, *12*, 627240. doi:10.3389/fpls.2021.627240 PMID:33747008

Adu-Gyamfi, S., & Brenya, E. (2015). The marijuana factor in a university in Ghana: A survey. *J Siberian Feder Univ*, *8*(11), 2162–2182. doi:10.17516/1997-1370-2015-8-11-2162-2182

Adu-Mireku, S. (2003). The prevalence of alcohol, cigarette, and marijuana use among Ghanaian senior secondary students in an urban setting. *Journal of Ethnicity in Substance Abuse*, *2*(1), 53–65. doi:10.1300/J233v02n01_05

Agarwal, C., Máthé, K., Hofmann, T., & Csoka, L. (2018). Ultrasound-Assisted Extraction of Cannabinoids from Cannabis Sativa L. Optimized by Response Surface Methodology. *Journal of Food Science*, *83*(3), 700–710. doi:10.1111/1750-3841.14075 PMID:29437231

Ahmad, A., Hadi, F., & Ali, N. (2015). Effective phytoextraction of cadmium (Cd) with increasingconcentration of total phenolics and free proline in Cannabis sativa (L.) plant under varioustreatments of fertilizers, plant growth regulators and sodium salt. *International Journal of Phytoremediation, 17*(1–6), 56–65. doi:10.1080/15226514.2013.828018 PMID:25174425

Ahmad, R., Tehsin, Z., Malik, S. T., Asad, S. A., Shahzad, M., Bilal, M., Shah, M. M., & Khan, S. A. (2015). S.A. Phytoremediation Potential of Hemp (Cannabis sativa L.): Identiðcation and Characterization of Heavy Metals Responsive Genes. *Clean-Soil Air Water, 44*(2), 195–201. doi:10.1002/clen.201500117

Ainsworth, C. (2000). Boys and girls come out to play: The molecular biology of dioecious plants. *Annals of Botany, 86*(2), 211–221. doi:10.1006/anbo.2000.1201

Akerman, S., Holland, P. R., Lasalandra, M. P., & Goadsby, P. J. (2013). Endocannabinoids in the brainstem modulate dural trigeminovascular nociceptive traffic via CB1 and "triptan" receptors: Implications in migraine. *The Journal of Neuroscience: The Official Journal of the Society for Neuroscience, 33*(37), 14869–14877. doi:10.1523/JNEUROSCI.0943-13.2013 PMID:24027286

Akhtar, N., Rashid, A., Murad, W., & Bergmeier, E. (2013). Diversity and use of ethnomedicinalplantsintheregionofSw at,NorthPakistan. *Journal of Ethnobiology and Ethnomedicine, 9*(1), 25. doi:10.1186/1746-4269-9-25 PMID:23587127

Aldington, S., Harwood, M., Cox, B., Weatherall, M., Beckert, L., Hansell, A., Pritchard, A., Robinson, G., & Beasley, R. (2008). Cannabis use and risk of lung cancer: A case- control study. *The European Respiratory Journal, 31*(2), 280–286. doi:10.1183/09031936.00065707 PMID:18238947

Aldrich, M. (1997). History of therapeutic cannabis. In: Mathre, M.L. (Ed.), Cannabis in Medical Practice: A Legal, Historical and Pharmacological Overview of the Therapeutic use of Marijuana. McFarland & Co.

Aldrich, M. (1997). History of Therapeutic Cannabis. In M. L. Mathre (Ed.), *Cannabis in Medical Practice: a Legal, Historical and Pharmacological Overview of the Therapeutic use of Marijuana* (pp. 35–55). McFarland & Co.

Alexander, T. (1987) Hepatitis outbreak linked to imported pot. *Sinsemilla Tips.*

Ali EM, Almagboul AZ, Khogali SM, et al. (2012) Antimicrobial Activity of Cannabis sativa L. *Chinese Medicine, 1;3*(1), 61.

Ali, A., & Akhtar, N. (2015). The safety and efficacy of 3% *Cannabis* seeds extract cream for reduction of human cheek skin sebum and erythema content. *Pakistan Journal of Pharmaceutical Sciences, 28*(4), 1389–1395. PMID:26142529

Ali, E. M., Almagboul, A. Z., Khogali, S. M., & Gergeir, U. M. (2012). Antimicrobial Activity of *Cannabis sativa* L. *Chinese Medicine, 3*(1), 61–64. doi:10.4236/cm.2012.31010

Aliferis, K. A., & Bernard-Perron, D. (2020). Cannabinomics: Application of Metabolomics in Cannabis (*Cannabis sativa* L.) Research and Development. *Frontiers in Plant Science, 11*, 554. doi:10.3389/fpls.2020.00554 PMID:32457786

Alkaseem, M., & Baron, M. (2018). SERS and DFT study of 5F-PB-22. *Journal of Raman Spectroscopy: JRS, 49*(10), 1594–1606. doi:10.1002/jrs.5444

Allan, G. M., Finley, C. R., Ton, J., Perry, D., Ramji, J., Crawford, K., Lindblad, A. J., Korownyk, C., & Kolber, M. R. (2018). Systematic review of systematic reviews for medical cannabinoids: Pain, nausea and vomiting, spasticity, and harms. *Canadian Family Physician Medecin de Famille Canadien, 64*, e78–e94. PMID:29449262

Allen, K. D., McKernan, K., Pauli, C., Roe, J., Torres, A., & Gaudino, R. (2019). Genomic characterization of the complete terpene synthase gene family from *Cannabis sativa. PLoS One, 14*(9), e0222363. doi:10.1371/journal.pone.0222363 PMID:31513654

Amaducci, S., & Gusovius, H. J. (2010). Cannabis sativa-cultivation, extraction and processing. In *Industrial Applications of Natural Fibers: Structure, Properties and Technical Applications* (pp. 109–134). John Wiley & Sons. doi:10.1002/9780470660324.ch5

Amar, M. B., & Léonard, L. (2002). Cannabis. In L. Léonard & M. B. Amar (Eds.), Les psychotropes: pharmacologie et toxicomania [Psychotropics: Pharmacology and Addiction] (pp. 571–627). Les Presses del'Université de Montréal.

Amin, S. S., & Sachdeva, S. (2013). Alopecia areata: A review. *Journal of the Saudi Society of Dermatology & Dermatologic Surgery*, *17*(2), 37–45. doi:10.1016/j.jssdds.2013.05.004

Anand, U., Jacobo-Herrera, N., Altemimi, A., & Lakhssassi, N. (2019). A Comprehensive Review on Medicinal Plants as Antimicrobial Therapeutics: Potential Avenues of Biocompatible Drug Discovery. *Metabolites*, *9*(11), 258. doi:10.3390/metabo9110258 PMID:31683833

Anderson, B. R., & Scurlock, J. (2005). *Diagnoses in Assyrian and Babylonian Medicine*. University of Illinois Press.

Andersson-Sköld, Y., Hagelqvist, A., Crutu, G., & Blom, S. (2014). Bioenergy grown on contaminated land—A sustainable bioenergy contributor? *Biofuels*, *5*(5), 487–498. doi:10.1080/17597269.2014.996728

Andre, C.M.; Hausman, J.F.; Guerriero, G., (2016). Cannabis sativa: The plant of the thousand and one molecules. *Front Plant Sci. 7*, 19.

Andreasson, S., Allebeck, P., Engström, A., & Rydberg, U. (1987). Cannabis and schizophrenia. A longitudinal study of Swedish conscripts. *Lancet*, *330*(8574), 1483–1486. doi:10.1016/S0140-6736(87)92620-1 PMID:2892048

Andre, C. M., Hausman, J.-F., & Guerriero, G. (2016). *Cannabis sativa*: The Plant of the Thousand and One Molecules. *Frontiers in Plant Science*, *7*, 19. doi:10.3389/fpls.2016.00019 PMID:26870049

Andries, A., Frystyk, J., Flyvbjerg, A., & Støving, R. K. (2014). Dronabinol in severe, enduringanorexia nervosa: A randomized controlled trial. *International Journal of Eating Disorders*, *47*(1), 18–23. doi:10.1002/eat.22173 PMID:24105610

Angelova, V., Ivanova, R., Delibaltova, V., & Ivanov, K. (2004). Bioaccumulation and distribution of heavy metals in fibre crops (flax, cotton, and Cannabis sativa). *Industrial Crops and Products*, *19*(3), 197–205. doi:10.1016/j.indcrop.2003.10.001

Anil, S. M., Shalev, N., Vinayaka, A. C., Nadarajan, S., Namdar, D., Belausov, E., Shoval, I., Mani, K. A., Mechrez, G., & Koltai, H. (2021). Cannabis compounds exhibit anti-inflammatory activity in vitro in COVID-19-related inflammation in lung epithelial cells and pro-inflammatory activity in macrophages. *Scientific Reports*, *11*(1), 1462. doi:10.103841598-021-81049-2 PMID:33446817

Anonymous. (2000) *Phytoremediation: using plants to clean soil.* McGraw Hill Botany. www.mhhe.com/biosci/pae/botany/botany_map/articles/article_10.html

Anwara, F., Latifa, S., Ashrafb, M., (2006). Analytical Characterization of Hemp (Cannabis sativa) *Seed Oil from Different Agro-Ecological Zones of Pakistan, 83*, 323–329. áhttps://doi:. doi:10.1007/s11746-006-1207-xñ

Anwar, F., Latif, S., & Ashraf, M. (2006). Analytical characterization of hemp (*Cannabis sativa*) seed oil from different agro-ecological zones of Pakistan. *Journal of the American Oil Chemists' Society*, *83*(4), 323–329. doi:10.100711746-006-1207-x

Apostol, L., Popa, M., & Mustatea, G. (2015). Cannabis sativa L partially skimmed flour as source of bio-compounds in the bakery industry. *Romanian Biotechnological Letters*, *20*(5), 10835–10844.

Armijos, C., Cota, I., & González, S. (2014). Traditional medicine applied by the Saraguro yachakkuna: A preliminary approach to the use of sacred and psychoactive plant species in the southern region of Ecuador. *Journal of Ethnobiology and Ethnomedicine*, *10*(1), 26. doi:10.1186/1746-4269-10-26 PMID:24565054

Arnaud, L., & Gourlay, E. (2012). Experimental study of parameters influencing mechanical properties of hemp concretes. *Construction & Building Materials*, *28*(1), 50–56. doi:10.1016/j.conbuildmat.2011.07.052

Arru, L.; Rognoni, S.; Baroncini, M.; Bonatti, P.M.; Perata, P., (2004). Copper localization in *Cannabis sativa* L. grown in a copper-rich solution. *Euphytica140*, 33–38.

Arru, L., Rognoni, S., Baroncini, M., Bonatti, P. M., & Perata, P. (2004). Copper localization in Cannabissativa L. grown in a copper-rich solution. *Euphytica*, *140*(1-2), 33–38. doi:10.100710681-004-4752-0

Arseneault, L., Cannon, M., Poulton, R., Murray, R., Caspi, A., & Mofðtt, T. E. (2002). Cannabis use in adolescence and risk for adult psychosis: Longitudinal prospective study. *BMJ (Clinical Research Ed.)*, *325*(7374), 1212–1213. doi:10.1136/bmj.325.7374.1212 PMID:12446537

Associated Press. (2016) Oregon, other states stop sales of pot pesticide due to labeling problem. *USA Today*.

Atakan, Z. (2012). Cannabis, a complex plant: Different compounds and different effects on individuals. *Therapeutic Advances in Psychopharmacology*, *2*(6), 241–254. doi:10.1177/2045125312457586 PMID:23983983

Atalay, S., Gęgotek, A., Wroński, A., Domigues, P., & Skrzydlewska, E. (2021). Therapeutic application of cannabidiol on UVA and UVB irradiated rat skin. A proteomic study. *Journal of Pharmaceutical and Biomedical Analysis*, *192*, 113656. doi:10.1016/j.jpba.2020.113656 PMID:33086172

Audu, B. S., Ofojekwu, P. C., Ujah, A., & Ajima, M. N. O. (2014). M.N.O. Phytochemical, proximate composition, amino acid profile and characterization of Marijuana (Cannabis sativa L.). *J. Phytopharm*, *3*(1), 35–43. doi:10.31254/phyto.2014.3106

Australian Access Clinic. (2021, August 5). *Medical Cannabis for Insomnia: Everything You Need to Know*. Australian Access Clinics. https://www.auscannabisclinics.com.au/medical-cannabis-insomnia/

Avila, C., Massick, S., Kaffenberger, B. H., Kwatra, S. G., & Bechtel, M. (2020). Cannabinoids for the treatment of chronic pruritus: A review. *Journal of the American Academy of Dermatology*, *82*(5), 1205–1212. doi:10.1016/j.jaad.2020.01.036 PMID:31987788

Băbău, A. M. C., Micle, V., Damian, G. E., & Sur, I. M. (2020). Preliminary investigations regarding the potential of *Robiniapseudoacacia* L. (leguminosae) in the phytoremediation of sterile dumps. *Journal of Environmental Protection and Ecology*, *21*, 46–55.

Băbău, A. M. C., Micle, V., Damian, G. E., & Sur, I. M. (2021). Sustainable ecological restoration of sterile dumps using *Robiniapseudoacacia*. *Sustainability*, *13*(24), 14021. doi:10.3390u132414021

Babson, K. A., Sottile, J., & Morabito, D. (2017). Cannabis, cannabinoids, and sleep: A review of the literature. *Current Psychiatry Reports*, *19*(4), 23. doi:10.100711920-017-0775-9 PMID:28349316

Baca, R., & Migoya, D. (2015) Denver issues ninth pot product recall in 10 weeks. *The Denver Post*.

Badowski, M. E. (2017). A review of oral cannabinoids and medical marijuana for the treatment of chemotherapy-induced nausea and vomiting: A focus on pharmacokinetic variability and pharmacodynamics. *Cancer Chemotherapy and Pharmacology*, *80*(3), 441–449. doi:10.100700280-017-3387-5 PMID:28780725

Bahji, A., & Stephenson, C. (2019). International Perspectives on the Implications of Cannabis Legalization: A Systematic Review & Thematic Analysis. *International Journal of Environmental Research and Public Health, 16*(17), 3095. doi:10.3390/ijerph16173095 PMID:31454942

Baker, A. J. M. (1981). Accumulators and excluders-strategies in the response of plants to heavy metals. *Journal of Plant Nutrition, 3*(1-4), 643–654. doi:10.1080/01904168109362867

Bakowska-Barczak, A., Esparza, Y., Kaur, H., & Popek, T. (2022). Industrial hemp-based dietary supplements and cosmetic products. In M. Pojić & B. K. Tiwari (Eds.), *Industrial Hemp: Food and Nutraceutical Applications* (pp. 247–299). Academic Press. doi:10.1016/B978-0-323-90910-5.00010-5

Baldino, L., Scognamiglio, M., & Reverchon, E. (2020). Supercritical fluid technologies applied to the extraction of compounds of industrial interest from Cannabis sativa L. and to their pharmaceutical formulations: A review. *The Journal of Supercritical Fluids, 165*, 104960. doi:10.1016/j.supflu.2020.104960

Baldino, L., Scognamiglio, M., & Reverchon, E. (2020). Supercritical fluid technologies applied to the extraction of compounds of industrialinterest fromCannabis sativaL. and to their pharmaceutical formulations: A review. *[PDF] [The Medicinal Natural Products of Cannabis sativa Linn.: A Review.*]. *J. Pharm. Fluids., 165*, 104960.

Banerjee-Dube, I. (2014). *A history of modern India*. Cambridge University Press. doi:10.1017/CBO9781107588387

Banerjee, S., Anand, U., Ghosh, S., Ray, D., Ray, P., Nandy, S., Dewaji Deshmukh, G., Tripathi, V., & Dey, A. (2019). Bacosides from Bacopa monnieri extract: An overview of the effects on neurological disorders. *Phytotherapy Research*, 1–12. doi:10.1002/ptr.7203 PMID:34254371

Bañuelos, G. S., & Ajwa, H. A. (1999). Trace elements in soils and plants: An overview. *Journal of Environmental Science and Health. Part A, Toxic/Hazardous Substances & Environmental Engineering, 34*(4), 951–974. doi:10.1080/10934529909376875

Bao, Q., Liu, H., Fu, K., Zhang, C., Wang, C., & Feng, Y. (2014). *Hemp Bast Fiber Extract with Antibacterial Activity, Preparation Method, and Application of Hemp Bast Fiber Extract.* Patent publication number CN104018343A. Washington, DC: U.S. Patent and Trademark Office.

Barak, S., & Baker, H. (2016). *Clinical Management of Male Infertility*. Endotext.

Baral, P., Bagul, V., & Gajbhiye, S. (2020). Hemp seed oil for skin care (non-drug *Cannabis sativa* L.): A review. *World Journal of Pharmaceutical Research, 9*(8), 2534–2556.

Baranović, G. (2021). Understanding the conformational, electronic and vibrational properties of Tetrahydrocannabinol (THC) and Cannabidiol (CBD). Pharmacophoric similarities and differences. *Journal of Molecular Structure, 1244*, 130945. doi:10.1016/j.molstruc.2021.130945

Barbosa, N. S. V., de Almeida Lima, E. R., & Tavares, F. W. (2017). *Molecular modeling in chemical engineering*.

Barkus, E., & Murray, R. M. (2010). Substance use in adolescence and psychosis: Clarifying the relationship. *Annual Review of Clinical Psychology, 6*(1), 365–389. doi:10.1146/annurev.clinpsy.121208.131220 PMID:20192802

Barratt, E. S., Beaver, W., & White, R. (1974). The effects of marijuana on human sleep patterns. *Biol. Psychiatry, 8*, 47–54. http://psycnet.apa.org/record/1974-24717001.

Baswan, S. M., Klosner, A. E., Glynn, K., Rajgopal, A., Malik, K., Yim, S., & Stern, N. (2020). Therapeutic Potential of Cannabidiol (CBD) for Skin Health and Disorders. *Clinical, Cosmetic and Investigational Dermatology, 13*, 927–942. doi:10.2147/CCID.S286411 PMID:33335413

Batalla, A., Janssen, H., Gangadin, S. S., & Bossong, M. G. (2019). The Potential of Cannabidiol as a Treatment for Psychosis and Addiction: Who Benefits Most? A Systematic Review. *Journal of Clinical Medicine*, *8*(7), E1058. doi:10.3390/jcm8071058 PMID:31330972

Bauddh, K., Singh, B., & Korstad, J. (2017). *Phytoremediation potential of bioenergy plants*. Springer. doi:10.1007/978-981-10-3084-0

Baxter, L. L., Miles, T. R., Miles, T. R. Jr, Jenkins, B. M., Milne, T., Dayton, D., Bryers, R. W., & Oden, L. L. (1998). The behavior of inorganic material in biomass-fired power boilers: Field and laboratory experiences. *Fuel Processing Technology*, *54*(1–3), 47–78. doi:10.1016/S0378-3820(97)00060-X

Bell J (1857) On the haschisch or cannabis indica. *Boston Med Surg J 56*(209–216), 229–236.

Benet, S. (1975). Early diffusion and folk uses of hemp. In: Vera Rubin (Ed.), Cannabis and Culture. Mouton Publishers. doi:10.1515/9783110812060.39

Bennett, C. (2011). Early/Ancient History. In J. Holland (Ed.), *The Pot Book: A Complete Guide to Cannabis* (pp. 17–26). Its Role in Medicine, Politics, Science, and Culture.

Bergamaschi, M. M., Barnes, A., Queiroz, R. H. C., Hurd, Y. L., & Huestis, M. A. (2013). Impact of enzymatic and alkaline hydrolysis on CBD concentration in urine. *Analytical and Bioanalytical Chemistry*, *405*(14), 4679–4689. doi:10.100700216-013-6837-x PMID:23494274

Betthauser, K., Pilz, J., & Vollmer, L. E. (2015). Use and effects of cannabinoids in military veterans with posttraumatic stress disorder. *American Journal of Health-System Pharmacy*, *72*(15), 1279–1284. doi:10.2146/ajhp140523 PMID:26195653

Bhattacharyya, S., Morrison, P. D., Fusar-Poli, P., Martin-Santos, R., Borgwardt, S., Winton-Brown, T., Nosarti, C., O' Carroll, C. M., Seal, M., Allen, P., Mehta, M. A., Stone, J. M., Tunstall, N., Giampietro, V., Kapur, S., Murray, R. M., Zuardi, A. W., Crippa, J. A., Atakan, Z., & McGuire, P. K. (2010). Opposite effects of D-9- tetrahydrocannabinol and cannabidiol on human brain function and psychopathology. *Neuropsychopharmacology*, *35*(3), 764–774.

Bifulco, M., & Pisanti, S. (2015). Medicinal use of cannabis in Europe: The fact that more countries legalize the medicinal use of cannabis should not become an argument for unfettered and uncontrolled use. *EMBO Reports*, *16*(2), 130–132. doi:10.15252/embr.201439742 PMID:25576303

Bijauliya, R. K., Alok, S., Kumar, M., Chanchal, D. K., & Yadav, S. (2017). A comprehensive review on herbal cosmetics. *International Journal of Pharmaceutical Sciences and Research*, *8*(12), 4930–4949. doi:10.13040/IJPSR.0975-8232.8(12).4930-49

Bindesri, S. D., Jebailey, R., Albarghouthi, N., Pye, C. C., & Brosseau, C. L. (2020). Spectroelectrochemical and computational studies of tetrahydrocannabinol (THC) and carboxy-tetrahydrocannabinol (THC-COOH). *Analyst (London)*, *145*(5), 1849–1857. doi:10.1039/C9AN02173F PMID:31967120

Birdsall, S. M., Birdsall, T. C., & Tims, L. A. (2016). The Use of Medical Marijuana in Cancer. *Current Oncology Reports*, *18*(7), 40. doi:10.100711912-016-0530-0 PMID:27215434

Bíró, T., Tóth, B. I., Haskó, G., Paus, R., & Pacher, P. (2009). The endocannabinoid system of the skin in health and disease: Novel perspectives and therapeutic opportunities. *Trends in Pharmacological Sciences*, *30*(8), 411–420. doi:10.1016/j.tips.2009.05.004 PMID:19608284

Birt, D. F., Hendrich, S., & Wang, W. (2001). Dietary agents in cancer prevention: Flavonoids and isoflavonoids. *Pharmacology & Therapeutics*, *90*(2-3), 157–177. doi:10.1016/S0163-7258(01)00137-1 PMID:11578656

Bitencourt, R. M., & Takahashi, R. N. (2018). Cannabidiol as a therapeutic alternative for post-traumatic stress disorder: From bench research to confirmation in human trials. *Frontiers in neuroscience*, 502.

Blade, S. F., Ampong-Nyarko, K., & Przybylski, R. (2006). Fatty acid and tocopherol profiles of industrial hemp cultivars grown in the high latitude prairie region of Canada. *Journal of Industrial Hemp*, *10*(2), 33–43. doi:10.1300/J237v10n02_04

Blake, A., & Nahtigal, I. (2019). The evolving landscape of cannabis edibles. *Current Opinion in Food Science*, *28*, 25–31. doi:10.1016/j.cofs.2019.03.009

Blanton, R. E. (2002). Empires: Perspectives from Archaeology and History. Latin American Antiquity, 13(2), 237–238.

Bona, E., Marsano, F., Cavaletto, M., & Berta, G. (2007). Proteomic characterization of copper stress response in *Cannabis sativa* roots. *Proteomics*, *7*(7), 1121–1130. doi:10.1002/pmic.200600712 PMID:17352425

Bonini, S. A., Mastinu, A., Maccarinelli, G., Mitola, S., Premoli, M., La Rosa, L. R., Ferrari Toninelli, G., Grilli, M., & Memo, M. (2016). Cortical structure alterations and social behavior impairment in p50-deðcient mice. *Cerebral Cortex (New York, N.Y.)*, *26*(6), 2832–2849. doi:10.1093/cercor/bhw037 PMID:26946128

Bonini, S. A., Premoli, M., Tambaro, S., Kumar, A., Maccarinelli, G., Memo, M., & Mastinu, A. (2018). *Cannabis sativa*: A comprehensive ethnopharmacological review of a medicinal plant with a long history. *Journal of Ethnopharmacology*, *227*, 300–315. doi:10.1016/j.jep.2018.09.004 PMID:30205181

Bonnie, R. J., & Whitebread, C. H. (1974). *The Marijuana Conviction: A History of Marijuana Prohibition in the United States*. University Press of Virginia.

Booth, J. K., & Bohlmann, J. (2019). Terpenes in Cannabis sativa - from plant genome to humans. *Plant Science*, *284*, 67–72. doi:10.1016/j.plantsci.2019.03.022 PMID:31084880

Booth, J. K., Page, J. E., & Jörg, B. (2017). Terpene synthases from Cannabis sativa. *PLoS One*, *12*(3), e0173911. doi:10.1371/journal.pone.0173911 PMID:28355238

Borges, R. S., Batista, J. Jr, Viana, R. B., Baetas, A. C., Orestes, E., Andrade, M. A., Honório, K., & Da Silva, A. B. (2013). Understanding the molecular aspects of tetrahydrocannabinol and cannabidiol as antioxidants. *Molecules (Basel, Switzerland)*, *18*(10), 12663–12674. doi:10.3390/molecules181012663 PMID:24129275

Borhade, S. S. (2013). Chemical Composition and Characterization of Hemp (*Cannabis sativa*) Seed oil and essential fatty acids by HPLC Method. *Archives of Applied Science Research*, *5*(1), 5–8.

Bornheim, L. M., & Grillo, M. P. (1998). Characterization of Cytochrome P450 3A Inactivation by Cannabidiol: Possible Involvement of Cannabidiol-Hydroxyquinone as a P450 Inactivator. *Chemical Research in Toxicology*, *11*(10), 1209–1216. doi:10.1021/tx9800598 PMID:9778318

Borougerdi, B. J. (2014). *Cord of empire, exotic intoxicant: Hemp and culture in the Atlantic world, 1600-1900*. The University of Texas at Arlington.

Borougerdi, B. J. (2018). *Commodifying Cannabis: A Cultural History of a Complex Plant in the Atlantic World*. Rowman & Littlefield.

Botanix Pharmaceuticals. (n.d.). *BTX 1503 Acne Phase 2 Study Results Presentation*. ASX. https://www.asx.com.au/asxpdf/20191023/pdf/449s36d2bz6vfr.pdf

Bouchentouf, S., Ghalem, S., Allali, H., & Missoum, N. (2017). Investigating the Inhibition of 5-LO Enzyme by Main Cannabinoids Contained in Cannabis safiva and Seized Resin Cannabis by Using Molecular Modeling. *Insights Enzyme Res*, *1*(1), 10.

Bowles, D. W., O'Bryant, C. L., Camidge, D. R., & Jimeno, A. (2012). The intersection between cannabis and cancer in the United States. *Critical Reviews in Oncology/Hematology*, *83*(1), 1–10. doi:10.1016/j.critrevonc.2011.09.008 PMID:22019199

Braich, S., Baillie, R. C., Jewell, L. S., Spangenberg, G. C., & Cogan, N. O. (2019). Generation of a Comprehensive Transcriptome Atlas and Transcriptome Dynamics in Medicinal Cannabis. *Scientific Reports*, *9*(1), 1–12. doi:10.103841598-019-53023-6 PMID:31719627

Brand, E.J. & Zhao, Z., (2017). Cannabis in Chinese medicine: Are some traditional indications referenced in ancient literature related to cannabinoids. *Front. Pharmacol*, *8*, 108.. doi:10.3389/fphar.2017.00108

Breijyeh, Z., Jubeh, B., Bufo, S. A., Karaman, R., & Scrano, L. (2021). Cannabis: A Toxin- Producing Plant with Potential Therapeutic Uses. *Toxins*, *13*(2), 117. doi:10.3390/toxins13020117 PMID:33562446

Bridgeman, M. B., & Abazia, D. T. (2017). Medicinal cannabis: History, pharmacology, and implications for the acute care setting. *Pharm. Therap.*, *42*(3), 180. PMID:28250701

Brischia, R., Piccioni, E., & Standardi, A. (2002). Micropropagation and synthetic seed in M.26 apple rootstock (II): A new protocol for production of encapsulated differentiating propagules. *Plant Cell Tiss Org*, *68*(2), 137–141. doi:10.1023/A:1013802723018

Brown, D. T. (1998). *Cannabis: The genus cannabis*. CRC Press.

Brown, D. T. (1998). Non-medical uses of cannabis sativa. In D. T. Brown (Ed.), *Cannabis: the genus cannabis*. Harwood academic publishers.

Bruce-Amartey, E. Jr, Amissah, E. R. K., & Safo-Ankama, K. (2014). The decline of Ghana's textile industry: Its effects on textile education in Ghana. *Arts Design Stud.*, *22*, 36–45.

Brunetti, P., Faro, A. F. L., Pirani, F., Berretta, P., Pacifici, R., Pichini, S., & Busardò, F. P. (2020). Pharmacology and legal status of cannabidiol. *Annali dell'Istituto Superiore di Sanita*, *56*(3), 285–291. doi:10.4415/ANN_20_03_06 PMID:32959794

Budney, A. J., & Borodovsky, J. T. (2017). The potential impact of cannabis legalization on the development of cannabis use disorders. *Preventive Medicine*, *104*, 31–36. doi:10.1016/j.ypmed.2017.06.034 PMID:28668544

Budney, A., Roffman, R., Stephens, R., & Walker, D. (2007). Marijuana dependence and its treatment. *Addiction Science & Clinical Practice*, *4*(1), 4–16. doi:10.1151/ASCP07414 PMID:18292704

Burczyk, H., Grabowska, L., Kolodziej, J., & Strybe, M. (2008). Industrial hemp as a raw material for energy production. *Journal of Industrial Hemp*, *13*(1), 37–48. doi:10.1080/15377880801898717

Burstein, S. (1997). Marijuana as a medicine. *Nature*, *386*(6623), 320. doi:10.1038/386320d0 PMID:9121543

Busse, F. P., Fiedler, G. P., Leichtle, A., Hentschel, H., & Stumvoll, M. (2008). Lead poisoning due toadulterated marijuana in Leipzig. *Deutsches Ärzteblatt International*, *105*, 757–762. PMID:19623274

Bussmann, R. W., Paniagua Zambrana, N. Y., Sikharulidze, S., Kikvidze, Z., Kikodze, D., Tchelidze, D., Khutsishvili, M., Batsatsashvili, K., & Hart, R. E. (2016). A comparative ethnobotany of Khevsureti, Samtskhe-Javakheti, Tusheti, Svaneti, and RachaLechkhumi, Republic of Georgia (Sakartvelo), Caucasus. *Journal of Ethnobiology and Ethnomedicine*, *12*(1), 43. doi:10.118613002-016-0110-2 PMID:27659258

Butrica, J. L. (2002). The medical use of cannabis among the Greeks and Romans. *Journal of Cannabis Therapeutics*, *2*(2), 51–70. doi:10.1300/J175v02n02_04

Buxton, O. M., Broussard, J. L., Zahl, A. K., & Hall, M. (2014). Impact of Sleep and Sleep Disturbances on Obesity and Cancer, pp. 25–50. Springer; Berlin/Heidelberg, Germany.

Cabral, G.A., Staab, A., (2005). Effects on the immune system. *Cannabinoids,* 385–423.. doi:10.1007/3-540-26573-2_13

Caffarel, M. M., Andradas, C., Mira, E., Pérez-Gómez, E., Cerutti, C., Moreno-Bueno, G., Flores, J. M., García-Real, I., Palacios, J., Mañes, S., Guzmán, M., & Sánchez, C. (2010). Cannabinoids reduce ErbB2-driven breast cancer progression through Akt inhibition. *Molecular Cancer*, *9*(1), 196. doi:10.1186/1476-4598-9-196 PMID:20649976

Caffarel, M. M., Andradas, C., Pérez-Gómez, E., Guzmán, M., & Sánchez, C. (2012). Cannabinoids: A new hope for breast cancer therapy? *Cancer Treatment Reviews*, *38*(7), 911–918. doi:10.1016/j.ctrv.2012.06.005 PMID:22776349

Caligiani, A., Palla, G., & Bernardelli, B. (2006). GC-MS analysis of hashish samples: A case ofadulteration with colophony. *Journal of Forensic Sciences*, *51*(5), 1096–1100. doi:10.1111/j.1556-4029.2006.00202.x PMID:17018088

Calignano, A., La Rana, G., Giuffrida, A., & Piomelli, D. (1998). Control of pain initiation by endogenous cannabinoids. *Nature*, *394*(6690), 277–281. doi:10.1038/28393 PMID:9685157

Calik, M. W., & Carley, D. W. (2017). Effects of cannabinoid agonists and antagonists on sleep and breathing in Sprague-Dawley rats. *Sleep (Basel)*, *40*(9), zsx112. Advance online publication. doi:10.1093leep/zsx112 PMID:28934522

Callaway, J. C. (2004). Hempseed as a nutritional resource: An overview. *Euphytica*, *140*(1-2), 65–72. doi:10.100710681-004-4811-6

Callaway, J., Schwab, U., Harvima, I., Halonen, P., Mykkänen, O., Hyvönen, P., & Järvinen, T. (2004). Efficacy of dietary hempseed oil on plasma lipids and skin quality in patients with atopic dermatitis. *The Journal of Dermatological Treatment.*

Callaway, J., Schwab, U., Harvima, I., Halonen, P., Mykkänen, O., Hyvönen, P., & Järvinen, T. (2005). Efficacy of dietary hempseed oil in patients with atopic dermatitis. *The Journal of Dermatological Treatment*, *16*(2), 87–94. doi:10.1080/09546630510035832 PMID:16019622

Calvi, L., Pavlović, R., Panseri, S., Giupponi, L., Leoni, V., & Giorgi, A. (2018). Quality traits of medical Cannabis sativa L. inflorescences and derived products based on comprehensive mass-spectrometry analytical investigation. Recent Advances in Cannabinoid Research. IntechOpen.

Calvi, L., Pentimalli, D., Panseri, S., Giupponi, L., Gelmini, F., Beretta, G., Vitali, D., Bruno, M., Zilio, E., Pavlovic, R., & Giorgi, A. (2018). Comprehensive quality evaluation of medical Cannabis sativa L. inflorescence and macerated oils based on HS-SPME coupled to GC–MS and LC-HRMS (q-exactive orbitrap) approach. *J.Pharm.Biomed.Anal*, *150*, 208–219.. doi:10.1016/j.jpba.2017.11.073

Calvi, L., Pentimalli, D., Panseri, S., Giupponi, L., Gelmini, F., Beretta, G., Vitali, D., Bruno, M., Zilio, E., Pavlovic, R., Giorgi, A., (2018). Comprehensive quality evaluation of medical Cannabis sativa L. inflorescence and macerated oils based on HS-SPME coupled to GC–MS and LC-HRMS (q-exactive orbitrap®) approach. *J. Pharm. Biomed. Anal.*, *150*, 208–219. doi:. jpba.2017.11.073. doi:10.1016/j

Calvi, L., Pavlovic, R., Panseri, S., Giupponi, L., Leoni, V., & Giorgi, A. (2018). Quality Traits of Medical *Cannabis sativa* L. Inflorescences and Derived Products Based on Comprehensive Mass-Spectrometry Analytical Investigation. In W. J. Costain & R. B. Laprairie (Eds.), *Recent Advances in Cannabinoid Research* (pp. 55–78). IntechOpen. doi:10.5772/intechopen.79539

Campbell, S., Paquin, D., Awaya, J. D., & Li, Q. X. (2002). Remediation of benzo[a]pyrene andchrysene-contaminated soil with industrial hemp (Cannabis sativa). *International Journal of Phytoremediation*, *4*(2), 157–158. doi:10.1080/15226510208500080 PMID:12655808

Campbell, S., Paquin, D., Awaya, J. D., & Li, Q. X. (2006). Remediation of Benzo[a]pyrene and chrysenecontaminated soil with industrial hemp (Cannabis sativa). *International Journal of Theoretical Physics*, *4*(2), 157–168. PMID:12655808

Cao, H. X., Schmutzer, T., Scholz, U., Pecinka, A., Schubert, I., & Vu, G. T. (2015). Metatranscriptomeanalysis reveals host-microbiome interactions in traps of carnivorous Genlisea species. *Frontiers in Microbiology*, *6*, 526. doi:10.3389/fmicb.2015.00526 PMID:26236284

Carod-Artal, F. J. (2013). Psychoactive plants in ancient Greece. *Neurosci. Hist. 1*, 28–38. áhttp://nah.sen.es/en/130-journals/volume-1/issue-1/241-psychoactive-plants-inancient-greeceñ.

Carpenter, D. E. (2018). Legal hemp in 2019 may be a boon for stressed out American farmers. *Forbes*. https://www.forbes.com/sites/davidcarpenter/2018/12/20/legal-hemp-in-2019-may-be-a-boon-for-stressed-out-american-farmers/

Cascini, F., Farcomeni, A., Migliorini, D., Baldassarri, L., Boschi, I., Martello, S., Amaducci, S., Lucini, L., & Bernardi, J. (2019). Highly Predictive Genetic Markers Distinguish Drug-Type from Fiber-Type Cannabis sativa L. *Plants*, *8*(11), 496. doi:10.3390/plants8110496 PMID:31718081

Cassano, R., Trombino, S., Ferrarelli, T., Nicoletta, F. P., Mauro, M. V., Giraldi, C., & Picci, N. (2013). Hemp fiber (*Cannabis sativa* L.) derivatives with antibacterial and chelating properties. *Cellulose (London, England)*, *20*(1), 547–557. doi:10.100710570-012-9804-3

Cassano, T., Villani, R., Pace, L., Carbone, A., Bukke, V. N., Orkisz, S., Avolio, C., & Serviddio, G. (2020). From *Cannabis sativa* to Cannabidiol: Promising Therapeutic Candidate for the Treatment of Neurodegenerative Diseases. *Frontiers in Pharmacology*, *11*, 124. doi:10.3389/fphar.2020.00124 PMID:32210795

Castleman, T. (2006). *Hemp biomass for energy*. Fuel and Fiber Company.

Cates, W. C., & Warren, J. W. (1975). Hepatitis B in Nuremberg, Germany. Epidemiology of adrug-associated epidemic among US Army soldiers. *Journal of the American Medical Association*, *234*(9), 930–934. doi:10.1001/jama.1975.03260220034014 PMID:1242490

CDA. (2016) *Pesticide use in Cannabis production information*. Colorado Department of Agriculture. https://www.colorado.gov/pacific/agplants/pesticide-use-cannabisproduction-information

Cervantes, J. (2006). *Marijuana horticulture: The indoor/outdoor medical grower's bible*. Van Patten.

Cescon, D. W., Page, A. V., Richardson, S., Moore, M. J., Boerner, S., & Gold, W. L. (2008). Invasive pulmonaryaspergillosis associated with marijuana use in a man with colorectal cancer. *Journal of Clinical Oncology*, *26*(13), 2214–2215. doi:10.1200/JCO.2007.15.2777 PMID:18445848

Chaffey, N. (2001). Hemp on the move. *Trends in Plant Science*, *6*, 505.

Chait, L. D. (1990). Subjective and behavioral effects of marijuana the morning after smoking. *Psychopharmacology*, *100*(3), 328–333. doi:10.1007/BF02244601 PMID:2315429

Chakrabarty, D. K. (2009). India: An archaeological history: palaeolithic beginnings to early historic foundations. Oxford University Press. doi:10.1093/acprof:oso/9780198064121.001.0001

Chalot, M., Blaudez, D., Rogaume, Y., Provent, A.-S., & Pascual, C. (2012). Fate of trace elements during the combustion of phytoremediation wood. *Environmental Science & Technology*, *46*(24), 13361–13369. doi:10.1021/es3017478 PMID:23153074

Chandra, S. H., Lata, I., Khan, A., & ElSohly, M. A. (2010). Propagation of elite Cannabis sativa for the production of Δ9-Tetrahydrocannabinol (THC) using biotechnological tools. In A. Rajesh (Ed.), *Medicinal plant biotechnology* (pp. 98–114). CABI. doi:10.1079/9781845936785.0098

Chandra, S., Lata, H., & ElSohly, M. A. (2017). *Cannabis sativa L.—Botany and Biotechnology*. Springer. doi:10.1007/978-3-319-54564-6

Chandra, S., Lata, H., ElSohly, M. A., Walker, L. A., & Potter, D. (2017). Cannabis cultivation: Methodological issues for obtaining medicalgrade product. *Epilepsy & Behavior*, *70*, 302–312. doi:10.1016/j.yebeh.2016.11.029 PMID:28202406

Chandra, S., Lata, H., Khan, I. A., & ElSohly, M. A. (2017). *Cannabis sativa* L.: Botany and Horticulture. In S. Chandra, H. Lata, & M. ElSohly (Eds.), *Cannabis sativa L. - Botany and Biotechnology* (pp. 79–100). Springer. doi:10.1007/978-3-319-54564-6_3

Charkowski, E. (1998). *Cannabis sativa* "eats" Chernobyl waste offers hope for Hanford. *Rediscover Cannabis sativa.* sativa.com/inspire/Cannabis sativa-eats-chernobyl-waste-offers-hope-for-hanford/

Charles W. Webb and Sandra M. Webb RN, (2014), Therapeutic Benefits of Cannabis: A Patient Survey, *Hawai'i Jour. Of Med. & Pub. Health,73*(4).

Chattopadhyaya, D. (1978). *Science and society in ancient India* (Vol. 22). John Benjamins Publishing.

Chemat, F., Vian, M. A., & Cravotto, G. (2012). Green Extraction of Natural Products: Concept and Principles. *International Journal of Molecular Sciences*, *13*(7), 8615–8627. doi:10.3390/ijms13078615 PMID:22942724

Chen, C., & Pan, Z. (2021). Cannabidiol and terpenes from hemp–ingredients for future foods and processing technologies. *Journal of Future Foods*, *1*(2), 113–127. doi:10.1016/j.jfutfo.2022.01.001

Cherney, J.; Small, E., (2016). Industrial *Cannabis sativa* in North America: Production, politics, and potential. *Agronomy*, *6*, 58.

Cherney, J. H., & Small, E. (2016). Industrial hemp in North America:production,politicsand potential. *Agronomy (Basel)*, *6*(4), 58. doi:10.3390/agronomy6040058

Chopra, R. N. (1940). Use of hemp drugs in India. *Indian Medical Gazette*, *75*(6), 356. PMID:29013991

Chouvy, P.-A. (2019). Cannabis cultivation in the world: Heritages, trends and challenges. *EchoGéo*, (48). doi:10.4000/echogeo.17591

Christinat, N., Savoy, M.-C., & Mottier, P. (2020). Development, validation, and application of a LC-MS/MS method for quantification of 15 cannabinoids in food. *Food Chemistry*, *318*, 126469. doi:10.1016/j.foodchem.2020.126469 PMID:32143130

Chundawat, S. P. S., Beckham, G. T., Himmel, M. E., & Dale, B. E. (2011). Deconstruction of lignocellulosic biomass to fuels and chemicals. *Annual Review of Chemical and Biomolecular Engineering*, *2*(1), 121–145. doi:10.1146/annurev-chembioeng-061010-114205 PMID:22432613

Chung, S. C., Hammarsten, P., Josefsson, A., Stattin, P., Granfors, T., Egevad, L., Mancini, G., Lutz, B., Bergh, A., & Fowler, C. J. (2009). A high cannabinoid CB(1) receptor immunoreactivity is associated with disease severity and outcome in prostate cancer. *European Journal of Cancer (Oxford, England: 1990)*, *45*(1), 174–182. doi:10.1016/j.ejca.2008.10.010

Chusid, M. J., Gelfand, J. A., Nutter, C., & Fauci, A. S. (1975). Pulmonary aspergillosis, inhalation ofcontaminated marijuana smoke, chronic granulomatous disease. *Annals of Internal Medicine*, *82*(5), 682–683. doi:10.7326/0003-4819-82-5-682 PMID:1094876

Cinti, S. (2009). Medical marijuana in HIV-positive patients: What do we know? *Journal of the International Association of Physicians in AIDS Care*, *8*(6), 342–346. doi:10.1177/1545109709351167 PMID:19952287

Cirimele, V., Kintz, P., Jamey, C., & Ludes, B. (1999). Are Cannabinoids Detected in Hair After Washing With Cannabio® Shampoo? *Journal of Analytical Toxicology*, *23*(5), 349–351. doi:10.1093/jat/23.5.349 PMID:10488922

Citterio, S., Prato, N., Fumagalli, P., Aina, R., Massa, N., Santagostino, A., Sgorbati, G., & Berta, G. (2005). The arbuscular mycorrhizal fungus Glomus mosseae induces growth and metal accumulationchanges in Cannabis sativa L. *Chemosphere*, *59*(1), 21–29. doi:10.1016/j.chemosphere.2004.10.009 PMID:15698640

Citterio, S., Santagostino, A., Fumagalli, P., Prato, N., Ranalli, P., & Sgorbati, S. (2003). Heavy metal tolerance and accumulation of Cd, Cr and Ni by *Cannabis sativa* L. *Plant and Soil*, *256*(2), 243–252. doi:10.1023/A:1026113905129

Ciurli, A., Alpi, A., & Perata, P. (2002). Impiegodellacanapanellafitodepurazione da metallipesanti [Use of hemp in phytodepuration from heavy metals]. *Agroindustria*, *1*(1), 64–60.

Clarke, R. C., & Merlin, M. D. (2015). Letter to the editor: Small, Ernest. 2015. Evolution and Classification of Cannabis sativa (Marijuana, Hemp) in relation to human utilization. Botanical Review 81(3), 189-294.

Clarke, R. C., & Merlin, M. (2013). *Cannabis: evolution and ethnobotany*. University of California Press.

Clarke, R. C., & Merlin, M. D. (2013). *Cannabis, Evolution and Ethnobotany*. University of California press.

Clarke, R. C., & Merlin, M. D. (2016). *Cannabis* Domestication, Breeding History, Present-day Genetic Diversity, and Future Prospects. *Critical Reviews in Plant Sciences*, *35*(5-6), 293–327. doi:10.1080/07352689.2016.1267498

Clarke, R., & Merlin, M. (2013). 1. Introduction to the Multipurpose Plant Cannabis. In *Cannabis* (pp. 1–12). University of California Press.

Colizzi, M., McGuire, P., Giampietro, V., Williams, S., Brammer, M., & Bhattacharyya, S. (2018). Modulation of acute effects of delta-9-tetrahydrocannabinol on psychotomimetic effects, cognition and brain function by previous cannabis exposure. *European Neuropsychopharmacology*, *28*(7), 850–862. doi:10.1016/j.euroneuro.2018.04.003 PMID:29935939

Commission, I. H. D. (1894). *Report of the Indian Hemp Drug Commission, 1893-94*. Government Central Printing Office, Simla.

Compton, W. M., Han, B., Hughes, A., Jones, C. M., & Blanco, C. (2017). Use of Marijuana for Medical Purposes Among Adults in the United States. *Journal of the American Medical Association*, *317*(2), 209–211. doi:10.1001/jama.2016.18900 PMID:27992636

Console-Bram, L., Marcu, J., & Abood, M. E. (2012). Cannabinoid receptors: Nomenclature and pharmacological principles. *Progress in Neuro-Psychopharmacology & Biological Psychiatry, 38*(1), 4–15. doi:10.1016/j.pnpbp.2012.02.009 PMID:22421596

Cooper, S. (2020). *4 Reasons to use CBD oil for healthy hair.* American Spa. https://www.americanspa.com/cbd/4-reasons-use-cbd-oil-healthy-hair

Cooper, Z. D., & Haney, M. (2009). Comparison of subjective, pharmacokinetic, and physiological effects of marijuana smoked as joints and blunts. *Drug and Alcohol Dependence, 103*(3), 107–113. doi:10.1016/j.drugalcdep.2009.01.023 PMID:19443132

Cota, D., Marsicano, G., Luts, B., Vicennati, V., Stalla, G. K., Pasquali, R., & Pagotto, U. (2003). Endogenous cannabinoid system as a modulator of food intake. *International Journal of Obesity and Related Metabolic Disorders, 27*(3), 289–301. doi:10.1038j.ijo.0802250 PMID:12629555

Couch, D. G., Maudslay, H., Doleman, B., Lund, J. N., & O'Sullivan, S. E. (2018). The use of cannabinoids in colitis: A systematic review and meta-analysis. *Inñamm. Bowel Dis., 24*(4), 680–697. doi:10.1093/ibd/izy014 PMID:29562280

Couper, A. S. (1858). On a new chemical theory. *Philosophical Magazine, 4*(16), 104–116.

Crippa, J. A., Zuardi, A. W., Martín-Santos, R., Bhattacharyya, S., Atakan, Z., McGuire, P., & Fusar-Poli, P. (2009). Cannabis and anxiety: A critical review of the evidence. *Human Psychopharmacology, 24*(7), 515–523. doi:10.1002/hup.1048 PMID:19693792

Crocioni, E. (2021). *Raman spectroscopy of Cannabis Sativa trichomes and selected cannabinoids.* Politecnico Milano1863.

Crum Brown, A. (1864). On the theory of isomeric compounds. *Transactions of the Royal Society of Edinburgh, 23*, 234.

Crum Brown, A. (1867). On the Classification of chemical substances, by means of generic radicals. *Transactions of the Royal Society of Edinburgh, 24*(2), 331–339. doi:10.1017/S0080456800018597

Cunningham, S. D., & Berti, W. R. (1993). Remediation of contaminated soils with green plants: An overview. *Vitr. Cell. Dev. Biol. Plant, 29*(4), 207–212. doi:10.1007/BF02632036

Cunningham, S. D., Berti, W. R., & Huang, J. W. (1995). Phytoremediation of contaminated soils. *Trends in Biotechnology, 13*(9), 393–397. doi:10.1016/S0167-7799(00)88987-8

Dabija, A., Codină, G. G., Gâtlan, A.-M., Sănduleac, E. T., & Rusu, L. (2018). Effects of some vegetable proteins addition on yogurt quality. *Scientific Study & Research. Chemistry & Chemical Engineering, Biotechnology. Food Industries, 19*(2), 181–192.

Dalton, J. C. (1808). *A New System of Chemical Philosophy.* doi:10.5479il.324338.39088000885681

Das, L., Liu, E., Saeed, A., Williams, D. W., Hu, H., Li, C., Ray, A. E., & Shi, J. (2017). Industrial hemp as a potential bioenergy crop in comparison with kenaf, switchgrass and biomass sorghum. *Bioresource Technology, 244*, 641–649. doi:10.1016/j.biortech.2017.08.008 PMID:28810219

Davis, M. P. (2014). Cannabinoids in pain management: CB1, CB2 and non-classic receptor ligands. *Expert Opinion on Investigational Drugs, 23*(8), 1123–1140. doi:10.1517/13543784.2014.918603 PMID:24836296

Davis, M. P. (2016). Cannabinoids for symptom management and cancer therapy: The evidence. *Journal of the National Comprehensive Cancer Network: JNCCN, 14*(7), 915–922. doi:10.6004/jnccn.2016.0094 PMID:27407130

Dawidowicz, A. L., Olszowy-Tomczyk, M., & Typek, R. (2021). CBG, CBD, Δ9-THC, CBN, CBGA, CBDA and Δ9-THCA as antioxidant agents and their intervention abilities in antioxidant action. *Fitoterapia*, *152*, 104915. doi:10.1016/j.fitote.2021.104915 PMID:33964342

de Meijer, E. P., Bagatta, M., Carboni, A., Crucitti, P., Moliterni, V. M., Ranalli, P., & Mandolino, G. (2003). The inheritance of chemical phenotype in Cannabis sativa L. *Genetics*, *163*(1), 335–346. doi:10.1093/genetics/163.1.335 PMID:12586720

De Petrocellis, L., Ligresti, A., Moriello, A. S., Allarà, M., Bisogno, T., Petrosino, S., Stott, C. G., & Di Marzo, V. (2011). Effects of cannabinoids and cannabinoid-enriched Cannabis extracts on TRP channels and endocannabinoid metabolic enzymes. *British Journal of Pharmacology*, *163*(7), 1479–1494. doi:10.1111/j.1476-5381.2010.01166.x PMID:21175579

DeFilippis, E. M., Bajaj, N. S., Singh, A., Malloy, R., Givertz, M. M., Blankstein, R., Bhatt, D. L., & Vaduganathan, M. (2020). Marijuana use in patients with cardiovascular disease: JACC review topic of the week. *Journal of the American College of Cardiology*, *75*(3), 320–332. doi:10.1016/j.jacc.2019.11.025 PMID:31976871

Degenhardt, F., Stehle, F., & Kayser, O. (2017). The Biosynthesis of Cannabinoids. In V. R. Preedy (Ed.), *Handbook of Cannabis and Related Pathologies: Biology, Pharmacology, Diagnosis, and Treatment* (pp. 13–23). Elsevier. doi:10.1016/B978-0-12-800756-3.00002-8

Degenhardt, L., Hall, W., & Lynskey, M. (2001). Alcohol, cannabis and tobacco use among Australians: A comparison of their associations with other drug use and use disorders, affective and anxiety disorders, and psychosis. *Addiction (Abingdon, England)*, *96*(11), 1603–1614. doi:10.1046/j.1360-0443.2001.961116037.x PMID:11784457

Deguchi, M., Kane, S., Potlakayala, S., George, H., Proano, R., Sheri, V., Curtis, W. R., & Rudrabhatla, S. (2020). Metabolic Engineering Strategies of Industrial Hemp (Cannabis sativa L.): A Brief Review of the Advances and Challenges. *Front. Plant Sci.*, *11*, 580621. Advance online publication. doi:10.3389/fpls.2020.580621 PMID:33363552

del Río, C., Millán, E., García, V., Appendino, G., DeMesa, J., & Muñoz, E. (2018). The endocannabinoid system of the skin. A potential approach for the treatment of skin disorders. *Biochemical Pharmacology*, *157*, 122–133. doi:10.1016/j.bcp.2018.08.022 PMID:30138623

Demuth, D. G., & Molleman, A. (2006). Cannabinoid signalling. *Life Sciences*, *78*(6), 549–563. doi:10.1016/j.lfs.2005.05.055 PMID:16109430

Desanlis, F., Cerruti, N., & Warner, P. (2013). *Cannabis sativa* agronomics and cultivation. In P. Bouloc, S. Allegret, & L. Arnaud (Eds.), *Cannabis sativa: Industrial Production and Uses* (pp. 98–124). CABI. doi:10.1079/9781845937935.0098

Devi, M., Thalkari, A. B., & Thorat, V. M. (2022). Overview of Herbal Cosmetics. *Research Journal of Topical and Cosmetic Sciences*, *13*(1), 27–34. doi:10.52711/2321-5844.2022.00005

Devinsky, O., Marsh, E., Friedman, D., Thiele, E., Laux, L., Sullivan, J, & Filloux, F. (2016). Cannabidiol in patients with treatment-resistant epilepsy: An open-label interventional trial. *Lancet Neurology*, *15*(3), 270–278. doi:10.1016/S1474-4422(15)00379-8 PMID:26724101

Diabetes.co.uk. (2019, January 15). Cannabis, or marijuana, is a drug derived from the cannabis plant that is used for recreational use, medicinal purposes and religious or spiritual rites. *Diabetes*. https://www.diabetes.co.uk/recreational-drugs/cannabis.html

DiMarzo, V., Fontana, A., Cadas, H., Schinelli, S., Cimino, G., Schwartz, J. C., & Piomelli, D. (1994). Formation and inactivation of endogenous cannabinoid anandamide in central neurons. *Nature*, *372*(6507), 686–691. doi:10.1038/372686a0 PMID:7990962

Dobrosi, N., Tóth, B. I., Nagy, G., Dózsa, A., Géczy, T., Nagy, L., Zouboulis, C. C., Paus, R., Kovács, L., & Bíró, T. (2008). Endocannabinoids enhance lipid synthesis and apoptosis of human sebocytes *via* cannabinoid receptor-2-mediated signaling. *The FASEB Journal, 22*(10), 3685–3695. doi:10.1096/fj.07-104877 PMID:18596221

Doctor, B. (1993). Stash alert: How to preserve pot potency. *High Times, 213*, 75–79.

Do, E. P. B. (2018). Medicinal Properties of Cannabinoids, Terpenes, and Flavonoids in Cannabis, and Benefits in Migraine, Headache, and Pain: An Update on Current Evidence and Cannabis Science. *Wiley Online Library, 58*(7), 1139–1186. doi:10.1111/head.13345

Doğan, N., & Doğan, C. (2021). Mucizevi Bitki Kenevir'in (Cannabis sativa L.) Gıda Endüstrisinde Kullanımı. *Bozok Veterinary Sciences, 2*(2), 47–56.

Draelos, Z. D. (2012). Cosmetics, categories, and the future. *Dermatologic Therapy, 25*(3), 223–228. doi:10.1111/j.1529-8019.2012.01498.x PMID:22913438

Dragone, D., Prarolo, G., Vanin, P., Zanella, G., (2018). Crime and the legalization of recreational marijuana. *J. Econ. Behav. Organ.* doi:. 02.005. doi:10.1016/j.jebo.2018

Dubald, M., Bourgeois, S., Andrieu, V., & Fessi, H. (2018). Ophthalmic Drug Delivery Systems for Antibiotherapy—A Review. *Pharmaceutics, 10*(1), 10. doi:10.3390/pharmaceutics10010010 PMID:29342879

Dunford, N. (2015). Hemp and flaxseed oil: properties and applications for use in food. In *Specialty oils and fats in food and nutrition* (pp. 39–63). Elsevier. doi:10.1016/B978-1-78242-376-8.00002-8

Eagleston, L. R., Kalani, N. K., Patel, R. R., Flaten, H. K., Dunnick, C. A., & Dellavalle, R. P. (2018). Cannabinoids in dermatology: A scoping review. *Dermatology Online Journal, 24*(6), 1–17. doi:10.5070/D3246040706 PMID:30142706

Eboh, L. O., & Thomas, B. E. (2005). Analysis of heavy metal content in Cannabis leaf and seedcultivated in southern part of Nigeria. *Pakistan Journal of Nutrition, 4*(5), 349–351. doi:10.3923/pjn.2005.349.351

Eisenstein, M. (2015). Medical marijuana: Showdown at the cannabis corral. *Nature, 525*(7570), S15–S17. doi:10.1038/525S15a PMID:26398734

Elisa, B., Marsano, F., Cavaletto, M., & Berta, G. (2007). Copper stress in *Cannabis sativa* roots: Morphological and pro-teomic analysis. *Caryologia, 60*(1-2), 96–101. doi:10.1080/00087114.2007.10589553

Ellickson, P. L., D'Amico, E. J., Collins, R. L., & Klein, D. J. (2005). Marijuana use and later problems: When frequency of recent use explains age of initiation effects (and when it does not). *Substance Use & Misuse, 40*(3), 343–359. doi:10.1081/JA-200049356 PMID:15776981

Ellis, R. J., Toperoff, W., Vaida, F., van den Brande, G., Gonzales, J., Gouaux, B., Bentley, H., & Atkinson, J. H. (2009). Smoked medicinal cannabis for neuropathic pain in HIV: A randomized, crossover clinical trial. *Neuropsychopharmacology: Official Publication of the American College of Neuropsychopharmacology, 34*(3), 672–680. doi:10.1038/npp.2008.120 PMID:18688212

Elsohly, M. A., & Slade, D. (2005). Chemical constituents of marijuana: The complex mixture of natural cannabinoids. Elsevier. https://doi.org/ 10.1016/j.lfs.2005.09.011.

Elsohly, M. A., Radwan, M. M., Gul, W., Chandra, S., & Galal, A. (2017). Phytochemistry of Cannabis sativa L. *Phytocannabinoids, 103*, 1–36. doi:10.1007/978-3-319-45541-9_1 PMID:28120229

EPA. (2015) *Active ingredients eligible for minimum risk pesticide products*. United States Environmental Protection Agency. https://www.epa.gov/sites/production/files/ 2015-12/document s/minrisk-active-ingredients-tolerances-2015-12-15.pdf

EPA. (2016) *Pesticide use on marijuana*. United States Environmental Protection Agency. https://www.epa.gov/pesticide-registration/pesticide-use-mar ijuana

Epstein, H. A. (2010). A natural approach to soothing atopic skin. *Skinmed*, *8*, 95–97. PMID:20527141

Erukainure, O. L., Matsabisa, M. G., Muhammad, A., Abarshi, M. M., Amaku, J. F., Katsayal, S. B., & Nde, A. L. (2021). [b]). Targeting of Protein's Messenger RNA for Viral Replication, Assembly and Release in SARS-CoV-2 Using Whole Genomic Data From South Africa: Therapeutic Potentials of Cannabis Sativa L. *Frontiers in Pharmacology*, *12*, 2314. doi:10.3389/fphar.2021.736511

Erukainure, O., Matsabisa, M., Salau, V., Oyedemi, S., Oyenihi, O., Ibeji, C., & Islam, M. (2021). [a]). Cannabis sativa L.(var. indica) Exhibits Hepatoprotective Effects by Modulating Hepatic Lipid Profile and Mitigating Gluconeogenesis and Cholinergic Dysfunction in Oxidative Hepatic Injury. *Frontiers in Pharmacology*, *12*, 12. doi:10.3389/fphar.2021.705402 PMID:34992528

European Patent Office. (2019). *European publication server* [European publication server]. Composition Containing Cannabinoids for Use in a Method for the Treatment of Vitiligo. https://data.epo.org/publication-server/document?iDocId=5865 308&iFormat=2

Farinon, B., Molinari, R., Costantini, L., & Merendino, N. (2020). The seed of industrial hemp (Cannabis sativa L.): Nutritional quality and potential functionality for human health and nutrition. *Nutrients*, *12*(7), 1935. doi:10.3390/nu12071935 PMID:32610691

Farnsworth, N. R., & Cordell, G. A. (1976). New potential hazard regarding use of marijuana treatmentof plants with liquid fertilizers. *Journal of Psychedelic Drugs*, *8*(2), 151–155. doi:10.1080/02791072.1976.10471844

Farrer, D. G. (2015). *Technical report: Oregon health authority's process to determine which types ofcontaminants to test for in cannabis products*. Oregon Health Authority.

Faux, A. M., Draye, X., Lambert, R., Andrimont, R., Raulier, P., & Bertin, P. (2013). The relationship of stem and seed yields to flowering phenology and sex expression in monoecious hemp (*Cannabis sativa* L.). *European Journal of Agronomy*, *47*, 11–22. doi:10.1016/j.eja.2013.01.006

FDA. (2020). FDA and Cannabis: Research and Drug Approval Process. *FDA*. https://www.fda.gov/news-events/public-health-focus/fda-and-cannabis-research-and-drug-approval-process

Feeney, M., & Punja, Z. K. (2003). Tissue culture and Agrobacterium-mediated transformation of hemp (Cannabis sativa L.). *In Vitro Cellular & Developmental Biology. Plant*, *39*(6), 578–585. doi:10.1079/IVP2003454

Feldman, J. (2015). Pesticide use in marijuana production: Safety issues and sustainable options. *Pesticides You*, *34*(4), 14–23.

Feng, X., Sun, G., & Fang, Z. (2022). Effect of Hempseed Cake (Cannabis sativa L.) Incorporation on the Physicochemical and Antioxidant Properties of Reconstructed Potato Chips. *Foods*, *11*(2), 211. doi:10.3390/foods11020211 PMID:35053943

Feng, Z., Bartholomew, E. S., Liu, Z., Cui, Y., Dong, Y., Li, S., Wu, H., Ren, H., & Liu, X. (2021). Glandular trichomes: New focus on horticultural crops. *Horticulture Research*, *8*(1), 158. doi:10.103841438-021-00592-1 PMID:34193839

Ferrante, C., Recinella, L., Ronci, M., Menghini, L., Brunetti, L., Chiavaroli, A., Leone, S., Di Iorio, L., Carradori, S., Tirillini, B., Angelini, P., Covino, S., Venanzoni, R., & Orlando, G. (2019). Multiple pharmacognostic characterization on hemp commercial cultivars: Focus on inflorescence water extract activity. *Food and Chemical Toxicology*, *125*, 452–461. doi:10.1016/j.fct.2019.01.035 PMID:30711720

Filer, C. N. (2022). Cannabinoids as Cocrystals. *Medical Cannabis and Cannabinoids*, *5*(1), 7–8. doi:10.1159/000521137 PMID:35224435

Finnan, J., & Styles, D. (2013). Hemp: A more sustainable annual energy crop for climate and energy policy. *Energy Policy*, *58*, 152–162. doi:10.1016/j.enpol.2013.02.046

Finn, D. P., Haroutounian, S., Hohmann, A. G., Krane, E., Soliman, N., & Rice, A. S. (2021). Cannabinoids, the endocannabinoid system, and pain: A review of preclinical studies. *Pain*, *162*, S5–S25. doi:10.1097/j.pain.0000000000002268 PMID:33729211

Fisse, J., Braut, F., Cosson, L., & Paris, M. (1981). E ́tude in vitro des capacite ́s organoge ́ne ́tiques de tissus de Cannabis sativa L.; Effet de diffe ́rentes substances de croissance [In vitro study of the organoge netic capacities of Cannabis sativa L. tissues; Effect of different growth substances]. *Plantes Me ́dicinales et Phytotherapie*, *15*, 217–223.

Fitzgerald, K. T., Bronstein, A. C., & Newquist, K. L. (2013). Marijuana Poisoning. *Topical Review Marijuana Poisoning. Elsevier*, *28*(1), 8–12. doi:10.1053/j.tcam.2013.03.004 PMID:23796481

Flachenecker, P., Henze, T., & Zettl, U. K. (2014). Spasticity in patients with multiple sclerosis–clinical characteristics, treatment and quality of life. *Acta Neurologica Scandinavica*, *129*(3), 154–162. doi:10.1111/ane.12202 PMID:24256407

Fleischhauer, W. (1956). The old man of the mountain: The growth of a legend. Symp. *Q. J. Mod. Lit*, *9*(1), 79–90. doi:10.1080/00397709.1956.10113536

Flygare, J., & Sander, B. (2008). The endocannabinoid system in cancer—Potential therapeutic target? *Seminars in Cancer Biology*, *3*(3), 176–189. doi:10.1016/j.semcancer.2007.12.008 PMID:18249558

Fogli, S., & Breschi, M. C. (2008). The molecular bases of cannabinoid action in cancer. *Cancer Therapy*, *6*, 103–116.

Fort, J. (2012). Demic and cultural neolithic diffusion. *Proceedings of the National Academy of Sciences of the United States of America*, *109*, 18669–18673. doi:10.1073/pnas.1200662109 PMID:23112147

Frankland, E. (1852). On a New Series of Organic Bodies Containing Metals. *Philosophical Transactions of the Royal Society.*, *142*, 417–444. doi:10.1098/rstl.1852.0020

Freeman, T. P., Hindocha, C., Green, S. F., & Bloomfield, M. A. P. (2019). Medicinal use of cannabis based products and cannabinoids. *BMJ (Clinical Research Ed.)*, *365*, l1141. doi:10.1136/bmj.l1141 PMID:30948383

Freemon, F. R. (1982). The effect of chronically administered delta-9-tetrahydrocannabinol upon the polygraphically monitored sleep of normal volunteers. *Drug and Alcohol Dependence*, *10*(4), 345–353. doi:10.1016/0376-8716(82)90036-9 PMID:6299682

Gabros, S., Nessel, T. A., & Zito, P. M. (2022). *Sunscreens And Photoprotection*. StatPearls Publishing. https://www.ncbi.nlm.nih.gov/books/NBK537164/

Gagliano, M. (2013). Persons as plants: ecopsychology and the return to the dream of nature. Landsc.*: J. Int. Cent. Landsc. Lang.* *5*(2). áhttp://ro.ecu.edu.au/landscapes/ vol5/iss2/14ñ.

Gagne, S. J., Stout, J. M., Liu, E., Boubakir, Z., Clark, S. M., & Page, J. E. (2012). Identification of olivetolic acid cyclase from *Cannabis sativa* reveals a unique catalytic route to plant polyketides. *Proceedings of the National Academy of Sciences of the United States of America*, *109*(31), 12811–12816. doi:10.1073/pnas.1200330109 PMID:22802619

Gakuubi, M. M., & Wanzala, W. (2012). A survey of plants and plant products traditionally used in livestock health management in Buuri district, Meru County, Kenya. *Journal of Ethnobiology and Ethnomedicine*, *8*(1), 39. doi:10.1186/1746-4269-8-39 PMID:23044218

Galán-Ávila, A., Gramazio, P., Ron, M., Prohens, J., & Herraiz, F. J. (2021). A novel and rapid method for Agrobacterium-mediated production of stably transformed Cannabis sativa L. plants. *Industrial Crops and Products*, *170*, 113691. doi:10.1016/j.indcrop.2021.113691

Gaoni, Y., & Mechoulam, R. (1964). Isolation, Structure, and Partial Synthesis of an Active Constituent of Hashish. *Journal of the American Chemical Society*, *86*(8), 1646–1647. doi:10.1021/ja01062a046

Garbisu, C., & Alkorta, I. (2001). Phytoextraction: A cost-effective plant-based technology for the removal of metals from the environment. *Bioresource Technology*, *77*(3), 229–236. doi:10.1016/S0960-8524(00)00108-5 PMID:11272009

Garcia-Jaldon, C., Dupeyre, D., & Vignon, M. R. (1998). Fibers from semiretted hemp bundles by steam explosion treatment. *Biotechnology and Bioengineering*, *14*, 251–260.

Gautam, A. K., Kant, M., & Thakur, Y. (2013). Isolation of endophytic fungi from Cannabis sativa andstudy their antifungal potential. *Archiv für Phytopathologie und Pflanzenschutz*, *46*(6), 627–635. doi:10.1080/03235408.2012.749696

Gęgotek, A., Biernacki, M., Ambrożewicz, E., Surażyński, A., Wroński, A., & Skrzydlewska, E. (2016). The cross-talk between electrophiles, antioxidant defence and the endocannabinoid system in fibroblasts and keratinocytes after UVA and UVB irradiation. *Journal of Dermatological Science*, *81*(2), 107–117. doi:10.1016/j.jdermsci.2015.11.005 PMID:26674123

Gérard, N., Pieters, G., Goffin, K., Bormans, G., & Van Laere, K. (2011). Brain type 1 cannabinoid receptor availability in patients with anorexia and bulimia nervosa. *Biological Psychiatry*, *70*(8), 777–784. doi:10.1016/j.biopsych.2011.05.010 PMID:21718968

Ghosh, M., & Singh, S. P. (2005). A review on phytoremediation of heavy metals and utilization of its byproducts. *Applied Ecology and Environmental Research*, *3*(1), 1–18. doi:10.15666/aeer/0301_001018

Giacoppo, S., Mandolino, G., Galuppo, M., Bramanti, P., Mazzon, E., (2014). Cannabinoids: new promising agents in the treatment of neurological diseases. *Molecules*. doi:. doi:10.3390/molecules191118781

Giammona, C. (2018). Trendy hemp compound CBD set for big boost from U.S. *Farm Bill*. https://www.bloomberg.com/news/articles/2018-12-19/trendy-hemp-compound-cbd-set-for-big-boost-from-u-s-farm-bill

Giovanardi, R., Marchiol, L., Mazzocco, G. T., & Zuliani, F. (2002). Possibilità di impiegodellacanapanellafitoestrazione di metallipesanti in terrenicontaminati: Primirisultati [Possibility of using hemp in the phytoextraction of heavy metals in contaminated soils: First results.]. *Agroindustria*, *1*(1), 69–73.

Gleason, K. A., Birnbaum, S. G., Shukla, A., & Ghose, S. (2012). Susceptibility of the adolescent brain to cannabinoids: Long-term hippocampal effects and relevance to schizophrenia. *Translational Psychiatry*, *2*(11), e199. doi:10.1038/tp.2012.122 PMID:23188199

Glé, P., Gourdon, E., & Arnaud, L. (2011). Acoustical properties of materials made of vegetable particles with several scales of porosity. *Applied Acoustics*, *72*(5), 249–259. doi:10.1016/j.apacoust.2010.11.003

Glivar, T., Eržen, J., Kreft, S., Zagožen, M., Čerenak, A., Čeh, B., & Benković, E. T. (2020). Cannabinoid content in industrial hemp (Cannabis sativa L.) varieties grown in Slovenia. *Industrial Crops and Products, 145*, 112082. doi:10.1016/j.indcrop.2019.112082

GLOBOCAN. (2020). *Cancer today*. GCO. https://gco.iarc.fr/today/home

Glogauer, J. & Blay, J. (2021). Cannabinoids, their cellular receptors, and effects on the invasive phenotype of carcinoma and metastasis. *Cancer Reports,* e1475.

Gohad, P., McCoy, J., Wambier, C., Kovacevic, M., Situm, M., Stanimirovic, A., & Goren, A. (2021). Novel cannabidiol sunscreen protects keratinocytes and melanocytes against ultraviolet B radiation. *Journal of Cosmetic Dermatology, 20*(4), 1350–1352. doi:10.1111/jocd.13693 PMID:32964699

Gonçalves, E. C., Baldasso, G. M., Bicca, M. A., Paes, R. S., Capasso, R., & Dutra, R. C. (2020). Terpenoids, cannabimimetic ligands, beyond the cannabis plant. *Molecules (Basel, Switzerland), 25*(7), 1567. doi:10.3390/molecules25071567 PMID:32235333

González-García, S., Hospido, A., Feijoo, G., & Moreira, M. T. (2010). Life cycle assessment of raw materials for non-wood pulp mills: *Cannabis sativa* and flax. *Resources, Conservation and Recycling, 54*(11), 923–930. doi:10.1016/j.resconrec.2010.01.011

González-García, S., Luo, L., Moreira, M. T., Feijoo, G., & Huppes, G. (2012). Life cycle assessment of *Cannabis sativa* hurds use in second generation ethanol production. *Biomass and Bioenergy, 36*, 268–279. doi:10.1016/j.biombioe.2011.10.041

Gopal, L. (1961). Textiles in ancient India. *Journal of Economic and Social History of the Orient, 4*(1), 53–69. doi:10.1163/156852061X00132

Government Central Printing Office, Simla-Jurgensen C.W., & Madsen, A. (2009). Exposure to the airborne mould Botrytis and its health effects. *Annals of Agricultural and Environmental Medicine, 16*, 183–186. PMID:20047250

Grant, C. N., Lalor, G. C., & Vutchkov, M. K. (2004). Trace elements in Jamaican tobacco. *The West Indian Medical Journal, 53*(2), 66–70. PMID:15199713

Grassa, C. J., Wenger, J. P., Dabney, C., Poplawski, S. G., Motley, S. T., Michael, T. P., & Weiblen, G. D. (2018). A complete *Cannabis* chromosome assembly and adaptive admixture for elevated cannabidiol (CBD) content. *bioRxiv, 458083*. doi:10.1101/458083

Griffith, R. T. H. (1917). *The Hymns of the Atharva-veda* (Vol. 2). EJ Lazarus.

Grifoni, M., Rosellini, I., Angelini, P., Petruzzelli, G., & Pezzarossa, B. (2020). The efect of residual hydrocarbons in soil following oil spillages on the growth of Zea mays plants. *Environmental Pollution, 265*, 114950. doi:10.1016/j.envpol.2020.114950 PMID:32554092

Grof, C. P. (2018). Cannabis, from plant to pill. *British Journal of Clinical Pharmacology, 84*(11), 2463–2467. doi:10.1111/bcp.13618 PMID:29701252

Grucza, R. A., & Bierut, L. J. (2006). Cigarette smoking and the risk for alcohol use disorders among adolescent drinkers. *Alcoholism, Clinical and Experimental Research, 30*(12), 2046–2054. doi:10.1111/j.1530-0277.2006.00255.x PMID:17117970

Gu, L. F. (2006). *Surgical Sewing Free Zipper Made of Antibiotic Material Hemp Fiber.* Patent publication number CN 2829641 Y. Washington, DC: U.S. Patent and Trademark Office.

Guindon, J., & Hohmann, A. G. (2009). The endocannabinoid system and pain. *CNS & Neurological Disorders - Drug Targets*, *8*(6), 403–421. doi:10.2174/187152709789824660 PMID:19839937

Gunnarsson, I. B., Kuglarz, M., Karakashev, D., & Angelidaki, I. (2015). Thermochemical pretreatments for enhancing succinic acid production from industrial *Cannabis sativa* (*Cannabis sativa* L.). *Bioresource Technology*, *182*, 58–66. doi:10.1016/j.biortech.2015.01.126 PMID:25682224

Guo, T., Liu, Q., Hou, P., Li, F., Guo, S., Song, W., Zhang, H., Liu, X., Zhang, S., Zhang, J., Ho, C.-T., & Bai, N. (2018). Stilbenoids and cannabinoids from the leaves of Cannabis sativa f. sativa with potential reverse cholesterol transport activity. *Food & Function*, *9*(12), 6608–6617. doi:10.1039/C8FO01896K PMID:30500001

Gupta, P. L., Rajput, M., Oza, T., Trivedi, U., & Sanghvi, G. (2019). Eminence of Microbial Products in Cosmetic Industry. *Natural Products and Bioprospecting*, *9*(4), 267–278. doi:10.100713659-019-0215-0 PMID:31214881

Gurukkal, R. (2018). *History and Theory of Knowledge Production: An Introductory Outline*. Oxford University Press.

Gururajan, A., & Malone, D. T. (2016). Does cannabidiol have a role in the treatment of schizophrenia? *Schizophrenia Research*, *176*(2–3), 281–290. doi:10.1016/j.schres.2016.06.022 PMID:27374322

Gutiérrez, A., & del Río, J. C. (2005). Chemical characterization of pitch deposits produced in the manufacturing of high-quality paper pulps from hemp fibers. *Bioresource Technology*, *96*(13), 1445–1450. doi:10.1016/j.biortech.2004.12.008 PMID:15939271

Gzebenyuk, N. V. (1984). The occurrence of fungi on hemp stems. *Mikologiâ i Fitopatologiâ*, *18*(4), 322–326.

Hajar EW, Sulaiman AZ, Sakinah AM., (2014). Assessment of heavy metals tolerance in leaves, stems and flowers of *Stevia rebaudiana* plant. *Procedia Environmental Sciences, 20*, 386–93.

Halder, S., Anand, U., Nandy, S., Oleksak, P., Qusti, S., Alshammari, E.M., El-Saber Batiha, G., Koshy, E.P. & Dey, A. (2021). Herbal drugs and natural bioactive products as potential therapeutics: A review on pro-cognitives and brain boosters' perspectives. *Saudi Pharm. J. 29* (8), 879–907. doi:. jsps.2021.07.003. doi:10.1016/j

Hall, W.D., (2008). The contribution of research to the development of a national cannabis policy in Australia. *Addiction 103*, 712–720. doi:. doi:10.1111/j.1360-0443

Hall, A. (2008). Denis J. Murphy. People, Plants & Genes: The Story of Crops and Humanity. xxiv+ 402 pages, 54 figures, 12 tables. 2007. Oxford: Oxford University Press. *Antiquity*, *82*(316), 505–506. doi:10.1017/S0003598X00097040

Hallak, J., Teixeira, T. A., Pariz, J. R., Iori, I., Costa, E., & Saldiva, P. H. (2019). MP75-09 Marijuana consumption has a direct deleterious effect on spermatozoa by increasing intracellular reactive oxygen species levels 20 times more than tobacco smoking: Reasons for concern on widespread use. *The Journal of Urology*, *201*(4).

Hall, J., Bhattarai, S. P., & Midmore, D. J. (2012). Review of flowering control in industrial Cannabis sativa. *Journal of Natural Fibers*, *9*(1), 23–36. doi:10.1080/15440478.2012.651848

Hammond, C. T., & Mahlberg, P. G. (1994). Phloroglucinol glucoside as a natural constituent of *Cannabis sativa*. *Phytochemistry*, *37*(3), 755–756. doi:10.1016/S0031-9422(00)90352-2

Han, B., Compton, W. M., Blanco, C., & Jones, C. M. (2018). Trends in and correlates of medical marijuana use among adults in the United States. *Drug and Alcohol Dependence*, *186*, 120–129. doi:10.1016/j.drugalcdep.2018.01.022 PMID:29567626

Hand, A., Blake, A., Kerrigan, P., Samuel, P., & Friedberg, J. (2016). History of medical cannabis. *Journal of Pain Management*, *9*(4), 387–394.

Haney, M., Hart, C. L., Vosburg, S. K., Comer, S. D., Reed, S. C., & Foltin, R. W. (2008). Effects of THC and lofexidine in a human laboratory model of marijuana withdrawal and relapse. *Psychopharmacology 197* (1), 157–168. s00213-007-1020-8. doi:10.1007/

Haney, M., Hart, C. L., Vosburg, S. K., Nasser, J., Bennett, A., Zubaran, C., & Foltin, R. W. (2004). Marijuana withdrawal in humans: effects of oral THC or divalproex. *Neuropsychopharmacology 29* (1), 158–170. . npp.1300310. doi:10.1038/sj

Hao X. M., Yang Y., An L. X., Wang J. M., Han L. (2014). Study on antibacterial mechanism of hemp fiber. *Adv. Mat. Res.* doi:10.4028/www.scientific.net/AMR.887-888.610

Hao, Y. J., & Deng, X. X. (2003). Genetically stable regeneration of apple plants from slow growth. *Plant Cell Tiss Org, 72*(3), 253–260. doi:10.1023/A:1022388728497

Happyana, N., Agnolet, S., Muntendam, R., Van Dam, A., Schneider, B., & Kayser, O. (2013). Analysis of cannabinoids in laser-microdissected trichomes of medicinal Cannabis sativa using LCMS and cryogenic NMR. *Phytochemistry, 87*, 51–59. doi:10.1016/j.phytochem.2012.11.001 PMID:23280038

Hara, M., Ma, T., & Verkman, A. S. (2002). Selectively Reduced Glycerol in Skin of Aquaporin-3-deficient Mice May Account for Impaired Skin Hydration, Elasticity, and Barrier Recovery. *The Journal of Biological Chemistry, 277*(48), 46616–46621. doi:10.1074/jbc.M209003200 PMID:12270942

Hasenoehrl, C., Storr, M., & Schicho, R. (2017). Cannabinoids for treating inñammatory bowel diseases: Where are we and where do we go? *Expert Review of Gastroenterology & Hepatology, 11*(4), 329–337. doi:10.1080/17474124.2017.1292851 PMID:28276820

Hawthorne, S. B., Yang, Y., & Miller, D. J. (1994). Extraction of Organic Pollutants from Environmental Solids with Sub- and Supercritical Water. *Analytical Chemistry, 66*(18), 2912–2920. doi:10.1021/ac00090a019

Hazekamp, A. (2006). An evaluation of the quality of medicinal grade cannabis in the Netherlands. *Cannabinoids, 1*(1), 1–9.

Hazekamp, A. (2016). Evaluating the effects of gamma-irradiation for decontamination of medicinalcannabis. *Frontiers in Pharmacology, 7*, 108. doi:10.3389/fphar.2016.00108 PMID:27199751

Health Canada. (2008) *Product information sheet on dried marihuana (cannabis).* Health Canada. www.hc-sc.gc.ca/dhp-mps/marihuana/about-apropos/dried-information-sechee-eng.php

Heinrich, J., & Mathre, M. L. (2001). Policy Perspectives: Therapeutic Cannabis. *The American Journal of Nursing, 101*(4), 61–69. PMID:11301687

Herer, J. (1990). The forgotten history of hemp. *Earth Island Journal, 5*(4), 35–38.

Herer, J. (1992). *Hemp & the Marijuana Conspiracy: The Emperor Wears No Clothes: the Authoritative Historical Record of the Cannabis Plant, Marijuana Prohibition & how Hemp Can Still Save the World.* Help End Marijuana Prohibition.

Hernandez, C. M., Orsini, C. A., Blaes, S. L., Bizon, J. L., Febo, M., Bruijnzeel, A. W., & Setlow, B. (2021). Effects of repeated adolescent exposure to cannabis smoke on cognitive outcomes in adulthood. *Journal of Psychopharmacology (Oxford, England), 35*(7), 848–863. doi:10.1177/0269881120965931 PMID:33295231

Herzog, S., Shanahan, M., Grimison, P., Tran, A., Wong, N., Lintzeris, N., Simes, J., Stockler, M., & Morton, R. L. (2018). Systematic review of the costs and beneðts of prescribed cannabis-based medicines for the management of chronic illness: Lessons from multiple sclerosis. *PharmacoEconomics, 36*(1), 67–78. doi:10.100740273-017-0565-6 PMID:28866778

Hesami, M., Baiton, A., Alizadeh, M., Pepe, M., Torkamaneh, D., & Jones, A. M. P. (2021). Advances and Perspectives in Tissue Culture and Genetic Engineering of Cannabis. *International Journal of Molecular Sciences*, *22*(11), 5671. doi:10.3390/ijms22115671 PMID:34073522

Hesami, M., & Jones, A. M. P. (2021). Modeling and optimizing callus growth and development in Cannabis sativa using random forest and support vector machine in combination with a genetic algorithm. *Applied Microbiology and Biotechnology*, *105*(12), 5201–5212. doi:10.100700253-021-11375-y PMID:34086118

Hoch, E., Niemann, D., von Keller, R., Schneider, M., Friemel, C. M., Preuss, U. W., Hasan, A., & Pogarell, O. (2019). How effective and safe is medical cannabis as a treatment of mental disorders? A systematic review. *European Archives of Psychiatry and Clinical Neuroscience*, *269*(1), 87–105. doi:10.100700406-019-00984-4 PMID:30706168

Holland, K. (2020). CBD vs. THC: properties, benefits, and side effects. *Healthline*. https://www.healthline.com/health/cbd-vs-thc

Holmes M, Vyas JM, Steinbach W, McPartland J (2015) *Microbiological safety testing of cannabis*.

Horne, M. R. (2020). Bast fibres: hemp cultivation and production. In R. M. Kozłowski & M. Mackiewicz-Talarczyk (Eds.), *Handbook of Natural Fibres* (2nd ed., Vol. 1, pp. 163–196). Woodhead Publishing., doi:10.1016/B978-0-12-818398-4.00007-4

Horn, H., Böhme, B., Dietrich, L., & Koch, M. (2018). Endocannabinoids in body weight control. *Pharmaceuticals*, *11*(2), E55. doi:10.3390/ph11020055 PMID:29849009

Hoseini, P. S., Poursafa, P., Moattar, F., Amin, M. M., & Rezaei, A. H. (2012). Ability of phytoremediation forabsorption of strontium and cesium from soils using Cannabis sativa. *International Journal of Environmental Health Engineering*, *1*(1), 17. doi:10.4103/2277-9183.96004

Hou, D., O'Connor, D., Igalavithana, A. D., Alessi, D. S., Luo, J., Tsang, D. C. W., Sparks, D. L., Yamauchi, Y., Rinklebe, J., & Ok, Y. S. (2020). Metal contamination and bioremediation of agricultural soils for food safety and sustainability. *Nat. Rev. Earth Environ.*, *1*(7), 366–381. doi:10.103843017-020-0061-y

House, J. D., Neufeld, J., & Leson, G. (2010). Evaluating the quality of protein from hemp seed (Cannabis sativa L.) products through the use of the protein digestibility-corrected amino acid score method. *Journal of Agricultural and Food Chemistry*, *58*(22), 11801–11807. doi:10.1021/jf102636b PMID:20977230

Huang, H., Yao, W., Li, R., Ali, A., Du, J., Guo, D., Xiao, R., Guo, Z., Zhang, Z., & Awasthi, M. K. (2018). Effect of pyrolysis temperature on chemical form, behavior, and environmental risk of Zn, Pb and Cd in biochar produced from phytoremediation residue. *Bioresource Technology*, *249*, 487–493. doi:10.1016/j.biortech.2017.10.020 PMID:29073559

Huestis, M. (2007). Human cannabinoid pharmacokinetics. *Chemistry & Biodiversity*, *4*(8), 1770–1804. doi:10.1002/cbdv.200790152 PMID:17712819

Hu, R., & Lim, J.-K. (2016). Fabrication and mechanical properties of completely biodegradable *Cannabis sativa* fiber reinforced polylactic acid composites. *Journal of Composite Materials*, *41*(13), 1655–1669. doi:10.1177/0021998306069878

Husain, R., Weeden, H., Bogush, D., Deguchi, M., Soliman, M., Potlakayala, S., Katam, R., Goldman, S., & Rudrabhatla, S. (2019). Enhanced tolerance of industrial hemp (Cannabis sativa L.) plants on abandoned mine land soil leads to overexpression of cannabinoids. *PLoS One*, *14*(8), e0221570. doi:10.1371/journal.pone.0221570 PMID:31465423

Hussain, S. H. F. (2014). *Cannabinoids production in Cannabis sativa L. An In Vitro Approach*. [Ph.D. Thesis, Technischen Universitat Dortmund, Dortmund, Germany].

Hussain, T., Jeena, G., Pitakbut, T., Vasilev, N., & Kayser, O. (2021). *Cannabis sativa* research trends, challenges, and new-age perspectives. *iScience, 24*(12), 103391. doi:10.1016/j.isci.2021.103391

Ibrahim, T. A. (2012). Chemical composition and biological activity of extracts from Salvia bicolor Desf. growing in Egypt. *Molecules (Basel, Switzerland), 17*(10), 11315–11334. doi:10.3390/molecules171011315 PMID:23011275

Ikarashi, N., Shiseki, M., Yoshida, R., Tabata, K., Kimura, R., Watanabe, T., Kon, R., Sakai, H., & Kamei, J. (2021). Cannabidiol Application Increases Cutaneous Aquaporin-3 and Exerts a Skin Moisturizing Effect. *Pharmaceuticals, 14*(9), 879. doi:10.3390/ph14090879 PMID:34577578

Ingrao, C., Giudice, A. L., Bacenetti, J., Tricase, C., Dotelli, G., Fiala, M., & Mbohwa, C. (2015). Energy and environmental assessment of industrial hemp for building applications: A review. *Renewable & Sustainable Energy Reviews, 51*, 29–42. doi:10.1016/j.rser.2015.06.002

Inui, A. (2002). Cancer anorexia-cachexia syndrome: Current issues in research and management. *CA: a Cancer Journal for Clinicians, 52*(2), 72–91. doi:10.3322/canjclin.52.2.72 PMID:11929007

Iqbal, A., Arshad, M., Hashmi, I., Karthikeyan, R., Gentry, T. J., & Schwab, A. P. (2018). Biodegradation of phenol and benzene by endophytic bacterial strains isolated from refnery wastewater-fed Cannabis sativa. *Environmental Technology, 39*(13), 1705–1714. doi:10.1080/09593330.2017.1337232 PMID:28562230

Ireland, T. (1893). Indian hemp as a cause of insanity. *British Medical Journal, 2*(1710), 813.

Iványi, I. (2006). Effect of genotype and environmental on the oil content and fatty acid composition of hempseed. *Cereal Research Communications, 34*(1), 493–496. doi:10.1556/CRC.34.2006.1.123

Jae-We, C., Yeon-Su, J., Ji-Won, H., Young-Jin, C., Hyun-Kyu, K., Min-Young, K., Beom-Joon, K., Ki-Moon, P., Jong-Keun, K., Jae-Hyun, K., & Soo-Muk, C. (2011). Skin Hydration and Collagen Synthesis of AF-343 in HS68 Cell Line and NC/Nga Mice by Filaggrin Expression and Suppression of Matrix Metallopreteinase. *Toxicological Research, 27*(4), 225–229. doi:10.5487/TR.2011.27.4.225 PMID:24278576

Jakubovski, E., & Müller-Vahl, K. (2017). Speechlessness in Gilles de la Tourette syndrome: Cannabis-based medicines improve severe vocal blocking tics in two patients. *International Journal of Molecular Sciences, 18*(8), E1739. doi:10.3390/ijms18081739 PMID:28796166

Janeczek, A., Zawadzki, M., Szpot, P., & Niedzwiedz, A. (2018). Marijuana intoxication in a cat. *Acta Veterinaria Scandinavica, 60*(1), 1–4. doi:10.118613028-018-0398-0 PMID:29996908

Jarai, M. (2022, March 29). HIV neuropathy: Causes, symptoms, treatment, and more. *Medical News Today.* https://www.medicalnewstoday.com/articles/hiv-neuropathy

Jarocka-Karpowicz, I., Biernacki, M., Wroński, A., Gęgotek, A., & Skrzydlewska, E. (2020). Cannabidiol Effects on Phospholipid Metabolism in Keratinocytes from Patients with Psoriasis Vulgaris. *Biomolecules, 10*(3), 367. doi:10.3390/biom10030367 PMID:32121131

Järup, L. (2003). Hazards of heavy metal contamination. *British Medical Bulletin, 68*(1), 167–182. doi:10.1093/bmb/ldg032 PMID:14757716

Jarzębski, M., Fathordoobady, F., Guo, Y., Xu, M., Singh, A., Kitts, D. D., Kowalczewski, P. Ł., Jeżowski, P., & Pratap Singh, A. (2019). Pea protein for hempseed oil nanoemulsion stabilization. *Molecules (Basel, Switzerland), 24*(23), 4288. doi:10.3390/molecules24234288 PMID:31775277

Jauregui, X., Clavo, Z. M., Jovel, E. M., & Pardo-de-Santayana, M. (2011). "Plantas con madre": plants that teach and guide in the shamanic initiation process in the EastCentral Peruvian Amazon. *J. Ethnopharmacol. 134*, 739–752. doi:1016/j.jep.2011.01.042.

Javid FA, Phillips RM, Afshinjavid S, Verde R, Ligresti A., (2016). Cannabinoid pharmacology in cancer research: a new hope for cancer patients? *Eur J Pharmacol.* 2775:1–14. doi:. 02.010. doi:10.1016/j.ejphar

Jeong, M., Cho, J., Shin, J. I., Jeon, Y. J., Kim, J. H., Lee, S. J., Kim, E. S., & Lee, K. (2014). Hempseed oil induces reactive oxygen species- and C/EBP homologous proteinmediated apoptosis in MH7A human rheumatoid arthritis ðbroblast-like synovial cells. *Journal of Ethnopharmacology*, *154*(3), 745–752. doi:10.1016/j.jep.2014.04.052 PMID:24814038

Jiang, H. E., Li, X., Zhao, Y. X., Ferguson, D. K., Hueber, F., Bera, S., Wang, Y. F., Zhao, L. C., Liu, C. J., & Li, C. S. (2006). A new insight into Cannabis sativa (Cannabaceae) utilization from 2500-year-old Yanghai Tombs, Xinjiang, China. *Journal of Ethnopharmacology*, *108*(3), 414–422. doi:10.1016/j.jep.2006.05.034 PMID:16879937

Jin, D., Dai, K., Xie, Z., & Chen, J. (2020). Secondary metabolites profiled in cannabis inflorescences, leaves, stem barks, and roots formedicinal purposes. *Scientific Reports*, *10*, 1–14.

Jin, D., Jin, S., Yu, Y., Lee, C., & Chen, J. (2017). Classification of Cannabis Cultivars Marketed in Canada for Medical Purposes by Quantification of Cannabinoids and Terpenes Using HPLC-DAD and GC-MS Analytical & Bioanalytical Techniques. *Journal of Analytical & Bioanalytical Techniques*, *8*(01), 1. doi:10.4172/2155-9872.1000349

Johnson, R. (2018). Hemp as an agricultural commodity (CRS report no. RL32725; p. 48). *Congressional research service*. https://fas.org/sgp/crs/misc/RL32725.pdf

Johnson, N. (2017). Workers' weed: Cannabis, sugar beets, and landscapes of labour in the American West, 1900–1946. *Agricultural History*, *91*(3), 320–341. doi:10.3098/ah.2017.091.3.320

John, W. S., Martin, T. J., Solingapuram Sai, K. K., Nader, S. H., Donald Gage, H., Mintz, A., & Nader, M. A. (2018). Chronic d9-THC in rhesus monkeys: Effects on cognitive performance and dopamine D2/D3 receptor availability. *The Journal ofPharmacology and Experimental Therapeutics*, *364*(2), 300–310. doi:10.1124/jpet.117.244194 PMID:29203575

Jones, D. I. H. (1970). Cell-wall constituents of some grass species and varieties. *Journal of the Science of Food and Agriculture*, *21*(11), 559–562. doi:10.1002/jsfa.2740211104

Jones, N. A., Hill, A. J., Smith, I., Bevan, S. A., Williams, C. M., Whalley, B. J., & Stephens, G. J. (2010). Cannabidiol displays antiepileptiform and antiseizure properties in vitro and in vivo. *The Journal of Pharmacology and Experimental Therapeutics*, *332*(2), 569–577. doi:10.1124/jpet.109.159145 PMID:19906779

Jourdan, T., Djaouti, L., Demizieux, L., Gresti, J., Vergès, B., & Degrace, P. (2010). CB1 Antagonism exerts speciðc molecular effects on visceral and subcutaneous fat and reversesliver steatosisindiet-inducedobesemice. *Diabetes*, *59*(4), 926–934. doi:10.2337/db09-1482 PMID:20110567

Jurkowska, H., Rogóz, A., & Wojciechowicz, T. (1990). The content of lithium in some species of plantsfollowing differentiated doses of nitrogen. *Polish Journal of Soil Science*, *23*, 195–199.

Kagen, S. L., Kurup, V. P., Sohnle, P. G., & Fink, J. N. (1983). Marijuana smoking and fungal sensitization. *The Journal of Allergy and Clinical Immunology*, *71*(4), 389–3893. doi:10.1016/0091-6749(83)90067-2 PMID:6833678

Kala CP, Farooquee NA, Dhar U. (2004). Prioritization of medicinal plants on the basis of available knowledge, existing practices and use value status in Uttaranchal. *India Biodiv Conser. 13*(2), 453–469. doi:: BIOC.0000006511.67354.7f. doi:10.1023/B

Kalant, O. J. (1972). Report of the Indian Hemp Drugs Commission, 1893-94: A critical review. *The International Journal of the Addictions*, *7*(1), 77–96. doi:10.3109/10826087209026763 PMID:4557840

Kanwar, V. S., Sharma, A., Srivastav, A. L., & Rani, L. (2020). Phytoremediation of toxic metals present in soil and water environment: A critical review. *Environmental Science and Pollution Research International*, *27*(36), 44835–44860. doi:10.100711356-020-10713-3 PMID:32981020

Karadjov, J. (2014) Eliminating heavy-metal toxicity in medical marijuana. *Advanced Nutrients*. www.advancednutrients.com/heavymetal//Eliminating-Heavy-Metal-Toxicity-in-Medical-Marijuana.pdf

Kasman, A. M., Thoma, M. E., McLain, A. C., & Eisenberg, M. L. (2018b). Association between use of marijuana and time to pregnancy in men and women: Findings from the National Survey of Family Growth. *Fertility and Sterility*, *109*(5), 866–871.

Kavousi, P., Giamo, T., Arnold, G., Alliende, M., Huynh, E., Lea, J., & Yee, A. (2022). What do we know about opportunities and challenges for localities from Cannabis legalization? *The Review of Policy Research*, *39*(2), 143–169. doi:10.1111/ropr.12460

Kazemi, F., Karimi, I., & Yousofvand, N. (2021). Molecular docking study of lignanamides from Cannabis sativa against P-glycoprotein. *In Silico Pharmacology*, *9*(1), 1–7. doi:10.100740203-020-00066-7 PMID:33442533

Keating, G. M. (2017). Delta-9-tetrahydrocannabinol/cannabidiol oromucosal spray (Sativex (®)): A review in multiple sclerosis-related spasticity. *Drugs*, *77*(5), 563–574. doi:10.100740265-017-0720-6 PMID:28293911

Keller, C., Ludwig, C., Davoli, F., & Wochele, J. (2005). Thermal treatment of metal-enriched biomass produced from heavy metal phytoextraction. *Environmental Science & Technology*, *39*(9), 3359–3367. doi:10.1021/es0484101 PMID:15926590

Khan, B. A., Wang, J., Warner, P., & Wang, H. (2015). Antibacterial properties of hemp hurd powder against *E. coli*. *Journal of Applied Polymer Science*, *132*(10), 41588. doi:10.1002/app.41588

Khattab, M. M., & Dahman, Y. (2019). Production and recovery of poly-3-hydroxybutyrate bioplastics using agro-industrial residues of *Cannabis sativa* hurd biomass. *Bioprocess and Biosystems Engineering*, *42*(7), 1115–1127. doi:10.100700449-019-02109-6 PMID:30993443

Kilmer, B., & Pacula, R. L. (2017). Understanding and learning from the diversification of cannabis supply laws. *Addiction (Abingdon, England)*, *112*(7), 1128–1135. doi:10.1111/add.13623 PMID:27891693

King, J. W. (2019). The relationship between cannabis/hemp use in foods and processing methodology. *Current Opinion in Food Science*, *28*, 32–40. doi:10.1016/j.cofs.2019.04.007

Kiprono, P. C., Kaberia, F., Keriko, J. M., & Karanja, J. N. (2000). The in vitro anti-fungal and anti-bacterial activities of beta-sitosterol from *Senecio lyratus* (Asteraceae). *Z. Naturforsch. C*, *55*(5-6), 485–488. doi:10.1515/znc-2000-5-629 PMID:10928565

Kladar, N., Čonić, B. S., Božin, B., & Torović, L. (2021). European hemp-based food products–Health concerning cannabinoids exposure assessment. *Food Control*, *129*, 108233. doi:10.1016/j.foodcont.2021.108233

Koch, M. (2017). Cannabinoid receptor signaling in central regulation of feeding behavior: A mini review. *Frontiers in Neuroscience*, *11*, 293. doi:10.3389/fnins.2017.00293 PMID:28596721

Ko, G. D., Bober, S. L., Mindra, S., & Moreau, J. M. (2016). Medical cannabis—The Canadian perspective. *Journal of Pain Research*, *9*, 735–744. doi:10.2147/JPR.S98182 PMID:27757048

Koltai, H., & Namdar, D. (2020). Cannabis Phytomolecule 'Entourage': From Domestication to Medical Use. *Trends in Plant Science*, *25*(10), 976–984. doi:10.1016/j.tplants.2020.04.007 PMID:32417167

Koppel, B.S., Brust, J.C., Fife, T., Bronstein, J., Youssof, S., Gronseth, G., Gloss, D., (2014). Systematic review: efficacy and safety of medical marijuana in selected neurologic disorders: report of the Guideline Development Subcommittee of the American Academy of Neurology. *Neurology 82*, 1556–1563. doi:.0000000000000363. doi:10.1212/WNL

Kors, A. C., & Peters, E. (2000). *Witchcraft in Europe, 400–1700: A Documentary History*. University of Pennsylvania Press.

Korus, A., Gumul, D., Krystyjan, M., Juszczak, L., & Korus, J. (2017). Evaluation of the quality, nutritional value and antioxidant activity of gluten-free biscuits made from corn-acorn flour or corn-hemp flour composites. *European Food Research and Technology*, *243*(8), 1429–1438. doi:10.100700217-017-2853-y

Korus, J., Witczak, M., Ziobro, R., & Juszczak, L. (2017). Hemp (Cannabis sativa subsp. sativa) flour and protein preparation as natural nutrients and structure forming agents in starch based gluten-free bread. *Lebensmittel-Wissenschaft + Technologie*, *84*, 143–150. doi:10.1016/j.lwt.2017.05.046

Kowal, M. A., Hazekamp, A., Colzato, L. S., van Steenbergen, H., van der Wee, N. J., Durieux, J., Manai, M., & Hommel, B. (2015). Cannabis and creativity: Highly potent cannabis impairs divergent thinking in regular cannabis users. *Psychopharmacology*, *232*(6), 1123–1134. doi:10.100700213-014-3749-1 PMID:25288512

Kozlowski, R. (1995). Interview with Professor R. Kozlowski, director of the Institute of NaturalFibres. *J Int Hemp Assoc*, *2*(2), 86–87.

Kraenzel, D. G., Petry, T. A., Nelson, B., Anderson, M. J., Mathern, D., & Todd, R. (1998). Industrial hemp as an alternative crop in North Dakota. *Agricultural Economics Report*, *402*. doi:10.22004/ag.econ.23264

Kriese, U., Schumann, E., Weber, W. E., Beyer, M., Bruhl, L., & Matthäus, B. (2004). Oil content, tocopherol composition and fatty acid patterns of the seeds of 51 Cannabis sativa L. genotypes. *Euphytica*, *137*(3), 339–351. doi:10.1023/B:EUPH.0000040473.23941.76

Kruger, D. J., Moffet, I. M., Seluk, L. C., & Zammit, L. A. (2020). A content analysis of internet information sources on medical cannabis. *J Cannabis Res.*, *2*(1), 1–6. doi:10.118642238-020-00041-1 PMID:33526127

Kuddus, M., Ginawi, I. A., & Al-Hazimi, A. (2013). *Cannabis sativa*: An ancient wild edible plant of India. *Emirates Journal of Food and Agriculture*, *25*(10), 736–745. doi:10.9755/ejfa.v25i10.16400

Ku, H., Wang, H., Pattarachaiyakoop, N., & Trada, M. (2011). A review on the tensile properties of natural fiber reinforced polymer composites. *Composites. Part B, Engineering*, *42*(4), 856–873. doi:10.1016/j.compositesb.2011.01.010

Kunwar, R.M., Shrestha, K.P., Bussmann, R.W., (2010). Traditional herbal medicine in farwest Nepal: a pharmacological appraisal. J. Ethnobiol. Ethnomed. 6, 35. doi:. doi:10.1186/1746-4269-6-35

Küpper, H., & Zhao, J. (1999). Cellular compartmentation of zinc in leaves of the hyperaccumulator *Thlaspicaerulescens*. *Plant Physiology*, *119*(1), 305–312. doi:10.1104/pp.119.1.305 PMID:9880373

Kurup, V. P., Resnick, A., Kagen, S. L., Cohen, S. H., & Fink, J. N. (1983). Allergenic fungi and actinomycetesin smoking materials and their health implications. *Mycopathologia*, *82*(1), 61–64. doi:10.1007/BF00436948 PMID:6348548

Kusari, P., Kusari, S., Spiteller, M., & Kayser, O. (2013). Endophytic fungi harbored in Cannabis sativaL.: Diversity and potential as biocontrol agents against host plant-specific phytopathogens. *Fungal Biodiversity*, *60*(1), 137–151. doi:10.100713225-012-0216-3

Lachenmeier, D. (2004). Hemp food products-A problem? *Deutsche Lebensmittel-Rundschau, 100*(12), 481–490.

Lammert, S., Harrison, K., Tosun, N., & Allen, S. (2018). Menstrual Cycle in Women Who Co-use Marijuana and Tobacco. *Journal of Addiction Medicine, 12*(3), 207–211.

Lash, R. (2010). Industrial Hemp: The crop for the seventh generation. *Am Indian Law Rev., 27*(1), 313–356. doi:10.2307/20070692

Lata, H., Chandra, S., Khan, I. A., & ElSohly, M. (2010). ElSohly, M.A. High Frequency Plant Regeneration from Leaf Derived Callus of HighΔ9Tetrahydrocannabinol Yielding Cannabis sativa L. *Planta Medica, 76*(14), 1629–1633. doi:10.1055-0030-1249773 PMID:20354950

Lata, H., Chandra, S., Khan, I. A., & ElSohly, M. A. (2008). Propagation of Cannabis sativa L. using synthetic seed technology. *Planta Medica, 74*(3), 328–328. doi:10.1055-2008-1075214

Lata, H., Chandra, S., Khan, I. A., & ElSohly, M. A. (2009). Propagation through alginate encapsulation of axillary buds of Cannabis sativa L. an important medicinal plant. *Physiology and Molecular Biology of Plants, 15*(1), 79–86. doi:10.100712298-009-0008-8 PMID:23572915

Lata, H., Chandra, S., Khan, I., & ElSohly, M. (2010a). Cannabis sativa L. Micropropagation in temporary immersion bioreactor system. *Planta Medica, 76*(05, P9). doi:10.1055-0030-1251771

Latif, S., & Anwar, F. (2009). Physicochemical studies of hemp (Cannabis sativa) seed oil using enzymeassisted cold pressing. *European Journal of Lipid Science and Technology, 111*(10), 1042–1048. doi:10.1002/ejlt.200900008

Latta, R. P., & Eaton, B. J. (1975).. . *Economic Botany, 29*, 153. doi:10.1007/BF02863315

Lawrence, R. G. (2019). *Pot in Pans: A History of Eating Cannabis*. The Rowman & Littleðeld Publishing Group.

Lazzari, P., Pau, A., Tambaro, S., Asproni, B., Ruiu, S., Pinna, G., Mastinu, A., Curzu, M. M., Reali, R., Bottazzi, M. E., Pinna, G. A., & Murineddu, G. (2012). Synthesis and pharmacological evaluation of novel 4-alkyl-5-thien-2¢-yl pyrazole carboxamides. *Central Nervous System Agents in Medicinal Chemistry, 12*, 254–276. doi:10.2174/187152412803760636 PMID:22931442

Lazzari, P., Sanna, A., Mastinu, A., Cabasino, S., Manca, I., & Pani, L. (2011). Weight loss induced by rimonabant is associated with an altered leptin expression and hypothalamic leptin signaling in diet-induced obese mice. *Behavioural Brain Research, 217*(2), 432–438. doi:10.1016/j.bbr.2010.11.022 PMID:21074566

Lazzari, P., Serra, V., Marcello, S., Pira, M., & Mastinu, A. (2017). Metabolic side effects induced by olanzapine treatment are neutralized by CB1 receptor antagonist compounds co-administration in female rats. *European Neuropsychopharmacology, 27*(7), 667–678. doi:10.1016/j.euroneuro.2017.03.010 PMID:28377074

Lee, M. A. (2013). *Smoke Signals: A Social History of Marijuana: Medical, Recreational and Scientiðc*. Scribner Paperback Edition.

Leizer, C., Ribnicky, D., Poulev, A., Dushenkov, S., & Raskin, I. (2000). The composition of hemp seed oil and its potential as an important source of nutrition. *J Nutraceuticals Funct Med Foods. 2*(4), 35–53. doi:10.1300/J133v02n04_04

Levinthal, C. F. (2012). *Drugs, Behavior, and Modern Society*. Pearson College Div.

Levitz, S. M., & Diamond, R. D. (1991). Aspergillosis and marijuana. *Annals of Internal Medicine, 115*(7), 578–579. doi:10.7326/0003-4819-115-7-578_2 PMID:1652910

Leweke, F. M., Piomelli, D., Pahlisch, F., Muhl, D., Gerth, C. W., Hoyer, C., Klosterkötter, J., Hellmich, M., & Koethe, D. (2012). Cannabidiol enhances anandamide signaling and alleviates psychotic symptoms of schizophrenia. *Translational Psychiatry*, *2*(3), e94.

Lewis, M. M., Yang, Y., Wasilewski, E., Clarke, H. A., & Kotra, L. P. (2017). Chemical profiling of medical Cannabis extracts. *ACS Omega*, *2*(9), 6091–6103. doi:10.1021/acsomega.7b00996 PMID:30023762

Leyva, D. R., McCullough, R. S., & Pierce, G. N. (2011). Medicinal Use of Hempseeds (Cannabis sativa L.): Effects on Platelet Aggregation. In V. R. Preedy, R. R. Watson, & V. B. Patel (Eds.), *Nuts and Seeds in Health and Diseases Prevention*. Elsevier. doi:10.1016/B978-0-12-375688-6.10074-X

Liao, J., Zhang, S., & Tang, X. (2020). Sound absorption of hemp fibers (cannabis sativa L.) based nonwoven fabrics and composites: A review. *Journal of Natural Fibers*, 1–13.

Li, H. (1974). Anarchaeological and historical account of Cannabis in China. *Economic Botany*, *28*(4), 437–448. doi:10.1007/BF02862859

Lim, K., See, Y.M., Lee, J., (2017). A systematic review of the effectiveness of medical cannabis for psychiatric, movement and neurodegenerative disorders. *Clin. Psychopharmacol. Neurosci.* 15, 301–312. doi:. 301. doi:10.9758/cpn.2017.15.4

Lim, M., & Kirchhof, M. G. (2019). Dermatology-Related Uses of Medical Cannabis Promoted by Dispensaries in Canada, Europe, and the United States. *Journal of Cutaneous Medicine and Surgery*, *23*(2), 178–184. doi:10.1177/1203475418808761 PMID:30380925

Linde, M., Jakobsson, E. L., Galbe, M., & Zacchi, G. (2008). Steam pretreatment of dilute H2SO4 – impregnated wheat straw and SSF with low yeast and enzyme loadings for bioethanol production. *Biotechnology and Bioengineering*, *32*, 326–332.

Linger, P., Müssig, J., Fischer, H., & Kobert, J. (2002). Industrial *Cannabis sativa* (*Cannabis sativa* L.) growing on heavy metal contaminated soil: Fiber quality and phytoremediation potential. *Industrial Crops and Products*, *16*, 33–42. doi:10.1016/S0926-6690(02)00005-5

Linger, P., Ostwald, A., & Haensler, J. (2005). *Cannabis sativa* L. growing on heavy metal contaminated soil: Growth, cadmium uptake and photosynthesis. *Biologia Plantarum*, *49*(4), 567–576. doi:10.100710535-005-0051-4

Lintner, K. (2009). Cosmetic ingredients: Definitions, legal requirements, and an attempt to harmonize (global?) characterization. In K. Lintner (Ed.), *Global Regulatory Issues for the Cosmetics Industry* (pp. 31–53). Elsevier. doi:10.1016/B978-0-8155-1569-2.50009-9

Liu Y., Wheaton A.G., Chapman D.P., Cunningham T.J., Lu H., Croft J.B., (2014). Prevalence of healthy sleep duration among adults—United States. *Morb. Mortal. Wkly.*

Liu, C. F., Li, Y. H., & Shi, G. R. (2012). Utilize heavy metal-contaminated farmland to develop bioenergy. *Advanced Materials Research*, *414*, 254–261. doi:10.4028/www.scientific.net/AMR.414.254

Liu, Y., Liu, H.-Y., Li, S.-H., Ma, W., Wu, D.-T., Li, H.-B., Xiao, A.-P., Liu, L.-L., Zhu, F., & Gan, R.-Y. (2022). Cannabis sativa bioactive compounds and their extraction, separation, purification, and identification technologies: An updated review. *Trends in Analytical Chemistry*, *149*, 116554. doi:10.1016/j.trac.2022.116554

Llamas, R., Hart, D. R., & Schneider, N. S. (1978). Allergic bronchopulmonary aspergillosis associatedwith smoking moldy marihuana. *Chest*, *73*(6), 871–872. doi:10.1378/chest.73.6.871 PMID:657864

Llewellyn, G. C., & O'Rear, C. O. (1977). Examination of fungal growth and aflatoxin production onmarijuana. *Mycopathologia*, *62*(2), 109–112. doi:10.1007/BF01259400 PMID:414138

Löser, C., Zehnsdorf, A., Fussy, M., & Stärk, H. J. (2002). Conditioning of heavy metal-polluted riversediment by Cannabis sativa L. *International Journal of Phytoremediation*, *4*(1), 27–45. doi:10.1080/15226510208500071

Lowe, H., Toyang, N., Steele, B., Bryant, J., Ngwa, W., & Nedamat, K. (2021). The Current and Potential Application of Medicinal Cannabis Products in Dentistry. *Dentistry Journal*, *9*(9), 106. doi:10.3390/dj9090106 PMID:34562980

Lozano, I. (2001, January). (201). The therapeutic use of Cannabis sativa (L.) in Arabic medicine. *Journal of Cannabis Therapeutics*, *1*(1), 63–70. doi:10.1300/J175v01n01_05

Lubman, D. I., Cheetham, A., & Yücel, M. (2015). Cannabis and adolescent brain development. *Pharmacology & Therapeutics*, *148*, 1–16. doi:10.1016/j.pharmthera.2014.11.009 PMID:25460036

Lucas, P. G. (2008). Regulating compassion: An overview of Canada's federal medical cannabispolicy and practice. *Harm Reduction Journal*, *5*(1), 5. doi:10.1186/1477-7517-5-5 PMID:18226254

Lu, G. W. (2010). Recent Advances in Developing Ophthalmic Formulations: A Patent Review. *Recent Patents on Drug Delivery & Formulation*, *4*(1), 49–57. doi:10.2174/187221110789957246 PMID:19807679

Luna, L. E. (1984). The concept of plants as teachers among four mestizo shamans of Iquitos, northeastern Peru. *Journal of Ethnopharmacology*, *11*(2), 135–156. doi:10.1016/0378-8741(84)90036-9 PMID:6492831

Lu, X., & Clarke, R. C. (1995). The cultivation and use of hemp (Cannabis sativa L.) in ancient China. *Journal of the International Hemp Association*, *2*(1), 26–30.

Machado Bergamaschi, M., Helena Costa Queiroz, R., Waldo Zuardi, A., & Crippa, A. S. (2011). Safety and Side Effects of Cannabidiol, a *Cannabis sativa* Constituent. *Current Drug Safety*, *6*(4), 237–249. doi:10.2174/157488611798280924 PMID:22129319

Mack, A., & Joy, J. (2000). *Marijuana as Medicine? The Science Beyond the Controversy*. National Academies Press (US). https://www.ncbi.nlm.nih.gov/books/NBK224394/

Maðmisebi, T. E., & Oguntade, A. E. (2010). Preparation and use of plant medicines for farmers' health in Southwest Nigeria: Socio-cultural, magico-religious and economic aspects. *Journal of Ethnobiology and Ethnomedicine*, *6*(1), 1. doi:10.1186/1746-4269-6-1 PMID:20089149

Małgorzata, L., Dominika, W., Aleksandra, T., Kamila, J., & Adam, R. (2016). Natural cold pressed oils as cosmetic products. *Family Medicine and Primary Care Review*, *4*, 443–447. doi:10.5114/fmpcr.2016.63699

Malik, R. N., Husain, S. Z., & Nazir, I. (2010). Heavy metal contamination and accumulation in soil and wild plant species from industrial area of Islamabad, Pakistan. *Pakistan Journal of Botany*, *42*, 291–301.

Manach, C., Mazur, A., & Scalbert, A. (2005). Polyphenols and prevention of cardiovascular diseases. *Current Opinion in Lipidology*, *16*(1), 77–84. doi:10.1097/00041433-200502000-00013 PMID:15650567

Manca, I., Mastinu, A., Olimpieri, F., Falzoi, M., Sani, M., Ruiu, S., Loriga, G., Volonterio, A., Tambaro, S., Bottazzi, M.E., Zanda, M., Pinna, G.A., Lazzari, P., (2013). Novel pyrazole derivatives as neutral CB_1 antagonists with signiðcant activity towards food intake. *Eur. J. Med. Chem.* 62, 256–269. doi:. 056. doi:10.1016/j.ejmech.2012.12

Mandelbaum, D. E., & Suzanne, M. (2017). Adverse structural and functional effects of marijuana on the brain: Evidence reviewed. *Pediatric Neurology*, *66*, 12–20. doi:10.1016/j.pediatrneurol.2016.09.004 PMID:27789118

Mandolino, G., & Ranalli, P. (1999). Advances in biotechnological approaches for hemp breeding and industry. In P. Ranalli (Ed.), *Advances in hemp research* (pp. 185–212). The Haworth Press.

Manzanares, J., Julian, M., & Carrascosa, A. (2006). Role of the Cannabinoid System in Pain Control and Therapeutic Implications for the Management of Acute and Chronic Pain Episodes. *Current Neuropharmacology*, *4*(3), 239–257. doi:10.2174/157015906778019527 PMID:18615144

Mao, J., Price, D. D., Lu, J., Keniston, L., & Mayer, D. J. (2000). Two distinctive antinociceptive systems in rats with pathological pain. *Neuroscience Letters*, *280*(1), 13–16. doi:10.1016/S0304-3940(99)00998-2 PMID:10696800

Marcu, J. P., Christian, R. T., Lau, D., Zielinski, A. J., Horowitz, M. P., Lee, J., Pakdel, A., Allison, J., Limbad, C., Moore, D. H., Yount, G. L., Desprez, P.-Y., & McAllister, S. D. (2010). Cannabidiol enhances the inhibitory effects of Δ9-tetrahydrocannabinol on human glioblastoma cell proliferation and survival. *Molecular Cancer Therapeutics*, *9*(1), 180–189. doi:10.1158/1535-7163.MCT-09-0407 PMID:20053780

Marks, M. D., Tian, L., Wenger, J. P., Omburo, S. N., Soto-Fuentes, W., He, J., Gang, D. R., Weiblen, G. D., & Dixon, R. A. (2009). Identification of candidate genes affecting Δ^9-tetrahydrocannabinol biosynthesis in *Cannabis sativa. Journal of Experimental Botany*, *60*(13), 3715–3726. doi:10.1093/jxb/erp210 PMID:19581347

Martin, B. R., & Lichtman, A. H. (1998). Cannabinoid transmission and pain perception. *Neurobiology of Disease*, *5*(6, 6 Pt B), 447–461. doi:10.1006/nbdi.1998.0218 PMID:9974177

Martin-Diana, A. B., Izquierdo, N., Albertos, I., Sanchez, M. S., Herrero, A., Sanz, M. A., & Rico, D. (2017). Valorization of carob's germ and seed peel as natural antioxidant ingredients in gluten-free crackers. *Journal of Food Processing and Preservation*, *41*(2), e12770. doi:10.1111/jfpp.12770

Martínez, V., Iriondo De-Hond, A., Borrelli, F., Capasso, R., Del Castillo, M. D., & Abalo, R. (2020). Cannabidiol and Other Non-Psychoactive Cannabinoids for Prevention and Treatment of Gastrointestinal Disorders: Useful Nutraceuticals. *International Journal of Molecular Sciences*, *21*(9), 3067.

Martin, J. H., Hill, C., Walsh, A., Efron, D., Taylor, K., Kennedy, M., & Irving, H. (2020). Clinical trials with cannabis medicines—guidance for ethics committees, governance officers and researchers to streamline ethics applications and ensuring patient safety: Considerations from the Australian experience. *Trials*, *21*(1), 1–7. doi:10.118613063-020-04862-6 PMID:33203469

Martin, M., Svensson, N., Fonseca, J., & Eklund, M. (2014). Quantifying the environmental performance of integrated bioethanol and biogas production. *Renewable Energy*, *61*, 109–116. doi:10.1016/j.renene.2012.09.058

Martins, A. M., Gomes, A. L., Vilas Boas, I., Marto, J., & Ribeiro, H. M. (2022). Cannabis-Based Products for the Treatment of Skin Inflammatory Diseases: A Timely Review. *Pharmaceuticals*, *15*(2), 210. doi:10.3390/ph15020210 PMID:35215320

Martyny, J. W., Serrano, K. A., Schaeffer, J. W., & Van Dyke, M. V. (2013). Potential exposures associatedwith indoor marijuana growing operations. *Journal of Occupational and Environmental Hygiene*, *10*(11), 622–639. doi:10.1080/15459624.2013.831986 PMID:24116667

Massi, P., Vaccani, A., Bianchessi, S., Costa, B., Macchi, P., & Parolaro, D. (2006). The non-psychoactive cannabidiol triggers caspase activation and oxidative stress in human glioma cells. *Cellular and Molecular Life Sciences CMLS*, *63*(17), 2057–2066. doi:10.100700018-006-6156-x PMID:16909207

Mastinu, A., Pira, M., Pinna, G.A., Pisu, C., Casu, M.A., Reali, R., Marcello, S., Murineddu, G., Lazzari, P., (2013). NESS06SM reduces body weight with an improved proðle relative to SR141716A. *Pharmacol. Res.* 74, 94–108. doi:. 2013.06.001. doi:10.1016/j.phrs

Mastinu, A., Pira, M., Pani, L., Pinna, G. A., & Lazzari, P. (2012). NESS038C6, a novel selective CB1 antagonist agent with anti-obesity activity and improved molecular prof̈le. *Behavioural Brain Research*, *234*(2), 192–204. doi:10.1016/j.bbr.2012.06.033 PMID:22771813

Mastinu, A., Premoli, M., Ferrari-Toninelli, G., Tambaro, S., Maccarinelli, G., Memo, M., & Bonini, S. A. (2018). Cannabinoids in health and disease: Pharmacological potential inmetabolic syndrome andneuroinñammation. *Hormone Molecular Biology and Clinical Investigation*, *36*(2). Advance online publication. doi:10.1515/hmbci-2018-0013 PMID:29601300

Mathur, J., Ahuja, P. S., Lal, N., & Mathur, A. K. (1989). Propagation of Valeriana-Wallichii Dc using encapsulated apical and axial shoot buds. *Plant Science*, *60*(1), 111–116. doi:10.1016/0168-9452(89)90050-2

Matsuda, L. A., Lolait, S. J., Brownstein, M. J., Young, A. C., & Bonner, T. I. (1990). Structure of a cannabinoid receptor and functional expression of the cloned cDNA. *Nature*, *346*(6284), 561–564. doi:10.1038/346561a0 PMID:2165569

Matthäus, B., & Brühl, L. (2008). Why it is so difficult to produce high quality virgin rapeseed oil for human consumption? *European Journal of Lipid Science and Technology*, *110*(7), 611–617. doi:10.1002/ejlt.200700275

Mattila, P. H., Pihlava, J.-M., Hellström, J., Nurmi, M., Eurola, M., Mäkinen, S., Jalava, T., & Pihlanto, A. (2018). Contents of phytochemicals and antinutritional factors in commercial protein-rich plant products. *Food Quality and Safety*, *2*(4), 213–219. doi:10.1093/fqsafe/fyy021

Mattsson, J. E., & Briere, D. M. (1984) External biomass characteristics for efficient energy conversionsome considerations. Biomass characteristics for efficient energy conversion. In: R.L. Gambles (ed) *Proceedings of joint workshop of IEA/FE programme Groups B, C and D, Uppsala, Sweden.* Canadian Forestry Service, Ottawa, Canada

McGinty, E. E., Niederdeppe, J., Heley, K., & Barry, C. L. (2017). Public perceptions of arguments supporting and opposing recreational marijuana legalization. *Preventive Medicine*, *99*, 80–86. doi:10.1016/j.ypmed.2017.01.024 PMID:28189806

McGrath, S. P., Zhao, J., & Lombi, E. (2002). Phytoremediation of metals, metalloids, and radionuclides. *Advances in Agronomy*, *75*, 1–56. doi:10.1016/S0065-2113(02)75002-5

McKenna, T. (1992). *Food of the Gods: The Search for the Original Tree of Knowledge – A Radical History of Plants, Drugs, and Human Evolution.* Bantam.

McKernan, K., Spangler, J., Zhang, L., Tadogotla, V., Helbert, Y., Foss, T., & Smith, D. (2015). Cannabismicrobiome sequencing reveals several mycotoxic fungi native to dispensary grade cannabisflowers. *bioRxiv*.

Mclean, K. (2010). Pot and pesticides: A bustling illegal trade. The Bay Citizen.

McPartland JM, West D (1999) Killing Cannabis with mycoherbicides. *J Int Hemp Assoc 6*(1), 1,4–8

McPartland, J. M. (2004). Phylogenomic and chemotaxonomic analysis of the endocannabinoid system. *Brain Res. Rev.* 45, 18–29. . 1016/j.brainresrev.2003.11.005.

McPartland, J., Di Marzo, V., De Petrocellis, L., Mercer, A., & Glass, M. (2001). Cannabinoid receptors are absent in insects. J. *Comp. Neurol.* 436, 423–429. . 1002/cne.1078.

McPartland, J. M. (1984). Pathogenicity of Phomopsis ganjae on Cannabis sativa and the fungistaticeffect of cannabinoids produced by the host. *Mycopathologia*, *87*, 149–153.

McPartland, J. M. (1989). Storage molds associated with post-harvest Cannabis decay. CoverIllustration. *Mycol Soc Am Newsl*, *40*(1), 1.

McPartland, J. M. (1992). The Cannabis pathogen project: Report of the second five-year plan. *MycolSoc Am Newsl*, *43*(1), 43.

McPartland, J. M. (1994a). Microbiological contaminants of marijuana. *J Int Hemp Assoc*, *1*, 41–44.

McPartland, J. M. (1994b). Cannabis pathogens X: Phoma, Ascochyta and Didymella species. *Mycologia*, *86*(6), 870–878. doi:10.1080/00275514.1994.12026492

McPartland, J. M. (2002). Contaminants and adulterants in herbal Cannabis. In F. Grotenhermen & E. Russo (Eds.), *Cannabis and Cannabinoids pharmacology, toxicology and therapeuticpotential* (pp. 337–343).

McPartland, J. M. (2003). Byssinosis in hemp mill workers. *J Int Hemp Assoc*, *8*(1), 33–44. doi:10.1300/J237v08n01_04

McPartland, J. M. (2018). *Cannabis* Systematics at the Levels of Family, Genus, and Species. *Cannabis and Cannabinoid Research*, *3*(1), 203–212. doi:10.1089/can.2018.0039 PMID:30426073

McPartland, J. M., Blanchon, D., & Musty, R. E. (2008). Cannabimimetic effects modulated by cholinergic compounds. *Addiction Biology*, *13*(3-4), 411–415. doi:10.1111/j.1369-1600.2008.00126.x PMID:18782385

McPartland, J. M., Clarke, R. C., & Watson, D. P. (2000). *Hemp diseases and pests management and biological control*. CABI Publishing.

McPartland, J. M., & Cubeta, M. A. (1997). New species, combinations, host associations and locationrecords of fungi associated with hemp (Cannabis sativa). *Mycological Research*, *101*(7), 853–857. doi:10.1017/S0953756297003584

McPartland, J. M., Hegman, W., & Long, T. (2019). Cannabis in Asia: Its center of origin and early cultivation, based on a synthesis of subfossil pollen and archaeobotanical studies. *Vegetation History and Archaeobotany*, *28*(6), 691–702. doi:10.100700334-019-00731-8

McPartland, J. M., & Pruitt, P. (1997). Medical marijuana and its use by the immunocompromised. *Alternative Therapies in Health and Medicine*, *3*(3), 39–45. PMID:9141290

Mead, A. (2017). The legal status of cannabis (marijuana) and cannabidiol (CBD) under US law. *Epilepsy & Behavior*, *70*, 288–291. doi:10.1016/j.yebeh.2016.11.021 PMID:28169144

Mechoulam, R., & Gaoni, Y. (1965). A total synthesis of dl-delta-1-tetrahydrocannabinol, the active constituent of hashish. *J. Am. Chem. Soc.* 87, 3273–3275. . 1021/ja01092a065.

Mechoulam, R. (2005). *Cannabinoids as therapeutics*. Springer. doi:10.1007/3-7643-7358-X

Mechoulam, R., Fride, E., & Di Marzo, V. (1998). Endocannabinoids. *European Journal of Pharmacology*, *359*(1), 1–18. doi:10.1016/S0014-2999(98)00649-9 PMID:9831287

Meers, E., Ruttens, A., Hopgood, M., Lesage, E., & Tack, F. M. (2005). Potential of Brassicrapa, Cannabissativa, Helianthus annuus and Zea mays for phytoextraction of heavy metals from calcareousdredged sediment derived soils. *Chemosphere*, *61*(4), 561–572. doi:10.1016/j.chemosphere.2005.02.026 PMID:16202810

Meers, E., Van Slycken, S., Adriaensen, K., Ruttens, A., Vangronsveld, J., Du Laing, G., Witters, N., Thewys, T., & Tack, F. M. G. (2010). The use of bio-energy crops (Zea mays) for 'phytoattenuation' of heavy metalson moderately contaminated soils: A fieldexperiment. *Chemosphere*, *78*(1), 35–41. doi:10.1016/j.chemosphere.2009.08.015 PMID:19837447

Meier, M. H., Caspi, A., Ambler, A., Harrington, H., Houts, R., Keefe, R. S. E., Mcdonald, K., Ward, A., Poulton, R., & Moffitt, T. E. (2012). Persistent cannabis users show neuropsychological decline from childhood to midlife. *Nat. Acad Sci.*, *109*, 15980. doi:10.1073/pnas.1206820109

Melamede, R. J. (2005). Cannabis and tobacco smoke are not equally carcinogenic. *Harm Reduction Journal*, *2*(1), 21. doi:10.1186/1477-7517-2-21 PMID:16232311

Mensah, K.B. & Adu-Gyamfi, P.K.T. (2019). To legalize cannabis in Ghana or not to legalize? Reviewing the pharmacological evidence. *Arch Pharm Pharm Sci.* 3(1):082–8.

Mercuri, A., Accorsi, C., & Bandini Mazzanti, M. (2002). The long history of Cannabis and its cultivation by theRomans in central Italy,shown by pollen recordsfromLago Albano and Lago di Nemi. *Vegetation History and Archaeobotany*, *11*(4), 263–276. doi:10.1007003340200039

Merlin, M.D., (2003). Archaeological evidence for the tradition of psychoactive plant use in the old world. *Econ. Bot. 57*, 295–323. doi: 057[0295:AEFTTO]2.0.CO;2. doi:10.1663/0013-0001(2003)

Metcalf, B. D., & Metcalf, T. R. (2006). *A concise history of modern India*. Cambridge University Press. doi:10.1017/CBO9780511812750

Mihoc, M., Pop, G., Alexa, E., & Radulov, I. (2012). Nutritive quality of romanian *Cannabis sativa* varieties (*Cannabis sativa* L.) with special focus on oil and metal contents of seeds. *Chemistry Central Journal*, *6*(1), 122. doi:10.1186/1752-153X-6-122 PMID:23088580

Mikulec, A., Kowalski, S., Sabat, R., Skoczylas, Ł., Tabaszewska, M., & Wywrocka-Gurgul, A. (2019). Hemp flour as a valuable component for enriching physicochemical and antioxidant properties of wheat bread. *Lebensmittel-Wissenschaft + Technologie*, *102*, 164–172. doi:10.1016/j.lwt.2018.12.028

Mikuriya, T. H., North, W., Lucido, F., Jaffee, R., & Weirick, J. (2005) Cerebrospinal delayed allergicreaction to pesticide residue. In: *Conference proceedings, international association forCannabis as medicine*, (p 14). Springer.

Miller, R. J., & Miller, R. E. (2017). Is cannabis an effective treatment for joint pain? *Clinical and Experimental Rheumatology*, *35*(5), 59–67. PMID:28967368

Mills, J. (2000). Madness, Cannabis and Colonialism. *The «Native Only» Lunatic Asylums of British India 1857-1900.*

Mills, J. (2009). Cannabis and the Cultures of Colonialism: Government, medicine, ritual and pleasures in the history of an Asian drug (c. 1800-c. 1895). *Zeitenblicke, 9*(3).

Mishra, S., Bharagava, R. N., More, N., Yadav, A., Zainith, S., & Mani, S. (2019). *Heavy Metal Contamination: An Alarming Threat to Environment and Human Health Environmental Biotechnology: For Sustainable Future*. Springer.

Mnekin, L., & Ripoll, L. (2021). Topical Use of Cannabis sativa L. Biochemicals. *Cosmetics*, *8*(3), 85. doi:10.3390/cosmetics8030085

Moir, D., Rickert, W. S., Levasseur, G., Larose, Y., Maertens, R., White, P., & Desjardins, S. (2008). Acomparison of nainstream and sidestream marijuana and tobacco cigarette smoke producedunder two machine smoking conditions. *Chemical Research in Toxicology*, *21*(2), 494–502. doi:10.1021/tx700275p PMID:18062674

Monthony, A. S., Page, S. R., Hesami, M., & Jones, A. M. P. (2021). A.M.P. The Past, Present and Future of Cannabis sativa Tissue Culture. *Plants*, *10*(1), 185. doi:10.3390/plants10010185 PMID:33478171

Montonya, D. (2016). *Hemp as Fibre and Food? Regulatory Developments and Current Issues; Breaðng Paper*. Parliamentary Research Service.

Moody, M., Wharton, R. C., Schnaper, N., & Schimpff, S. C. (1982). Do water pipes prevent transmission offungi from contaminated marijuana? *The New England Journal ofMedicine*, *306*(24), 1492–1493. doi:10.1056/NEJM198206173062424 PMID:7078603

Moore, T. H., Zammit, S., Lingford-Hughes, A., Barnes, T. R., Jones, P. B., Burke, M., & Lewis, G. (2007). Cannabis use and risk of psychotic or affective mental health outcomes: A systematic review. *Lancet*, *370*(9584), 319–328. https:// doi.org/ 10.1016/S0140-6736(07)61162-3

Moreau, J. J. (1973). *Hashish and Mental Illness (1845)*. Raven Press.

Morgan, M. (2022, March 11). *Can Medical Marijuana Help With HIV/AIDS?* Medical Marijuana Doctor | West Palm Beach Medical Marijuana. https://mmjhealth.com/can-medical-marijuana-help-with-hiv-aids/

Morin-Crini, N., Staelens, J. N., Loiacono, S., Martel, B., Chanet, G., & Crini, G. (2019). Simultaneous removal of Cd, Co, Cu, Mn, Ni, and Zn from synthetic solutions on a Cannabis sativa-based felt. III. Real discharge waters. *Journal of Applied Polymer Science*, *137*(24), 48823. doi:10.1002/app.48823

Movahedi, M., Ghasemi-Omran, V., & Torabi, S. (2014). The effect of different concentrations of TDZ and BA on in vitro regeneration of Iranian cannabis (Cannabis sativa) using cotyledon and epicotyl explants. *J. Plant Mol. Breed.*, *3*, 20–27.

Müller, L., Radtke, A., Decker, J., Koch, M., & Belge, G. (2017). The Synthetic Cannabinoid WIN 55,212-2 Elicits Death in Human Cancer Cell Lines. *Anticancer Research*, *37*(11), 6341–6345. doi:10.21873/anticanres.12086 PMID:29061818

Mulpuri, Y., Marty, V.N., Munier, J.J., Mackie, K., Schmidt, B.L., Seltzman, H.H., Spigelman, I., (2018). Synthetic peripherally restricted cannabinoid suppresses chemotherapy-induced peripheral neuropathy pain symptoms by CB1 receptor activation. *Neuropharmacology* 139, 85–97. doi:. 07.002. doi:10.1016/j.neuropharm.2018

Munson, A. E., Harris, L. S., Friedman, M. A., Dewey, W. L., & Carchman, R. A. (1975). Antineoplastic activity of cannabinoids. *Journal of the National Cancer Institute*, *55*(3), 597–602. doi:10.1093/jnci/55.3.597 PMID:1159836

Murawski, B., Wade, L., Plotnikoff, R. C., Lubans, D. R., & Duncan, M. J. (2018). A systematic review and meta-analysis of cognitive and behavioral interventions to improve sleep health in adults without sleep disorders. *Sleep Medicine Reviews*, *40*, 160–169. doi:10.1016/j.smrv.2017.12.003 PMID:29397329

Murkovic, M., Draxl, S., & Pfannhaeser, W. (1997). Vitamin B1 in Austrian cereals. *Ernaehrung*, *21*, 263–265.

Musio, S., Müssig, J., & Amaducci, S. (2018). Optimizing *Cannabis sativa* fiber production for high performance composite applications. *Front. Plant Sci.*, *9*, 1702. doi:10.3389/fpls.2018.01702 PMID:30532760

Nadar, R. M., Pathak, S., Ramesh, S., Govindarajulu, M., Moore, T., Agrawal, D. C., & Dhanasekaran, M. (2022). Cannabis-Based Cosmetic Products and Their Uses. In D. C. Agrawal, R. Kumar, & M. Dhanasekaran (Eds.), *Cannabis/Marijuana for Healthcare* (pp. 253–269). Springer., doi:10.1007/978-981-16-8822-5_13

Nadolska, K., & Goś, R. (2008). [The role of endocannabinoid system in physiological and pathological processes in the eye]. *Klinika Oczna*, *110*(10–12), 392–396. PMID:19195174

Naftali, T., Mechulam, R., Lev, L. B., & Konikoff, F. M. (2014). Cannabis for iñammatory bowel disease. *Digestive Diseases (Basel, Switzerland)*, *32*(4), 468–474. doi:10.1159/000358155 PMID:24969296

Nahas, G. G. (1982). Hashish in Islam 9th to 18th century. *Bulletin of the New York Academy of Medicine*, *58*(9), 814. PMID:6762898

Naim-Feil, E., Pembleton, L. W., Spooner, L. E., Malthouse, A. L., Miner, A., Quinn, M., Polotnianka, R. M., Baillie, R. C., Spangenberg, G. C., & Cogan, N. O. (2021). The characterization of key physiological traits of medicinal cannabis (*Cannabis sativa* L.) as a tool for precision breeding. *BMC Plant Biology*, *21*(1), 1–15. doi:10.118612870-021-03079-2 PMID:34174826

Nallathambi, R., Mazuz, M., Ion, A., Selvaraj, G., Weininger, S., Fridlender, M., Nasser, A., Sagee, O., Kumari, P., Nemichenizer, D., Mendelovitz, M., Firstein, N., Hanin, O., Konikoff, F., Kapulnik, Y., Naftali, T., & Koltai, H. (2017). Anti-inñammatory activity in colon models is derived from 9-tetrahydrocannabinolic acid that interacts with additional compounds in cannabis extracts. *Cannabis and Cannabinoid Research*, *2*(1), 167–182. doi:10.1089/can.2017.0027 PMID:29082314

Namsa, N. D., Mandal, M., Tangjang, S., & Mandal, S. C. (2011). Ethnobotany of the Monpa ethnic group at Arunachal Pradesh, India. J. Ethnobiol. Ethnomed. 7, 31. . Nichols, D.E., 2016. *Psychedelics. Pharmacol. Rev.* 68 (2), 264–355. doi:1124/pr.115.011478. doi:10.1186/1746-4269-7-31

Napimoga, M. H., Benatti, B. B., Lima, F. O., Alves, P. M., Campos, A. C., Pena-dos-Santos, D. R., Severino, F. P., Cunha, F. Q., & Guimarães, F. S. (2009). Cannabidiol decreases bone resorption by inhibiting RANK/RANKL expression and pro-inflammatory cytokines during experimental periodontitis in rats. *International Immunopharmacology*, *9*(2), 216–222. doi:10.1016/j.intimp.2008.11.010 PMID:19070683

Nath, M. K. (2022). Benefits of Cultivating Industrial Hemp (Cannabis sativa ssp. sativa)—A Versatile Plant for a Sustainable Future. *Chemistry Proceedings*, *10*(1), 14.

NCCEH. (2009). *Recommendations for safe re-occupancy of marijuana grow operations*. NationalCollaborating Centre for Environmental Health.

NCI. (2015, April 2). *Cancer Statistics*. NCI. https://www.cancer.gov/about-cancer/understanding/statistics

Nielsen, S., Germanos, R., Weier, M., Pollard, J., Degenhardt, L., Hall, W., Buckley, N., & Farrell, M. (2018). The use of cannabis and cannabinoids in treating symptoms of multiple sclerosis: A systematic review of reviews. *Current Neurology and Neuroscience Reports*, *18*(2), 8. doi:10.100711910-018-0814-x PMID:29442178

Nionelli, L., Montemurro, M., Pontonio, E., Verni, M., Gobbetti, M., & Rizzello, C. G. (2018). Pro-technological and functional characterization of lactic acid bacteria to be used as starters for hemp (Cannabis sativa L.) sourdough fermentation and wheat bread fortification. *International Journal of Food Microbiology*, *279*, 14–25. doi:10.1016/j.ijfoodmicro.2018.04.036 PMID:29715603

Nissen, L., Casciano, F., Babini, E., & Gianotti, A. (2021). Prebiotic potential and bioactive volatiles of hemp byproduct fermented by lactobacilli. *Lebensmittel-Wissenschaft + Technologie*, *151*, 112201. doi:10.1016/j.lwt.2021.112201

Nissen, L., di Carlo, E., & Gianotti, A. (2020). Prebiotic potential of hemp blended drinks fermented by probiotics. *Food Research International*, *131*, 109029. doi:10.1016/j.foodres.2020.109029 PMID:32247454

Nissen, L., Zatta, A., Stefanini, I., Grandi, S., Sgorbati, B., Biavati, B., & Monti, A. (2010). Characterization and antimicrobial activity of essential oils of industrial hemp varieties (Cannabis sativa L.). *Fitoterapia*, *81*(5), 413–419. doi:10.1016/j.fitote.2009.11.010 PMID:19969046

NJMMP. (2011) *Medicinal marijuana program rules.* New Jersey Medicinal Marijuana Program.: www.nj.gov/health/medicalmarijuana/documents/final_rules.pdf

Novak, J., Zitterl-Eglseer, K., Deans, S. G., & Franz, C. M. (2001). Essential oils of different cultivars ofCannabis sativa L. and their antimicrobial activity. *Flavour and Fragrance Journal*, *16*(4), 259–262. doi:10.1002/ffj.993

Nycz, J. E., Malecki, G., Zawiazalec, M., Pazdziorek, T., & Skop, P. (2010). 1-Pentyl-3-(4-methoxy-1-naphthoyl) indole and 2-(2-methoxy-phenyl)-1-(1-pentyl-1H-indol-3-yl)-ethanone: X-ray structures and computational studies. *Journal of Molecular Structure*, *984*(1-3), 125–130. doi:10.1016/j.molstruc.2010.09.016

O'Shaughnessy, W. B. 1843. On the preparations of the Indian hemp, or Gunjah. Prov. Med. J. *Retrosp. Med. Sci.* 5, 363–369. áhttps://www.ncbi.nlm.nih.gov/pmc/ articles/PMC2490264/ñ.

Odani, S., & Odani, S. (1998). Isolation and primary structure of a methionine-and cystine-rich seed protein of Cannabis sativa. *Bioscience, Biotechnology, and Biochemistry*, *62*(4), 650–654. doi:10.1271/bbb.62.650 PMID:9614695

Ogawa, E., Sato, Y., Minagawa, A., & Okuyama, R. (2018). Pathogenesis of psoriasis and development of treatment. *The Journal of Dermatology*, *45*(3), 264–272. doi:10.1111/1346-8138.14139 PMID:29226422

Oláh, A., Tóth, B. I., Borbíró, I., Sugawara, K., Szöllõsi, A. G., Czifra, G., Pál, B., Ambrus, L., Kloepper, J., Camera, E., Ludovici, M., Picardo, M., Voets, T., Zouboulis, C. C., Paus, R., & Bíró, T. (2014). Cannabidiol exerts sebostatic and antiinflammatory effects on human sebocytes. *The Journal of Clinical Investigation*, *124*(9), 3713–3724. doi:10.1172/JCI64628 PMID:25061872

Ondrej, M. (1991). Vyskyt hub nastonínchkonopi [Occurrence of hemp fungus]. *Len a Konopí*, *21*, 51–57.

Oomah, B. D., Busson, M., Godfrey, D. V., & Drover, J. C. G. (2002). Characteristics of hemp (Cannabis sativa L.) seed oil. *Food Chemistry*, *76*(1), 33–43. doi:10.1016/S0308-8146(01)00245-X

Pacula, R. L., & Smart, R. (2017). Medical Marijuana and Marijuana Legalization. *Annual Review of Clinical Psychology*, *13*(1), 397–419. doi:10.1146/annurev-clinpsy-032816-045128 PMID:28482686

Pagano, E., Romano, B., Iannotti, F. A., Parisi, O. A., D'Armiento, M., Pignatiello, S., Coretti, L., Lucafò, M., Venneri, T., Stocco, G., Lembo, F., Orlando, P., Capasso, R., Di Marzo, V., Izzo, A. A., & Borrelli, F. (2019). The non-euphoric phytocannabinoid cannabidivarin counteracts intestinal inflammation in mice and cytokine expression in biopsies from UC pediatric patients. *Pharmacological Research*, *149*, 104464. doi:10.1016/j.phrs.2019.104464 PMID:31553934

Pain, S. (2015). A potted history. *Nature*, *525*(7570), S10–S11. doi:10.1038/525S10a PMID:26398731

Palm, M. D., & O'Donoghue, M. N. (2007). Update on photoprotection: Photoprotection. *Dermatologic Therapy*, *20*(5), 360–376. doi:10.1111/j.1529-8019.2007.00150.x PMID:18045361

Pandey, A., Jatana, G. K., & Sonthalia, S. (2021). Cosmeceuticals. In *StatPearls*. StatPearls Publishing.

Panghal, M., Arya, V., Yadav, S., Kumar, S., & Yadav, J. P. (2010). Indigenous knowledge of medicinal plants used by Saperas community of Khetawas, Jhajjar District, Haryana, India. *Journal of Ethnobiology and Ethnomedicine*, *6*(1), 4. doi:10.1186/1746-4269-6-4 PMID:20109179

Pap, N., Hamberg, L., Pihlava, J.-M., Hellström, J., Mattila, P., Eurola, M., & Pihlanto, A. (2020). Impact of enzymatic hydrolysis on the nutrients, phytochemicals and sensory properties of oil hemp seed cake (Cannabis sativa L. FINOLA variety). *Food Chemistry*, *320*, 126530. doi:10.1016/j.foodchem.2020.126530 PMID:32222655

Pattnaik, S., & Chand, P. K. (2000). Morphogenic response of the alginate encapsulated axillary buds from in vitro shoot cultures of six mulberries. *Plant Cell Tiss Org*, *60*(3), 177–185. doi:10.1023/A:1006424626433

Paul, R., Williams, R., Hodson, V., & Peake, C. (2019). Detection of cannabinoids in hair after cosmetic application of hemp oil. *Scientific Reports*, *9*(1), 1–6. doi:10.103841598-019-39609-0 PMID:30796346

Pavisian, B., MacIntosh, B. J., Szilagyi, G., Staines, R. W., O'Connor, P., & Feinstein, A. (2014). Effects of cannabis on cognition in patients with MS: A psychometric and MRI study. *Neurology*, *82*(21), 1879–1887. doi:10.1212/WNL.0000000000000446 PMID:24789863

Pellati, F., Borgonetti, V., Brighenti, V., Biagi, M., Benvenuti, S., & Corsi, L. (2018). Cannabis sativa L. and nonpsychoactive cannabinoids: Their chemistry and role against oxidative stress, inflammation, and cancer. *BioMed Research International, 1691428*, 1–15. doi:10.1155/2018/1691428 PMID:30627539

Pellati, F., Brighenti, V., Sperlea, J., Marchetti, L., Bertelli, D., & Benvenuti, S. (2018). New Methods for the Comprehensive Analysis of Bioactive Compounds in Cannabis sativa L. (hemp). *Molecules (Basel, Switzerland), 23*(10), 2639. doi:10.3390/molecules23102639 PMID:30322208

Peltzer, K., & Pengpid, S. (2017). Cannabis and Amphetamine Use Among Adolescents in Five Asian Countries. *Central Asian Journal of Global Health, 6*(1). doi:10.5195/cajgh.2017.288 PMID:30881756

Pepe, M., Hesami, M., Small, F., & Jones, A. M. P. (2021). A.M.P. Comparative Analysis of Machine Learning and Evolutionary Optimization Algorithms for Precision Micropropagation of Cannabis sativa: Prediction and Validation of in vitro Shoot Growth and Development Based on the Optimization of Light and Carbohydrate Sources. *Front. Plant Sci., 12*, 757869. doi:10.3389/fpls.2021.757869 PMID:34745189

Pérez-Gómez, E., Andradas, C., Blasco-Benito, S., Caffarel, M. M., García-Taboada, E., Villa-Morales, M., Moreno, E., Hamann, S., Martín-Villar, E., Flores, J. M., Wenners, A., Alkatout, I., Klapper, W., Röcken, C., Bronsert, P., Stickeler, E., Staebler, A., Bauer, M., Arnold, N., & Sánchez, C. (2015). Role of cannabinoid receptor CB2 in HER2 pro-oncogenic signaling in breast cancer. *Journal of the National Cancer Institute, 107*(6), djv077. doi:10.1093/jnci/djv077 PMID:25855725

Perkins, J. A. (2005). A history of molecular representation. Part one: 1800 to the 1960s. *The Journal of Biocommunication, 31*(1), 1.

Perlín, C. (2002). Hemp as food. *Výživa a potraviny, 61*, 121-122.

Perry, D. C. (1977). Street drug analysis and drug use trends 1969-1975. Part II. *PharmChem Newsletter, 6*(4), 1–3.

Pertwee, R. (2008). The diverse CB_1 and CB_2 receptor pharmacology of three plant cannabinoids: Δ^9-tetrahydrocannabinol, cannabidiol and Δ^9-tetrahydrocannabivarin. *British Journal of Pharmacology, 153*(2), 199–215. doi:10.1038j.bjp.0707442 PMID:17828291

Pertwee, R. G. (2006). Cannabinoid pharmacology: The ðrst 66 years. *British Journal of Pharmacology, 147*(S1), S163–S171. doi:10.1038j.bjp.0706406 PMID:16402100

Peschel, W. (2016). Quality Control of Traditional Cannabis Tinctures: Pattern, Markers, and Stability. *Scientia Pharmaceutica, 84*(3), 567–584. doi:10.3390cipharm84030567 PMID:28117322

Petrović, M., Debeljak, Ž., Kezić, N., & Džidara, P. (2015). Relationship between cannabinoids content and composition of fatty acids in hempseed oils. *Food Chemistry, 170*, 218–225. doi:10.1016/j.foodchem.2014.08.039 PMID:25306338

Peyravian, N., Deo, S., Daunert, S., & Jimenez, J. J. (2022). The Anti-Inflammatory Effects of Cannabidiol (CBD) on Acne. *Journal of Inflammation Research, 15*, 2795–2801. doi:10.2147/JIR.S355489 PMID:35535052

Pittau, F., Krause, F., Lumia, G., & Habert, G. (2018). Fast-growing bio-based materials as an opportunity for storing carbon in exterior walls. *Building and Environment, 129*, 117–129. doi:10.1016/j.buildenv.2017.12.006

Placido, D. F., & Lee, C. C. (2022). Potential of Industrial *Cannabis sativa* for Phytoremediation of Heavy Metals. *Plants, 11*(5), 595. doi:10.3390/plants11050595 PMID:35270065

Plaza, M., & Turner, C. (2015). Pressurized hot water extraction of bioactives. *TrAC* [CrossRef] [Google Scholar]. *Trends in Analytical Chemistry, 71*, 39–54. doi:10.1016/j.trac.2015.02.022

Pollastro, F., Minassi, A., & Fresu, L. G. (2018). Cannabis Phenolics and their Bioactivities. *Current Medicinal Chemistry*, *25*(10), 1160–1185. doi:10.2174/0929867324666170810164636 PMID:28799497

Potter, D. J. (2004). Growth and morphology of medicinal Cannabis. In G. W. Guy, B. A. Whittle, & P. J. Robson (Eds.), *The medicinal uses of Cannabis and Cannabinoids* (pp. 17–54). Pharmaceutical Press.

Prade, T., Svensson, S.-E., & Mattsson, J. E. (2012). Energy balances for biogas and solid biofuel production from industrial Cannabis sativa. *Biomass and Bioenergy*, *40*, 36–52. doi:10.1016/j.biombioe.2012.01.045

Praspaliauskas, M., Žaltauskaitė, J., Pedišius, N., & Striūgas, N. (2020). Comprehensive evaluation of sewage sludge and sewage sludge char soil amendment impact on the industrial *Cannabis sativa* growth performance and heavy metal accumulation. *Industrial Crops and Products*, *150*, 112396. doi:10.1016/j.indcrop.2020.112396

Prohibition Partners. (2019). The African cannabis reports. *Prohibition Partners*. https://prohibitionpartners.com/reports/

Punyamurthula, N. S., Adelli, G. R., Gul, W., Repka, M. A., ElSohly, M. A., & Majumdar, S. (2017). Ocular Disposition of Δ^8-Tetrahydrocannabinol from Various Topical Ophthalmic Formulations. *AAPS PharmSciTech*, *18*(6), 1936–1945. doi:10.120812249-016-0672-2 PMID:27905004

Quan, P. M., Toan, T. Q., Hung, N. P., Nam, P. H., Kiet, N. T., Ha, N. X., & Thi, H. H. P. (2021). Cannabis sativa L. chemical compositions as potential plasmodium falciparum dihydrofolate reductase-thymidinesynthase enzyme inhibitors: An in silico study for drug development. *Open Chemistry*, *19*(1), 1244–1250. doi:10.1515/chem-2021-0102

Raderman, J.M., (2016). *Method for modifying THC content in a lipid-based extract of Cannabis.*

Radhakrishnan, R., Wilkinson, S. T., & D'Souza, D. C. (2014). Gone to pot-a review of the association between cannabis and psychosis. *Frontiers in Psychiatry*, 5. doi:10.3389/fpsyt.2014.00054 PMID:24904437

Radočaj, O., Dimić, E., & Tsao, R. (2014). Effects of hemp (Cannabis sativa L.) seed oil press-cake and decaffeinated green tea leaves (Camellia sinensis) on functional characteristics of gluten-free crackers. *Journal of Food Science*, *79*(3), C318–C325. doi:10.1111/1750-3841.12370 PMID:24527987

Radwan, M. M., Elsohly, M. A., Slade, D., Ahmed, S. A., Khan, I. A., & Ross, S. A. (2009). Biologically active cannabinoids from high-potency Cannabis sativa. *Journal of Natural Products*, *72*(5), 906–911. doi:10.1021/np900067k PMID:19344127

Raharjo, T. J., Chang, W.-T., Choi, Y. H., Peltenburg-Looman, A. M., & Verpoorte, R. (2004). Olivetol as product of a polyketide synthase in *Cannabis sativa* L. *Plant Science*, *166*(2), 381–385. doi:10.1016/j.plantsci.2003.09.027

Raimondi, G., Rodrigues, J., Maucieri, C., Borin, M., & Bona, S. (2020). Phytomanagement of chromium-contaminated soils using *Cannabis sativa* (L.). *Agronomy (Basel)*, *10*(9), 1223. doi:10.3390/agronomy10091223

Rajaei, A., Barzegar, M., & Yamini, Y. (2004). Supercritical fluid extraction of tea seed oil and its comparison with solvent extraction. *European Food Research and Technology*, *220*(3-4), 401–405. doi:10.100700217-004-1061-8

Rajak, N. (2022). Hemp Usage as a Green Building Material, Plastic, and Fuel. In *Revolutionizing the Potential of Hemp and Its Products in Changing the Global Economy* (pp. 157–167). Springer International Publishing. doi:10.1007/978-3-031-05144-9_8

Rajanahally, S., Raheem, O., Rogers, M., Brisbane, W., Ostrowski, K., Lendvay, T., & Walsh, T. (2019). The relationship between cannabis and male infertility, sexual health, and neoplasm: A systematic review. *Andrology*, *7*(2), 139–147. https:// doi.org/10.1111/andr.2019.7.issue-210.1111/andr.12585

Rajput, R., & Kumar, K. (2018). A Review on *Cannabis sativa*: Its Compounds and Their Effects. *International Journal of Pharmaceutical Sciences Review and Research, 53*(2), 59–63.

Ramar, K., Rosen, I.M., Kirsch, D.B., Chervin, R.D., Carden, K.A., Aurora, R.N., Kristo, D.A., Malhotra, R.K., Martin, J.L., Olson, E.J., Rosen, C.L., Rowley, J.A., American Academy of Sleep Medicine Board of Directors, (2018). Medical cannabis and the treatment of obstructive sleep apnea: an American academy of sleep medicine position statement. J. *Clin. Sleep. Med.* 14 (4), 679–681. doi:. 7070. doi:10.5664/jcsm

Ramírez J (1990) Acute pulmonary histoplasmosis: new recognized hazard of marijuana planthunters. *Am J Med 88*(5, Suppl.), 60 N.

Rampa, A., Bartolini, M., Bisi, A., Belluti, F., Gobbi, S., Andrisano, V., Ligresti, A., & Di Marzo, V. (2012). The ðrst dual ChE/FAAH inhibitors: New perspectives for alzheimer's disease? *ACS Medicinal Chemistry Letters, 3*(3), 182–186. doi:10.1021/ml200313p PMID:24900454

Ranalli, P. (1999). *Advances in hemp research.* CRC Press. doi:10.1201/9781498705820

Randall, M. D. (2007). Endocannabinoids and the haematological system. *British Journal of Pharmacology, 152*(5), 671–675. doi:10.1038j.bjp.0707420 PMID:17704826

Raskin, I., Smith, R. D., & Salt, D. E. (1997). Phytoremediation of metals: Using plants to remove pollutants from the environment. *Current Opinion in Biotechnology, 8*(2), 221–226. doi:10.1016/S0958-1669(97)80106-1 PMID:9079727

Reggio, P. (2010). Endocannabinoid Binding to the Cannabinoid Receptors: What Is Known and What Remains Unknown. *Current Medicinal Chemistry, 17*(14), 1468–1486. doi:10.2174/092986710790980005 PMID:20166921

Ren, G.; Zhang, X.; Li, Y.; Ridout, K.; Serrano-Serrano, M.L.; Yang, Y.; Liu, A.; Ravikanth, G.; Nawaz, M.A.; Mumtaz, A.S.; et al. (2021). Large-scale whole-genome resequencing unravels the domestication history of Cannabis sativa. *Sci. Adv.*,7, eabg 2286.

Renard, J., Rushlow, W. J., & LaViolette, S. R. (2018). Effects of Adolescent THC Exposure on the Prefrontal GABAergic System: Implications for Schizophrenia-Related Psychopathology. *Frontiers in Psychiatry, 9*, 281. doi:10.3389/fpsyt.2018.00281 PMID:30013490

Ren, M., Tang, Z., Wu, X., Spengler, R., Jiang, H., Yang, Y., & Boivin, N. (2019). The origins of cannabis smoking: Chemical residue evidence from the first millennium BCE in the Pamirs. *Science Advances, 205*(6), eaaw1391. doi:10.1126ciadv.aaw1391 PMID:31206023

Rice, B. (2008). Hemp as a feedstock for biomass-to-energy conversion. *Journal of Industrial Hemp, 13*(2), 145–156. doi:10.1080/15377880802391274

Rice, J., & Cameron, M. (2018). Cannabinoids for treatment of MS symptoms: State of the evidence. *Current Neurology and Neuroscience Reports, 18*(8), 50. doi:10.100711910-018-0859-x PMID:29923025

Richard, M., Ganguly, R., Steigerwald, S., Al-Khalifa, A., & Pierce, G. (2007). Dietary hempseed reduces platelet aggregation. *Journal of Thrombosis and Haemostasis, 5*(2), 424–425. doi:10.1111/j.1538-7836.2007.02327.x PMID:17155962

Riddle, J. M. (2011). *Dioscorides on Pharmacy and Medicine.* University of Texas Press.

Roberts, C. (2017). How Cannabis Cleans Up Nuclear Radiation and Toxic Soil. *High Times.* https://hightimes.com/news/how-cannabis-cleans-up-nuclear-radiation-and-toxic-soil/

Robinson, S. M., & Adinoff, B. (2016). The Classification of Substance Use Disorders: Historical, Contextual, and Conceptual Considerations. *Behavioral Sciences (Basel, Switzerland)*, *6*(3), E18. doi:10.3390/bs6030018 PMID:27548233

Rocky Mountain High Intensity Drug Trafficking Area. (2015). The legalization of marijuana in Colorado: *The impact, 3*. http://www.rmhidta.org/html/2015%20PREVIEW%20Legalization%20of%20MJ%20in%20Colorado%20the%20Impact.pdf (Retrieved 30 October 2020).

Rodriguez-Morrison, V., Llewellyn, D., & Zheng, Y. (2021). Cannabis Inflorescence Yield and Cannabinoid Concentration Are Not Increased With Exposure to Short-Wavelength Ultraviolet-B Radiation. *Frontiers in Plant Science*, *12*, 725078. doi:10.3389/fpls.2021.725078 PMID:34795683

Rohleder, C., Müller, J. K., Lange, B., & Leweke, F. M. (2016). Cannabidiol as a Potential New Type of an Antipsychotic. A Critical Review of the Evidence. *Frontiers in Pharmacology*, *7*, 422. doi:10.3389/fphar.2016.00422 PMID:27877130

Ross, S. A., & ElSohly, M. A. (1996). The volatile oil composition of fresh and air-dried buds of Cannabissativa. *Journal of Natural Products*, *59*(1), 49–51. doi:10.1021/np960004a PMID:8984153

Rough, L. (2017). 7 Must-Try Cannabis Topicals for Those Scorching Summer Days. *Leafly*. https://www.leafly.com/news/strains-products/cannabis-topicals-for-summer

Roychoudhury, P., Wang, N. N., & Narouze, S. N. (2021). Phytocannabinoids: Tetrahydrocannabinol (THC). In S. N. Narouze (Ed.), *Cannabinoids and Pain* (pp. 71–77). Springer. doi:10.1007/978-3-030-69186-8_10

Ruchlemer, R., Amit-Kohn, M., Raveh, D., & Hanuš, L. (2015). Inhaled medicinal cannabis and theimmunocompromised patient. *Supportive Care in Cancer*, *23*(3), 819–822. doi:10.100700520-014-2429-3 PMID:25216851

Rudroff, T., Honce, J.M., (2017). Cannabis and multiple sclerosis-the way forward. Front. Neurol. 8, 299. . Russo,E. B.,2007.History ofcannabis anditspreparations insaga,science,andsobriquet. *Chem. Biodivers.* 4, 1614–1648. . doi:10.3389/fneur.2017.00299

Rupasinghe, H. P., Davis, A., Kumar, S. K., Murray, B., & Zheljazkov, V. D. (2020). Industrial hemp (Cannabis sativa subsp. sativa) as an emerging source for value-added functional food ingredients and nutraceuticals. *Molecules (Basel, Switzerland)*, *25*(18), 4078. doi:10.3390/molecules25184078 PMID:32906622

Russo, E. (2016) Pesticide contamination of cannabis in the legal market. In: *Proceedings of the26th Annual Symposium on the Cannabinoids.* International Cannabinoid Research Society.

Russo, E. B. (2017). Cannabidiol Claims and Misconceptions. *Trends in Pharmacological Sciences*, *38*(3), 198–201. doi:10.1016/j.tips.2016.12.004 PMID:28089139

Russo, E. B., Jiang, H. E., Li, X., Sutton, A., Carboni, A., del Bianco, F., Mandolino, G., Potter, D. J., Zhao, Y. X., Bera, S., Zhang, Y. B., Lü, E. G., Ferguson, D. K., Hueber, F., Zhao, L. C., Liu, C. J., Wang, Y. F., & Li, C. S. (2008). Phytochemical and genetic analyses of ancient cannabis from Central Asia. *Journal of Experimental Botany*, *59*(15), 4171–4182. doi:10.1093/jxb/ern260 PMID:19036842

Russo, E. B., & Marcu, J. (2017). Cannabis pharmacology: The usual suspects and a few promising leads. *Advances in Pharmacology*, *80*, 67–134. doi:10.1016/bs.apha.2017.03.004 PMID:28826544

Russo, E., & Guy, G. W. (2006). A tale of two cannabinoids: The therapeutic rationale for combining tetrahydrocannabinol and cannabidiol. *Medical Hypotheses*, *66*(2), 234–246. doi:10.1016/j.mehy.2005.08.026 PMID:16209908

Ryz, N. R., Remillard, D. J., & Russo, E. B. (2017). Cannabis roots: A traditional therapy with future potential for treating inñammation and pain. *Cannabis and Cannabinoid Research*, *2*(1), 210–216. doi:10.1089/can.2017.0028 PMID:29082318

Safari Singani, A. A., & Ahmadi, P. (2012). Manure application and Cannabis cultivation influence onspeciation of lead and cadmium by selective sequential extraction. *Soil & Sediment Contamination*, *21*(3), 305–321. doi:10.1080/15320383.2012.664186

Salema, A., Valiathan, M. S., Malamound, C., Raghunathan, K., Wujastyk, D., & Walker, T. (2001). *Ayurveda at the crossroads of care and cure*. Indo-European Seminar on Ayurveda Held in Arrabida.

Salt, D. E., Blaylock, M., Kumar, N. P. B. A., Dushenkov, V., Ensley, B. D., Chet, I., & Raskin, I. (1995). Phytoremediation: A novel strategy for the removal of toxic metals from the environment using plants. *Nature Biotechnology*, *13*(5), 468–474. doi:10.1038/nbt0595-468 PMID:9634787

Salzet, M., Breton, C., Bisogno, T., & Di Marzo, V. (2000). Comparative biology of the endocannabinoid system possible role in the immune response. *European Journal of Biochemistry*, *267*(16), 4917–4927. doi:10.1046/j.1432-1327.2000.01550.x PMID:10931174

Samson, R. A., Hoekstra, E. S., & Frisvad, J. C. (Eds.). (2004). Introduction to food- and airborne fungi.Centraalbureau-voorSchimmelcultures, UtrechtScheel AH, Kraus D, Haars H, Schmitz I, Junker K (2012) Talcum induced pneumoconiosisfollowing inhalation of adulterated marijuana. *Diagnostic Pathology*, *7*, 26.

Sandle, T. (2020, November 24). *Cannabis For Medical And Pharmaceutical Purposes – Part 1: An Overview Of The Development And Application*. IVT Network. https://www.ivtnetwork.com/article/cannabis-medical-and-pharmaceutical-purposes-%E2%80%93-part-1-overview-development-an
d-application-0

Santos, C. B. R. D., Lobato, C. C., de Sousa, M. A. C., Macêdo, W. J. D. C., & Carvalho, J. C. T. (2014). Molecular modeling: Origin, fundamental concepts and applications using structure-activity relationship and quantitative structure-activity relationship. *Reviews in Theoretical Science*, *2*(2), 91–115. doi:10.1166/rits.2014.1016

Sarma, N. D., Waye, A., ElSohly, M. A., Brown, P. N., Elzinga, S., Johnson, H. E., & Deyton, L. (2020). Cannabis Inflorescence for Medical Purposes: USP Considerations for Quality Attributes. *Journal of Natural Products*, *83*(4), 1334–1351. doi:10.1021/acs.jnatprod.9b01200 PMID:32281793

Savonenko, A.V., Melnikova, T., Wang, Y., Ravert, H., Gao, Y., Koppel, J., Lee, D., Pletnikova, O., Cho, E., Sayyida, N., Hiatt, A., Troncoso, J., Davies, P., Dannals, R.F., Pomper, M.G., Horti, A.G., (2015). Cannabinoid CB2 receptors in a mouse model of Aβ amyloidosis: immune histochemical analysis and suitability as a PET biomarker of neuroinñammation. PLoS One 10, e0129618. doi:. 0129618. doi:10.1371/journal.pone

Savo, V., La Rocca, A., Caneva, G., Rapallo, F., & Cornara, L. (2013). Plants used in artisanal ðsheries on the Western Mediterranean coasts of Italy. *Journal of Ethnobiology and Ethnomedicine*, *9*(1), 9. doi:10.1186/1746-4269-9-9 PMID:23356937

Saxena, A., Wong, D., Diraviyam, K., & Sept, D. (2009). The basic concepts of molecular modeling. *Methods in Enzymology*, *467*, 307–334. doi:10.1016/S0076-6879(09)67012-9 PMID:19897098

Saxena, G., Purchase, D., Mulla, S. I., Saratale, G. D., & Bharagava, R. N. (2019). *Phytoremediation of Heavy Metal-Contaminated Sites: Eco-environmental Concerns, Field Studies, Sustainability Issues, and Future Prospects*. Springer.

Schenberg, E. E. (2018). Psychedelic-assisted psychotherapy: A paradigm shift in psychiatric research and development. *Frontiers in Pharmacology*, *9*, 733. doi:10.3389/fphar.2018.00733 PMID:30026698

Scherma, M., Satta, V., Collu, R., Boi, M. F., Usai, P., Fratta, W., & Fadda, P. (2017). Cannabinoid CB (1)/CB (2) receptor agonists attenuate hyperactivity and body weight loss in a rat model of activity-based anorexia. *British Journal of Pharmacology*, *174*(16), 2682–2695. doi:10.1111/bph.13892 PMID:28561272

Schluttenhofer, C., & Yuan, L. (2017). Challenges towards revitalizing hemp: A multifaceted crop. *Trends in Plant Science, 22*(11), 917–929. doi:10.1016/j.tplants.2017.08.004 PMID:28886910

Schofs, L., Sparo, M. D., & Sánchez Bruni, S. F. (2021). The antimicrobial effect behind *Cannabis sativa. Pharmacology Research & Perspectives, 9*(2). Advance online publication. doi:10.1002/prp2.761 PMID:33822478

Schreurs, E., Voets, T., & Thewys, T. (2011). GIS-based assessment of the biomass potential from phytoremediation of contaminated agricultural land in the Campine region in Belgium. *Biomass and Bioenergy, 35*(10), 4469–4480. doi:10.1016/j.biombioe.2011.09.005

Schröder, P., Beckers, B., Daniels, S., Gnädinger, F., Maestri, E., Marmiroli, N., Mench, M., Millan, R., Obermeier, M. M., Oustriere, N., Persson, T., Poschenrieder, C., Rineau, F., Rutkowska, B., Schmid, T., Szulc, W., Witters, N., & Sæbø, A. (2018). Intensify production, transform biomass to energy and novel goods and protect soils in Europe—A vision how to mobilize marginal lands. *The Science of the Total Environment, 616–617*, 1101–1123. doi:10.1016/j.scitotenv.2017.10.209 PMID:29132720

Schultes, R. E., Hoffman, A., & Ratsch, C. (1992). *Plants of the Gods – Their Sacred, Healing and Hallucinogenic Powers*. Healing Arts Press.

Schussel, V., Kenzo, L., Santos, A., Bueno, J., Yoshimura, E., de Oliveira Cruz Latorraca, C., Pachito, D. V., & Riera, R. (2018). Cannabinoids for nausea and vomiting related to chemotherapy: Overview of systematic reviews. *Phytotherapy Research, 32*(4), 567–576. doi:10.1002/ptr.5975 PMID:29168289

Secades-Villa, R., Garcia-Rodríguez, O., Jin, C. J., Wang, S., & Blanco, C. (2015). Probability and predictors of the cannabis gateway effect: A national study. *The International Journal on Drug Policy, 26*(2), 135–142. doi:10.1016/j.drugpo.2014.07.011 PMID:25168081

Seddon, T., & Floodgate, W. (2020). *Regulating Cannabis: A Global Review and Future Directions*. Palgrave Macmillan. doi:10.1007/978-3-030-52927-7

Seely, K. A., Prather, P. L., James, L. P., & Moran, J. H. (2011). Marijuana-based drugs: Innovative therapeutics or designer drugs of abuse. *Molecular Interventions, 11*(1), 36–51. doi:10.1124/mi.11.1.6 PMID:21441120

Shamir, R., & Hacker, D. (2001). Colonialism's civilizing mission: The case of the Indian Hemp Drug Commission. *Law & Social Inquiry, 26*(2), 435–461. doi:10.1111/j.1747-4469.2001.tb00184.x

Sharkey, K. A., Darmani, N. A., & Parker, L. A. (2014). Regulation of nausea and vomiting by cannabinoids and the endocannabinoid system. *European Journal of Pharmacology, 722*, 134–146. doi:10.1016/j.ejphar.2013.09.068 PMID:24184696

Sharma, A. (2017). Male infertility; evidences, risk factors, causes, diagnosis and management in human. *Annals of Clinical and Laboratory Research, 5*(3), 188.

Sharma, D., Kumar, S., & Narasimhan, B. (2018). Estrogen alpha receptor antagonists for the treatment of breast cancer: A review. *Chemistry Central Journal, 12*(1), 107. doi:10.118613065-018-0472-8 PMID:30361894

Sharma, P., Murthy, P., & Bharath, M. S. (2012). Chemistry, metabolism, and toxicology of cannabis: Clinical implications. *Iranian Journal of Psychiatry, 7*(4), 149. PMID:23408483

Sheng, W. S., Chauhan, P., Hu, S., Prasad, S., & Lokensgard, J. R. (2019). Antiallodynic effects of cannabinoid receptor 2 (CB2R) agonists on retrovirus infection-induced neuropathic pain. *Pain Research and Management*.

Shen, P., Gao, Z., Fang, B., Rao, J., & Chen, B. (2021). Ferreting out the secrets of industrial hemp protein as emerging functional food ingredients. *Trends in Food Science & Technology, 112*, 1–15. doi:10.1016/j.tifs.2021.03.022

Sheoran, V., Sheoran, A. S., & Poonia, P. (2013). Phytomining of gold: A review. *Journal of Geochemical Exploration*, *128*, 42–50. doi:10.1016/j.gexplo.2013.01.008

Sheriff, T., Lin, M. J., Dubin, D., & Khorasani, H. (2020). The potential role of cannabinoids in dermatology. *The Journal of Dermatological Treatment*, *31*(8), 839–845. doi:10.1080/09546634.2019.1675854 PMID:31599175

Shi, G., & Cai, Q. (2009). Cadmium tolerance and accumulation in eight potential energy crops. *Biotechnology Advances*, *27*(5), 555–561. doi:10.1016/j.biotechadv.2009.04.006 PMID:19393309

Sicurani, M., Piccioni, E., & Standardi, A. (2001). Micropropagation and preparation of synthetic seed in M.26 apple rootstock I: Attempts towards saving labor in the production of adventitious shoot tips suitable for encapsulation. *Plant Cell Tiss Org*, *66*(3), 207–216. doi:10.1023/A:1010627720368

Silva, T. B., Pereira, M. A., Malta, V. S., Bento, E. S., San-Miguel, M. A., Ziolli, R. L., & Taft, C. A. (2008). Study of the structure-activity relationship for theoretical molecular descriptors using density functional theory and chemometric methods in cannabinoid metabolites. *International Journal of Quantum Chemistry*, *108*(13), 2530–2539. doi:10.1002/qua.21696

Silver, R. J. (2019). The endocannabinoid system of animals. *Animals (Basel)*, *9*(9), 686. doi:10.3390/ani9090686 PMID:31527410

Sim, L. J., Hampson, R. E., Deadwyler, S. A., & Childers, S. R. (1996). Effects of chronic treatment with delta9-tetrahydrocannabinol on cannabinoid-stimulated [35S]GTP gamma S autoradiography in rat brain. *The Journal of Neuroscience: The Official Journal of the Society for Neuroscience*, *16*(24), 8057–8066. doi:10.1523/JNEUROSCI.16-24-08057.1996 PMID:8987831

Singh, B., & Sharma, R. A. (2015). Plant terpenes: defense responses, phylogenetic analysis, regulation and clinical applications. *3 Biotech, 5*(2), 129-151. doi:10.1007/s13205-014-0220-2

Singh, M., Mamania, D., & Shinde, V. (2018). *The scope of hemp (Cannabis sativa L.) use in Historical conservation in India*.

Singh, A., Saluja, S., Kumar, A., Agrawal, S., Thind, M., Nanda, S., & Shirani, J. (2018). Cardiovascular Complications of Marijuana and Related Substances: A Review. *Cardiology and Therapy*, *7*(1), 45–59. doi:10.100740119-017-0102-x PMID:29218644

Singh, M., & Sardesai, M. M. (2016). Cannabis sativa (Cannabaceae) in ancient clay plaster of Ellora Caves, India. *Current Science*, 884–891.

Sirikantaramas, S., Taura, F., Tanaka, Y., Ishikawa, Y., Morimoto, S., & Shoyama, Y. (2005). Tetrahydrocannabinolic acid synthase, the enzyme controlling marijuana psychoactivity, is secreted into the storage cavity of the glandular trichomes. *Plant & Cell Physiology*, *46*(9), 1578–1582. doi:10.1093/pcp/pci166 PMID:16024552

Slusarkiewicz-Jarzina, A., Ponitka, A., & Kaczmarek, Z. (2005). Influence of cultivar, explant source and plant growth regulator on callus induction and plant regeneration of *Cannabis sativa* L. *Acta Biologica Cracoviensia. Series; Botanica*, *47*(2), 145–151.

Slusarkiewicz-Jarzina, A., Ponitka, A., & Kaczmarek, Z. (2005). Inñuence of cultivar, explant source and plant growth regulator on callus induction and plant regeneration of Cannabis sativa L. *Acta Biologica Cracoviensia. Series; Botanica*, *47*, 145–151.

Small, E. (2015). Classification of *Cannabis sativa* (Marijuana, Hemp) in Relation to Human Utilization. *Botanical Review*, *81*(3), 189–294. doi:10.100712229-015-9157-3

Small, E. (2017). Classification of Cannabis sativa L. in Relation to agricultural, biotechnological, medical, and recreational utilization. In S. Chandra, H. Lata, & M. ElSohly (Eds.), *Cannabis sativa L. - Botany and Biotechnology*. Springer. doi:10.1007/978-3-319-54564-6_1

Small, E., & Cronquist, A. (1976). A Practical and Natural Taxonomy for Cannabis. *Taxon*, *25*(4), 405–435. doi:10.2307/1220524

Small, E., & Naraine, S. G. (2016). Size matters: Evolution of large drug-secreting resin glands in elite pharmaceutical strains of *Cannabis sativa* (marijuana). *Genetic Resources and Crop Evolution*, *63*(2), 349–359. doi:10.100710722-015-0254-2

Small, E., Pocock, T., & Cavers, P. B. (2003). The biology of Canadian weeds. 119. *Cannabis sativa* L. *Canadian Journal of Plant Science*, *83*(1), 217–237. doi:10.4141/P02-021

Smith, G. L., & Satino, J. (2021). Case Study of Hair Regrowth with Topical Cannabidiol (CBD). *International Society of Hair Restoration Surgery*, *31*(4), 140–142. doi:10.33589/31.4.140

Smýkalová, I., Vrbová, M., Cvečková, M., Plačková, L., Žukauskaitė, A., Zatloukal, M., Hrdlička, J., Plíhalová, L., Doležal, K., & Griga, M. (2019). Cvecˇková, M.; Placˇková, L.; Žukauskaitˇe, A.; Zatloukal, M.; Hrdlicˇka, J.; Plíhalová, L.; Doležal, K.; Griga, M. The effects of novel synthetic cytokinin derivatives and endogenous cytokinins on the in vitro growth responses of hemp (Cannabis sativa L.) explants. *Plant Cell, Tissue and Organ Culture*, *139*(2), 381–394. doi:10.100711240-019-01693-5

Soelberg Sorensen, P. (2017). Safety concerns and risk management of multiple sclerosis therapies. *Acta Neurologica Scandinavica*, *136*(3), 168–186. doi:10.1111/ane.12712 PMID:27891572

Solowij, N., & Battisti, R. (2008). The chronic effects of cannabis on memory in humans: A review. Curr. *Drug Abus. Rev*, *1*(1), 81–98. doi:10.2174/1874473710801010081 PMID:19630708

Song, H., & Lee, S. Y. (2006). Production of succinic acid by bacterial fermentation. *Enzyme and Microbial Technology*, *39*(3), 352–361. doi:10.1016/j.enzmictec.2005.11.043

Spindle, T. R., Bonn-Miller, M. O., & Vandrey, R. (2019). Changing landscape of cannabis: Novel products, formulations, and methods of administration. *Current Opinion in Psychology*, *30*, 98–102. doi:10.1016/j.copsyc.2019.04.002 PMID:31071592

Spitzer-Rimon, B., Duchin, S., Bernstein, N., & Kamenetsky, R. (2019). Architecture and Florogenesis in Female *Cannabis sativa* Plants. *Frontiers in Plant Science*, *10*, 350. doi:10.3389/fpls.2019.00350 PMID:31001293

Stahl, V., & Vasudevan, K. (2020). Comparison of Efficacy of Cannabinoids versus Commercial Oral Care Products in Reducing Bacterial Content from Dental Plaque: A Preliminary Observation. *Cureus*, *12*(1), e6809. doi:10.7759/cureus.6809 PMID:32038896

Starowicz, K., & Finn, D. P. (2017). Cannabinoids and pain: Sites and mechanisms of action. *Advances in Pharmacology (San Diego, Calif.)*, *80*, 437–475. doi:10.1016/bs.apha.2017.05.003 PMID:28826543

Stasiłowicz, A., Tomala, A., Podolak, I., & Cielecka-Piontek, J. (2021). Cannabis sativa L. as a natural drug meeting the criteria of a multitarget approach to treatment. *International Journal of Molecular Sciences*, *22*(2), 778. doi:10.3390/ijms22020778 PMID:33466734

Stein, M. A. (1989). *Kalhana's Rajatarangini: A Chronicle of the Kings of Kashmir* (Vol. 1 & 2). Motilal Banarsidass Publ.

Stella, A., Palmieri, B., Laurino, C., & Vadalà, M. (2019). A therapeutic effect of cbd-enriched ointment in inflammatory skin diseases and cutaneous scars. *La Clinica Terapeutica*, *170*(2), e93–e99. doi:10.7417/CT.2019.2116 PMID:30993303

Stevens, C. J., Murphy, C., Roberts, R., Lucas, L., Silva, F., & Fuller, D. Q. (2016). Between China and South Asia: A middle Asian corridor of crop dispersal and agricultural innovation in the bronze age. *The Holocene*, *26*(10), 1541–1555. doi:10.1177/0959683616650268 PMID:27942165

Stonehouse, G. C., McCarron, B. J., Guignardi, Z. S., El Mehdawi, A. F., Lima, L. W., Fakra, S. C., & Pilon-Smits, E. A. H. (2020). Selenium metabolism in *Cannabis sativa* (*Cannabis sativa* L.)—Potential for phytoremediation and biofortification. *Environmental Science & Technology*, *54*(7), 4221–4230. doi:10.1021/acs.est.9b07747 PMID:32182043

Storr, M., Devlin, S., Kaplan, G. G., Panaccione, R., & Andrews, C. N. (2014). Cannabis use provides symptom relief in patients with inflammatory bowel disease but is associated with worse disease prognosis in patients with Crohn's disease. *Inflammatory Bowel Diseases*, *20*(3), 472–480. doi:10.1097/01.MIB.0000440982.79036.d6 PMID:24407485

Stout, J. M., Boubakir, Z., Ambrose, S. J., Purves, R. W., & Page, J. E. (2012). The hexanoyl-CoA precursor for cannabinoid biosynthesis is formed by an acyl-activating enzyme in *Cannabis sativa* trichomes. *The Plant Journal*, *71*(3), 353–365. doi:10.1111/j.1365-313X.2012.04949.x PMID:22353623

Subramaniam. (2020). Cannabis industry to be worth just $5 billion by 2021 amid flat rollout, high costs. *Financial Post*. https://financialpost.com/cannabis/cannabis-industry-to-be-worth-just-5-billion-by-2021-amid-flat-rollout-high-costs

Sumiahadi, A., & Acar, R. (2018). A review of phytoremediation technology: Heavy metals uptake by plants. *IOP Conference Series. Earth and Environmental Science*, *142*, 012023. doi:10.1088/1755-1315/142/1/012023

Sun, H. Y., Youn-Jung, K., Ok, K. M., Mingyeong, K., & Woong, O. S. (2017). Cannabidiol upregulates melanogenesis through CB1 dependent pathway by activating p38 MAPK and p42/44 MAPK. *Chemico-Biological Interactions*, *273*, 107–114. doi:10.1016/j.cbi.2017.06.005 PMID:28601556

Suryavanshi, S. V., Kovalchuk, I., & Kovalchuk, O. (2020). Cannabinoids as Key Regulators of Inflammasome Signaling: A Current Perspective. *Frontiers in Immunology*, *11*, 613613. doi:10.3389/fimmu.2020.613613 PMID:33584697

Szabó, I. L., Lisztes, E., Béke, G., Tóth, K. F., Paus, R., Oláh, A., & Bíró, T. (2020). The Phytocannabinoid (–)-Cannabidiol Operates as a Complex, Differential Modulator of Human Hair Growth: Anti-Inflammatory Submicromolar versus Hair Growth Inhibitory Micromolar Effects. *The Journal of Investigative Dermatology*, *140*(2), 484–488. doi:10.1016/j.jid.2019.07.690 PMID:31369737

Tafelski, S., Häuser, W., & Schäfer, M. (2016). Efficacy, tolerability, and safety of cannabinoids for chemotherapy-induced nausea and vomiting–a systematic review of systematic reviews. *Schmerz (Berlin, Germany)*, *30*(1), 14–24. doi:10.100700482-015-0092-3 PMID:26787227

Taffe, M. A. (2012). d 9-Tetrahydrocannabinol attenuates MDMA-induced hyperthermia in rhesus monkeys. *Neuroscience*, *201*, 125–133. doi:10.1016/j.neuroscience.2011.11.040 PMID:22138434

Tahir, M. N., Shahbazi, F., Rondeau-Gagné, S., & Trant, J. F. (2021). The biosynthesis of the cannabinoids. *Journal of Cannabis Research*, *3*(1), 1–12. doi:10.118642238-021-00062-4 PMID:33722296

Tambaro, S., Casu, M. A., Mastinu, A., & Lazzari, P. (2014). Evaluation of selective cannabinoid CB (1) and CB(2) receptor agonists in a mouse model of lipopolysaccharide-induced interstitial cystitis. *European Journal of Pharmacology*, *729*, 67–74. doi:10.1016/j.ejphar.2014.02.013 PMID:24561047

Tanasescu, R., & Constantinescu, C.S. (2010). Cannabinoids and the immune system: An overview. *Elsevier,215*(8), 588–597.

Tangahu, B. V., Abdullah, S., Rozaimah, S., Basri, H., Idris, M., & Anuar, N. (2011). A review on heavy metals (As, Pb, and Hg) uptake by plants through phytoremediation. *International Journal of Chemical Engineering, 2011*, 1–31. doi:10.1155/2011/939161

Tang, C.-H., Ten, Z., Wang, X.-S., & Yang, X.-Q. (2006). Physicochemical and functional properties of hemp (Cannabis sativa L.) protein isolate. *Journal of Agricultural and Food Chemistry*, *54*(23), 8945–8950. doi:10.1021/jf0619176 PMID:17090145

Tashkin, D. P. & Roth, M.D. (2007). Effects of Marijuana on the Lung and Immune Defenses. *Marijuana and the Cannabinoids,* 253–275. . doi:10.1007/978-1-59259-947-9_11

Tashkin, D. P., & Roth, M. D. (2019). Pulmonary effects of inhaled cannabis smoke. *The American Journal of Drug and Alcohol Abuse*, *45*(6), 596–609. doi:10.1080/00952990.2019.1627366 PMID:31298945

Taskar, P. (2019). *Formulation development, preclinical testing, and primary packaging optimization for cannabinoids and other therapeutics*. University of Mississippi.

Taylor, D. N., Wachsmuth, I. K., Shangkuan, Y. H., Schmidt, E. V., Barrett, T. J., Schrader, J. S., Scherach, C. S., McGee, H. B., Feldman, R. A., & Brenner, D. J. (1982). Salmonellosis associated with marijuana: Amultistate outbreak traced by plasmid fingerprinting. *The New England Journal of Medicine*, *306*(21), 1249–1253. doi:10.1056/NEJM198205273062101 PMID:7070444

Telek, A., Bíró, T., Bodó, E., Tóth, B. I., Borbíró, I., Kunos, G., & Paus, R. (2007). Inhibition of human hair follicle growth by endo-and exocannabinoids. *The FASEB Journal*, *21*(13), 3534–3541. doi:10.1096/fj.06-7689com PMID:17567570

Thomas, G., Kloner, R. A., & Rezkalla, S. (2014). Adverse cardiovascular, cerebrovascular, and peripheral vascular effects of marijuana inhalation: What cardiologists need to know. *The American Journal of Cardiology*, *113*(1), 187–190. doi:10.1016/j.amjcard.2013.09.042 PMID:24176069

Thompson, G. R., Rosenkrantz, H., Schaeppi, U. H., & Braude, M. C. (1973). Comparison of acute oral toxicity of cannabinoids in rats, dogs and monkeys. *Toxicology and Applied Pharmacology*, *25*(3), 363–372. doi:10.1016/0041-008X(73)90310-4 PMID:4199474

Thompson, S. A., Patterson, K., & Hodges, J. R. (2003). Left/right asymmetry of atrophy in semantic dementia: Behavioral-cognitive implications. *Neurology*, *61*(9), 1196–1203. doi:10.1212/01.WNL.0000091868.28557.B8 PMID:14610120

Tian, N., Liu, F., Wang, P., Zhang, X., Li, X., & Wu, G. (2017). The molecular basis of glandular trichome development and secondary metabolism in plants. *Plant Gene*, *12*, 1–12. doi:10.1016/j.plgene.2017.05.010

Touwn, M. (1981). The religious and medicinal uses of Cannabis in China, India and Tibet. *Journal of Psychoactive Drugs*, *13*(1), 23–34. doi:10.1080/02791072.1981.10471447 PMID:7024492

Trezza, V., Cuomo, V., & Vanderschuren, L. J. (2008). Cannabis and the developing brain: Insights from behavior. *European Journal of Pharmacology*, *585*(2-3), 441–452. doi:10.1016/j.ejphar.2008.01.058 PMID:18413273

Tsou, K., Brown, S., Sañudo-Peña, M. C., Mackie, K., & Walker, J. M. (1998). Immuno histochemical distribution of cannabinoid CB1 receptors in the rat central nervous system. *Neuroscience*, *83*(2), 393–411. doi:10.1016/S0306-4522(97)00436-3 PMID:9460749

Turner, T. R., James, E. K., & Poole, P. S. (2013). The plant microbiome. *Genome Biology*, *14*(6), 209. doi:10.1186/gb-2013-14-6-209 PMID:23805896

Tuzun, B. (2020). Investigation of the molecules obtained from marijuana: Computational study of spectral, structural and docking. [IAU Iran]. *Journal of Physical & Theoretical Chemistry*, *16*, 59–74.

Tyrrell, S. (2019). *How Cannabis Eye Creams Can Help With Puffy-Looking Eyes*. Cannabis MD. https://cannabismd.com/beauty/skin-care/how-cannabis-eye-creams-can-help-with-puffy-looking-eyes/

Ungerleider, J. T., Andrysiak, T., Tashkin, D. P., & Gale, R. P. (1982). Contamination of marijuana cigaretteswith pathogenic bacteria. *Cancer Treatment Reports*, *66*(3), 589–590. PMID:7060050

UNODC. (2019). *World Drug Report. Cannabis and Hallucinogens*. UNODC.

Upton, R., Craker, L., ElSohly, M., Romm, A., Russo, E., & Sexton, M. (Eds.). (2013). *Cannabis inflorescence,Cannabis spp. Standards of identity, analysis, and quality control*. American HerbalPharmacopoeia.

Vaidya, M., Choudhury, A., Brumlik, C., Agrawal, D. C., & Kumar, R. (2022). A Complete Patent Analysis of Cannabis/Marijuana in Drug Delivery and Disease Conditions. In D. C. Agrawal, R. Kumar, & M. Dhanasekaran (Eds.), *Cannabis/Marijuana for Healthcare* (pp. 1–34). Springer. doi:10.1007/978-981-16-8822-5_1

Valizadehderakhshan, M., Shahbazi, A., Kazem-Rostami, M., Todd, M. S., Bhowmik, A., & Wang, L. (2021). Extraction of Cannabinoids from *Cannabis sativa* L. (Hemp)—. *Revista de Agricultura (Piracicaba)*, *11*(5), 384. doi:10.3390/agriculture11050384

Van Bakel, H., Stout, J. M., Cote, A. G., Tallon, C. M., Sharpe, A. G., Hughes, T. R., & Page, J. E. (2011). The draft genome and transcriptome of *Cannabis sativa*. *Genome Biology*, *12*(10), 1–18. doi:10.1186/gb-2011-12-10-r102 PMID:22014239

van Breemen, R. B., Muchiri, R. N., Bates, T. A., Weinstein, J. B., Leier, H. C., Farley, S., & Tafesse, F. G. (2022). Cannabinoids Block Cellular Entry of SARS-CoV-2 and the Emerging Variants. *Journal of Natural Products*, *85*(1), 176–184. doi:10.1021/acs.jnatprod.1c00946 PMID:35007072

Vandenhove, H., & Van Hees, M. (2005). Fiber crops as alternative land use for radioactively contaminated arable land. *Journal of Environmental Radioactivity*, *81*(2-3), 131–141. doi:10.1016/j.jenvrad.2005.01.002 PMID:15795030

Vanhove, W., Van Damme, P., & Meert, N. (2011). Factors determining yield and quality of illicit indoor cannabis (Cannabis spp.) production. *Forensic Science International*, *212*(1–3), 158–163. doi:10.1016/j.forsciint.2011.06.006 PMID:21737218

VanPool, C.S., (2009). The signs of the sacred: identifying shamans using archaeological evidence. *J. Anthropol. Archaeol.* 28, 177–190. doi:. 02.003. doi:10.1016/j.jaa.2009

Vasudevan, K., & Stahl, V. (2020). Cannabinoids infused mouthwash products are as effective as chlorhexidine on inhibition of total-culturable bacterial content in dental plaque samples. *Journal of Cannabis Research*, *2*(1), 1–9. doi:10.118642238-020-00027-z PMID:33526124

Vázquez, M. D., Barceló, J., Poschenrieder, C., Mádico, J., Hatton, P., Baker, A. J. M., & Cope, G. H. (1992). Localization of zinc and cadmium in *Thlaspicaerulescens* (Brassicaceae), a metallophyte that can hyperaccumulate both metals. *Journal of Plant Physiology*, *140*(3), 350–355. doi:10.1016/S0176-1617(11)81091-6

Velasco, G., Sánchez, C., & Guzmán, M. (2016). Anticancer mechanisms of cannabinoids. *Current Oncology (Toronto, Ont.)*, *23*(2), S23–S32. doi:10.3747/co.23.3080 PMID:27022311

Venhuis, B. J., & de Kaste, D. (2008). Sildenafil analogs used for adulterating marihuana. *Forensic Science International*, *182*(1-3), e23–e24. doi:10.1016/j.forsciint.2008.09.002 PMID:18945564

Vercelli, C., Barbero, R., Cuniberti, B., Racca, S., Abbadessa, G., Piccione, F., & Re, G. (2014). Transient receptor potential vanilloid 1 expression and functionality in mcf-7 cells: A preliminary investigation. *Journal of Breast Cancer*, *17*(4), 332–338. doi:10.4048/jbc.2014.17.4.332 PMID:25548580

Verma, R., Hoda, F., Arshad, M., Iqubal, A., Siddiqui, A. N., Khan, M. A., Haque, S. E., Akhtar, M., & Najmi, A. K. (2021). Cannabis, a Miracle Drug with Polyvalent Therapeutic Utility: Preclinical and Clinical-Based Evidence. *Medical Cannabis and Cannabinoids*, *4*(1), 43–60. doi:10.1159/000515042 PMID:34676349

Verotta, L., Macchi, M. P., & Venkatasubramanian, P. (2015). *Connecting Indian Wisdom and Western Science: Plant Usage for Nutrition and Health.*

Verweij, P. E., Kerremans, J. J., Voss, A., & Meis, J. F. (2000). Fungal contamination of tobacco andmarijuana. *Journal of the American Medical Association*, *284*(22), 2875. doi:10.1001/jama.284.22.2869 PMID:11147983

Vieira, G., Cavalli, J., Gonçalves, E. C., Braga, S. F., Ferreira, R. S., Santos, A. R., Cola, M., Raposo, N. R., Capasso, R., & Dutra, R. C. (2020). Antidepressant-like effect of terpineol in an inflammatory model of depression: Involvement of the cannabinoid system and D2 dopamine receptor. *Biomolecules*, *10*(5), 792. doi:10.3390/biom10050792 PMID:32443870

Vincenzi, C., & Tosti, A. (2020). Efficacy and Tolerability of a Shampoo Containing Broad-Spectrum Cannabidiol in the Treatment of Scalp Inflammation in Patients with Mild to Moderate Scalp Psoriasis or Seborrheic Dermatitis. *Skin Appendage Disorders*, *6*(6), 355–361. doi:10.1159/000510896 PMID:33313051

Vögeli-Lange, R., & Wagner, G. J. (1990). Subcellular localization of cadmium and cadmium-binding peptides in tobacco leaves: Implication of a transport function for cadmium-binding peptides. *Plant Physiology*, *92*(4), 1086–1093. doi:10.1104/pp.92.4.1086 PMID:16667375

Vogl, C. R., Mölleken, H., Lissek-Wolf, G., Surböck, A., & Kobert, J. (2004). Hemp (*Cannabis sativa* L.) as a resource for green cosmetics: Yield of seed and fatty acid compositions of 20 varieties under the growing conditions of organic farming in Austria. *Journal of Industrial Hemp*, *9*(1), 51–68. doi:10.1300/J237v09n01_06

Volkow, N. D., Baler, R. D., Compton, W. M., & Weiss, S. R. B. (2014a). Adverse health effects of marijuana use. *The New England Journal of Medicine*, *370*(23), 2219–2227. doi:10.1056/NEJMra1402309 PMID:24897085

Vonapartis, E., Aubin, M.-P., Seguin, P., Mustafa, A. F., & Charron, J.-B. (2015). Seed composition of ten industrial hemp cultivars approved for production in Canada. *Journal of Food Composition and Analysis*, *39*, 8–12. doi:10.1016/j.jfca.2014.11.004

Vulfsons, S., Minerbi, A., & Sahar, T. (2020). Cannabis and Pain Treatment—A Review of the Clinical Utility and a Practical Approach in Light of Uncertainty. *Rambam Maimonides Medical Journal*, *11*(1), e0002. doi:10.5041/RMMJ.10385 PMID:32017678

Wahby, I., Caba, J. M., & Ligero, F. (2013). *Agrobacterium* infection of *Cannabis sativa* (*Cannabis sativa* L.): Establishment of hairy root cultures. *Journal of Plant Interactions*, *38*(4), 312–320. doi:10.1080/17429145.2012.746399

Wang, Q., Jiang, J., & Xiong, Y. L. (2018). High pressure homogenization combined with pH shift treatment: A process to produce physically and oxidatively stable hemp milk. *Food Research International*, *106*, 487–494. doi:10.1016/j.foodres.2018.01.021 PMID:29579952

Wang, Q., & Xiong, Y. L. (2019). Processing, nutrition, and functionality of hempseed protein: A review. *Comprehensive Reviews in Food Science and Food Safety*, *18*(4), 936–952. doi:10.1111/1541-4337.12450 PMID:33336999

Wang, X., Li, Q. X., Heidel, M., Wu, Z., Yoshimoto, A., Leong, G., Pan, D., & Ako, H. (2021). Comparative evaluation of industrial hemp varieties: Field experiments and phytoremediation in Hawaii. *Industrial Crops and Products*, *170*, 113683. doi:10.1016/j.indcrop.2021.113683

Wang, X.-S., Tang, C.-H., Yang, X.-Q., & Gao, W.-R. (2008). Characterization, amino acid composition and in vitro digestibility of hemp (Cannabis sativa L.) proteins. *Food Chemistry*, *107*(1), 11–18. doi:10.1016/j.foodchem.2007.06.064

Warf, B. (2014). High points: An historical geography of cannabis. *Geographical Review*, *104*(4), 414–438. doi:10.1111/j.1931-0846.2014.12038.x

Wasim, K., Haq, I. U., & Ashraf, M. (1995). Antimicrobial Studies of the Leaf of Cannabis sativa L. *Pakistan Journal of Pharmaceutical Sciences*, *8*, 22–38. PMID:16414764

Watson, S. J., Benson, J. A., & Joy, J. E. (2000). Marijuana and medicine: Assessing the science base: a summary of the 1999 Institute of Medicine report. *Archives of General Psychiatry*, *57*(6), 547–552. doi:10.1001/archpsyc.57.6.547 PMID:10839332

Whiting, P. F., Wolff, R. F., Deshpande, S., Di Nisio, M., Duffy, S., Hernandez, A. V., Keurentjes, J. C., Lang, S., Misso, K., Ryder, S., Schmidlkofer, S., Westwood, M., & Kleijnen, J. (2015). Cannabinoids for medical use: A systematic review and metaanalysis. *Journal of the American Medical Association*, *313*(24), 2456–2473. doi:10.1001/jama.2015.6358 PMID:26103030

Wielgus, K., Luwanska, A., Lassocinski, W., & Kaczmarek, Z. (2008). Estimation of Cannabissativa L. Tissue Culture Conditions Essential for Callus Induction and Plant Regeneration. *Journal of Natural Fibers*, *5*(3), 199–207. doi:10.1080/15440470801976045

Wilkinson, S. T., Radhakrishnan, R., & D'Souza, D. C. (2016). A systematic review of the evidence for medical marijuana in psychiatric indications. *The Journal of Clinical Psychiatry*, *77*(08), 1050–1064. https://doi.org/10.4088/JCP.15r10036

Williams, H. C., Dellavalle, R. P., & Garner, S. (2012). Acne vulgaris. *Lancet*, *379*(9813), 361–372. doi:10.1016/S0140-6736(11)60321-8 PMID:21880356

Wilson, D. (2021). *Cannabidiol (CBD) in Hair Oil*. Science Senior Seminar.

Wilson, D., Steinegger, P., & Parkin, D. P. (1989). Effects of cannabis smoked together with a substancesold as Mandrax. *South African Medical Journal*, *76*(11), 636. PMID:2595497

Winston, M. E., Hampton-Marcell, J., Zarraonaindia, I., Owens, S. M., Moreau, C. S., Gilbert, J. A., Hartsel, J. A., Kennedy, S. J., & Gibbons, S. M. (2014). Understanding cultivar-specificity and soildeterminants of the cannabis microbiome. *PLoS One*, *9*(6), e99641. doi:10.1371/journal.pone.0099641 PMID:24932479

Wolff, V., & Jouanjus, E. (2017). Strokes are possible complications of cannabinoids use. *Epilepsy & Behavior: E&B*, *70*(Pt B), 355–363. doi:10.1016/j.yebeh.2017.01.031

World Health Organization (WHO). (2014). *Cancer country profile*. WHO. https://www.who.int/cancer/country-profiles/gha_en.pdf?ua=1

Wurzer, J. (2016) *Safety testing of medicinal cannabis*. In: Proceedings of the 2006 CannmedConference. Medical Genomics, Woburn, MA.

Wyatt, K. (2015). Marijuana subject to product liability claim in Colorado. *U.S. News & World Report.*

Xian-Sheng, W. (2007). Characterization. *Amino Acid Composition and in Vitro Digestibility of Hemp (Cannabis Sativa L.) Proteins. Food Chemistry*, *107*(1), 11–18.

Xiong, W., Cui, T., Cheng, K., Yang, F., Chen, S.-R., Willenbring, D., & Xu, Y. (2012). Cannabinoids suppress inflammatory and neuropathic pain by targeting α3 glycine receptors. *The Journal of Experimental Medicine*, *209*(6), 1121–1134. doi:10.1084/jem.20120242

Xu, J., Zhang, Y., Wang, W., & Li, Y. (2020). Advanced properties of gluten-free cookies, cakes, and crackers: A review. *Trends in Food Science & Technology*, *103*, 200–213. doi:10.1016/j.tifs.2020.07.017

Xu, X., Liu, Y., Huang, S., Liu, G., Xie, C., Zhou, J., Fan, W., Li, Q., Wang, Q., Zhong, D., & Miao, X. (2006). Overexpression of cannabinoid receptors CB1 and CB2 correlates with improved prognosis of patients with hepatocellular carcinoma. *Cancer Genetics and Cytogenetics, 171*(1), 31–38. doi:10.1016/j.cancergencyto.2006.06.014 PMID:17074588

Xu, X., Qiao, Y., Shi, B., & Dia, V. P. (2021). Alcalase and bromelain hydrolysis affected physicochemical and functional properties and biological activities of legume proteins. *Food Structure, 27*, 100178. doi:10.1016/j.foostr.2021.100178

Yan, Z. L., Wang, H., Lau, K. T., Pather, S., Zhang, J. C., Lin, G., & Ding, Y. (2013). Reinforcement of polypropylene with *Cannabis sativa* fibres. *Composites. Part B, Engineering, 46*, 221–226. doi:10.1016/j.compositesb.2012.09.027

Zagórska-Dziok, M., Bujak, T., Ziemlewska, A., & Nizioł-Łukaszewska, Z. (2021). Positive Effect of *Cannabis sativa* L. Herb Extracts on Skin Cells and Assessment of Cannabinoid-Based Hydrogels Properties. *Molecules (Basel, Switzerland), 26*(4), 802. doi:10.3390/molecules26040802 PMID:33557174

Zamberletti, E., Prini, P., Speziali, S., Gabaglio, M., Solinas, M., Parolaro, D., & Rubino, T. (2012). Gender-dependent behavioral and biochemical effects of adolescent delta-9-tetrahydrocannabinol in adult maternally deprived rats. *Neuroscience, 204*, 245–257. doi:10.1016/j.neuroscience.2011.11.038 PMID:22178986

Zhang, H., Zhong, Z., & Feng, L. (2016). Advances in the performance and application of hemp fiber. *Int J Simul Syst Sci Technol, 17*(9), 18.11-18.15.

Zhang, Q., Chen, X., Guo, H., Trindade, L. M., Salentijn, E. M., Guo, R., Guo, M., Xu, Y., & Yang, M. (2018). Latitudinal Adaptation and Genetic Insights Into the Origins of *Cannabis sativa* L. *Frontiers in Plant Science, 9*, 1876. doi:10.3389/fpls.2018.01876 PMID:30627133

Zhang, X., Xu, G., Cheng, C., Lei, L., Sun, J., Xu, Y., Deng, C., Dai, Z., Yang, Z., Chen, X., Liu, C., Tang, Q., & Su, J. (2021). Establishment of an Agrobacterium –mediated genetic transformation and CRISPR/Cas9-mediatedtargetedmutagenesisinHemp (CannabissativaL.). *Plant Biotechnology Journal, 19*(10), 1979–1987. doi:10.1111/pbi.13611 PMID:33960612

Zhao, J., Xu, Y., Wang, W., Griffin, J., Roozeboom, K., & Wang, D. (2020). Bioconversion of industrial *Cannabis sativa* biomass for bioethanol production: A review. *Fuel, 281*, 118725. doi:10.1016/j.fuel.2020.118725

Zimmer, A., Zimmer, A. M., Hohmann, A. G., Herkenham, M., & Bonner, T. I. (1999). Increased mortality, hypoactivity, and hypoalgesia in cannabinoid CB1receptor knock out mice. *Proceedings of the National Academy of Sciences of the United States of America, 96*(10), 5780–5785. doi:10.1073/pnas.96.10.5780 PMID:10318961

Zou, S., & Kumar, U. (2018). Cannabinoid receptors and the endocannabinoid system: Signalling and function in the central nervous system. *International Journal of Molecular Sciences, 19*(3), 833. doi:10.3390/ijms19030833 PMID:29533978

Zuardi, A. W. (2006). History of cannabis as a medicine: A review. *Revista Brasileira De Psiquiatria (Sao Paulo, Brazil: 1999), 28*(2), 153–157. doi:10.1590/s1516-44462006000200015

Zuardi, A. W. (2006). History of cannabis as a medicine: A review. Brazilian. *Journal of Psychiatry, 28*, 153–157. PMID:16810401

Zuardi, A. W. (2006). History of cannabis as a medicine: A review. *The British Journal of Psychiatry, 28*(2), 153–157. doi:10.1590/S1516-44462006000200015 PMID:16810401

Zuk-Golaszewska, K., & Golaszewski, J. (2018). *Cannabis sativa* L.–cultivation and quality of raw material. *Journal of Elementology, 23*(3), 971–984. doi:10.5601/jelem.2017.22.3.1500

Zwenger, S.R. *(2014). The biotechnology of* Cannabis sativa. *2*. Extreme Publications Inc.

Öhgren K, Galbe M, Zacchi G (2005) Optimization of steam pretreatment of SO2 impregnated corn stover for fuel ethanol production. *Appl Biochem Biotechnol*

About the Contributors

Rafiq Lone is presently working as Assistant Professor of Botany at Central University of Kashmir, Jammu and Kashmir- India. He has completed his M. Sc and Ph.D. in Botany from Jiwaji University, Gwalior, Madhya Pradesh, India. Dr. Lone has been awarded National Post-Doctoral Fellowship (NPDF) by SERB, DST, Government of India. Previously he was working as Assistant Professor in Botany at SBBS University, Khiala Jalandhar, Punjab, Lecturer (Academic arrangement) in higher education, Jammu and Kashmir, Teaching Assistant at School of Studies in Botany, Jiwaji University, Gwalior-India, and Project Fellow in a project funded by MPCST-Bhopal-(M.P)-India. Dr. Lone has five years of teaching and ten years of research experience. He has published more than 25 research papers in National and International journals and more than 16 book chapters, and four edited books are also to his credit. Dr. Lone has attended 25 national and international conferences and has presented papers on plant-microbe interaction and plant phenolics. His main research interest focuses on Plant-microbe interaction, Plant Nutrition, Plant Phenolics, and Invasion Biology.

Javid Manzoor is working as Assistant professor in the Department of Environmental Science, Shri JJT University, Jhunjhunu, Rajasthan India. He has obtained his Master's degree and doctorate from Jiwaji University, Gwalior, Madhya Pradesh. He has three five of teaching experience. He is an awardee of University Research Scholarship. He is a permanent member of people for animal. His areas of interest include Environmental pollution, Environmental monitoring and assessment. He has published research papers and book chapters in various national and international journals with impact factor. He has been working as editorial board member and reviewer of various national and international journals.

***

Irfan Bashir is a research scholar is working in the department of history university of Kashmir. The scholar has also qualified UGC NET JRF in History.

Sameena Bashir is research student in the Department of History, University of Kashmir Srinagar Jammu and Kashmir, India

Sajood Bhat is working as Assistant professor in the Department of Chemistry, GDC, Bhaderwah, J&K, India. He has obtained his doctorate from Awadhesh Pratap Singh University. Rewa, Madhya

Pradesh. He has three years of teaching experience. He has published research papers and book chapters in various national and international journals

Elif Cakir is an Assistant Professor at the Food Technology Department of Istanbul Aydın University (Turkey). Her research has focused on bioactive components in foods, antibacterial, antioxidant activities, food microbiology and fermentation studies. She has 6 scientific papers as SCI record.

Sefa Celik is an Associate Professor at the Physics Department of Istanbul University (Turkey). His research is focused on the elucidation of the structure of biomacromolecules using combined experimental (molecular spectroscopy) and theoretical methods (ab initio, molecular dynamics), particularly on the molecular docking studies for shedding light on new drug design. He has 38 scientific papers as SCI record.

Alev Er is an Associate Professor at the Physics Department of Istanbul University (Turkey). Her research is focused on the atomic and molecular physics, atom photon interactions and analysis of atomic structures. She has 13 scientific papers as SCI record.

Syed Javid Ahmad Andrabi is working as Assistant professor in the department of higher education, JKUT. He has pursued his PhD in the field of environmental science and engineering from Indian institute of technology, New Delhi India and qualified National Eligibility Test (NET). His teaching and research interests are in the areas of air pollution, water pollution control and treatment and also has research interests in environmental impact assessment. Dr Andrabi is author of more than thirty scientific articles of international repute. He has received various national and international awards related to publishing his work. Dr Andrabi has been working as editorial board member and reviewer of various international journals.

Priyanka Joshi Jain is a PhD scholar at Prin. K.M. Kundnani College of Pharmacy. She has 10 years of teaching experience in the subject of Pharmaceutics.

Nalini Kurup is an Assistant Professor (Department of Pharmaceutics) at Principal K. M. Kundnani College of Pharmacy, affiliated to University of Mumbai, India. She completed her Ph.D. in 2004 and has 17 years of experience in academics and research. She has handled research projects of Solubility enhancement, Development of Nano carriers and formulation of NDDS.

Nikhil Rajnani, a graduate in pharmacy specialized in pharmaceutics subject. Overall Rainani has six years of experience and has published 2 articles and 1 patent.

Malti Rajput is working as Senior Assistant professor in the Department of Chemistry, PSPS Govt. PG College for Women, Gandhi Nagar, Jammu, J&K, India. She has twelve years of teaching experience. She has published research papers in various national and international journals.

Sanjoy Sadhukhan obtained a B.Sc. from the University of Calcutta, Kolkata, West Bengal; M.Sc. in Botany from Visva Bharati, Santiniketan, West Bengal; and PhD from the IIT, Kharagpur. He pursued Postdoctoral research at Thomas Jefferson University, Philadelphia, USA and the University of Pittsburgh, Pittsburgh, USA for 5 years and 9 months. Dr. Sadhukhan is currently working as an Assistant Professor, Department of Botany, Raiganj University, Raiganj -733134, West Bengal. He is actively involved in teaching both UG and PG levels as well as research activities. His areas of research interest are seed germination, seed priming, abiotic stress, etc. At present five research scholars are pursuing PhD under his guidance. Dr. Sadhukhan has published several research papers in various international peer-reviewed journals. He has authored numerous book chapters. He is the Life Member of The Indian Science Congress Association Membership No # L40200.

Anup Sarkar is currently working as an Assistant Professor in the Department of Botany, Dukhulal Nibarna Chandra College, Murshidabad, India. He is pursuing his doctoral degree in the Department of Botany, at Raiganj University, India. He is actively involved in research activities in the area of Biological Science and Agriculture. He has published several book chapters as well as some articles in well-reputed journals.

Anuradha Sharma is working as Assistant professor in the Department of Environmental Sciences, GDC, Bhaderwah, J&K, India. She has obtained his Masters and M.Phil from University of Jammu J&K, India. She has seven years of teaching experience. She has published research papers and book chapters in various national and international journals

Khursheed Wani is Assistant Professor in the Department of Environmental Science, Government Degree College Thidim Kreeri, J&K. Dr. Wani served at ITM University Gwalior as Assistant Professor in the Department of Environmental Science from 2011 to 2017. He has completed his M. Sc. and Ph. D. in Environmental Science from Jiwaji University, Gwalior, Madhya Pradesh. He has also qualified Jammu and Kashmir State Level Eligibility Test (JKSET). His areas of interest include Environmental management, Environmental Impact Assessment and Occupational Health. He has published research papers in various national and international journals and is the author of three books on Environmental Science. He is a member of several national and international organizations and is in the editorial board of various journals. He has organized different programmes on Environmental Awareness and has completed research project sponsored by Madhya Pradesh Council of Science and Technology, Bhopal, India. Dr. Wani has organized various national and international conferences/seminars/ workshops as well.

Waseem Yaseen is presently serving as Assistant Professor in the Department of Environmental Sciences at Government Degree College Kangan, District Ganderbal, Jammu &Kashmir (UT).

Siraj Yousuf is a professor at GDC Bijbehara.

Index

A

Anemophilic 153
Atharvaveda 31, 35

B

Bioactive Compounds 82-84, 90, 102-104, 108, 154-156
Bioenergy 88, 116, 118, 122, 143, 146
Bioplastics 53, 88, 143-145, 147, 149

C

Cannabidiol 7, 43, 47, 53, 57, 63-65, 67, 70-74, 82, 84-86, 106-107, 144
Cannabinoids 9-13, 35-36, 45-47, 52-59, 63, 65-66, 68-71, 75, 82-89, 102-103, 105-107, 132, 144, 154, 156
Cannabis 1-13, 29-40, 43-50, 52-59, 63-71, 74-75, 81-91, 101-108, 115-122, 129-132, 134-135, 143-149, 153-156, 158-164
Cannabis Sativa 1-2, 5-6, 10, 13, 29-30, 32, 34-37, 39, 47, 49, 52-55, 57, 59, 63, 69, 74, 81-84, 89, 101-108, 115-122, 130, 132, 143-147, 153, 158
Climate Change 143, 145, 148-149
Contamination 117-118, 120, 129, 132-133, 160

D

drug 1, 12, 29, 32-40, 44, 46-48, 53, 63, 67, 69-70, 75, 83, 90, 106, 155, 157, 161

E

Emulsifying 101
Endocannabinoid System 6, 10, 12, 65-67, 70, 72, 82, 85

G

Gateway Drug 157

H

Heavy Metals 2, 115-118, 120-122, 129, 132-134, 136, 145-146
Hemp 1-3, 8-9, 14, 29-40, 44, 46, 49-50, 52-53, 59, 63-64, 71-72, 74-75, 82, 84-87, 90, 101-105, 108, 129-130, 132, 134, 143-150, 154
Hemp Drug Commission 33, 36-38, 40

I

Industrial Crop 89
Industrial Hemp 49-50, 90, 130, 146-147
Intoxicant 32, 35, 39-40

L

legal approaches 50

M

Marijuana 1-2, 6, 8, 35, 37, 40, 46, 48, 52, 54, 58-59, 63, 67-68, 75, 82, 90, 133, 135, 144, 153-157, 159-162
Medical Cannabis 3, 35, 44, 46, 48, 54, 67, 69, 86, 89, 102, 106, 135
Medicinal and Cosmetic Uses 65
Molecular Docking 106-108

N

Nanoemulsion 105

P

Pesticides 103, 117, 129, 132, 134-136, 145, 148
Pharmaceutical 3, 11, 46, 53, 63-64, 81-83, 88-90, 102, 154
Phytocannabinoids 2, 11, 64-65, 82, 132
Phytoremediation 115-122, 133-134, 146
Pollutants 115-116, 121, 132, 145
Psychoactive 1, 4, 6, 11, 13, 32, 36, 40, 43-44, 47-49, 68, 82, 102-103, 144, 156-157, 159-161

S

social impacts 40, 43

T

Tetrahydrocannabinol 4, 12, 37, 40, 47-48, 53, 63-64, 67, 72, 83, 107, 144, 155
Therapeutic 6, 11, 13, 29-31, 34-37, 39-40, 44, 46, 53-54, 64-65, 68, 74-75, 81, 83, 85, 87-89, 107, 144, 153, 161-162
Treatment 6, 10-13, 35-36, 44, 46, 48, 52-54, 57-59, 67, 70-71, 73-75, 87-88, 119-120, 146, 153-154, 164

www.ingramcontent.com/pod-product-compliance
Lightning Source LLC
LaVergne TN
LVHW080529300926
849162LV00007B/1570